Governing Health

GOVERNING HEALTH

The Politics of Health Policy

FOURTH EDITION

William G. Weissert
and
Carol S. Weissert

The Johns Hopkins University Press
Baltimore

© 1996, 2002, 2006, 2012 The Johns Hopkins University Press
All rights reserved. Published 2012
Printed in the United States of America on acid-free paper
9   8   7   6   5   4   3   2   1

The Johns Hopkins University Press
2715 North Charles Street
Baltimore, Maryland 21218-4363
www.press.jhu.edu

Library of Congress Cataloging-in-Publication Data

Weissert, William G.
  Governing health : the politics of health policy / William G. Weissert and
Carol S. Weissert. — 4th ed.
      p. ; cm.
  Carol S. Weissert's name appears first in earlier ed.
  Includes bibliographical references and index.
  ISBN 978-1-4214-0620-6 (hdbk. : alk. paper) —
ISBN 978-1-4214-0621-3 (pbk. : alk. paper) —
ISBN 1-4214-0620-9 (hdbk. : alk. paper) —
ISBN 1-4214-0621-7 (pbk. : alk. paper)
  I. Weissert, Carol S.   II. Weissert, Carol S. Governing health.   III. Title.
  [DNLM: 1. Health Policy—United States.   2. Politics—United States.
WA 540 AA1]

  362.10973—dc23

                                                        2011053062

A catalog record for this book is available from the British Library.

Special discounts are available for bulk purchases of this book. For more information,
please contact Special Sales at 410-516-6936 or specialsales@press.jhu.edu.

The Johns Hopkins University Press uses environmentally friendly book
materials, including recycled text paper that is composed of at least 30
percent post-consumer waste, whenever possible.

Contents

Abbreviations

AARP	AARP; formerly known as the American Association of Retired Persons
AFDC	Aid to Families with Dependent Children
AIDS	acquired immune deficiency syndrome
AMA	American Medical Association
CBO	Congressional Budget Office
CDC	Centers for Disease Control and Prevention
CMS	Centers for Medicare and Medicaid Services
DRG	diagnosis-related group
EPA	Environmental Protection Agency
ERISA	Employee Retirement Income Security Act
FDA	Food and Drug Administration
GAO	Government Accountability Office (formerly the General Accounting Office)
GDP	gross domestic product
HCFA	Health Care Financing Administration (became CMS in 2001)
HEW	(U.S. Department of) Health, Education, and Welfare; became HHS
HHS	(U.S. Department of) Health and Human Services
HIV	human immunodeficiency virus
HMO	health maintenance organization
IRS	Internal Revenue Service

MedPAC	Medicare Payment Advisory Commission
MMA	Medicare Modernization Act (in full, Medicare Prescription Drug, Improvement and Modernization Act of 2003)
NAFTA	North American Free Trade Agreement
OMB	Office of Management and Budget
OSHA	Occupational Safety and Health Administration
PAC	political action committee
PhRMA	Pharmaceutical Research and Manufacturers of America
PPACA	Patient Protection and Affordable Care Act
S-CHIP	State Children's Health Insurance Program
SEIU	Service Employees International Union

Governing Health

Introduction

A s the latest Obama administration health policy reform initiative heated up
in congressional debate, even though it was one of many such efforts over
the past 100 years, lobbyists and their clients began to think this one might actually become law. Although we'd not had real reform since Medicare and Medicaid were adopted 45 years earlier, this president seemed to have struck the right
note, at the right time, with the right majority in Congress. So the health care
industry took notice. Policy might change, and they wanted to do all they could
to make sure that the changes were favorable to their particular type of business.
So they did what any red-blooded American industry does when threatened with
a change in government policy: they hired lobbyists, 3,300 health care lobbyists
to be exact, at least six for every member of Congress. Many were successful in
negotiating smaller and less destructive—or later rather than sooner—cuts in
their payments or removal of protections from competition. And so the reforms
were much weaker than promised, because Congress never forgets that every
dollar of health care spending—whether as a nation we can afford it or not—is a
dollar of income to someone, someone who does business and provides jobs in
congressional members' districts (hospitals, for example), or is a big contributor
to their campaigns (Pharmaceutical Research and Manufacturers of America,
for example), or is very popular with a key voting block that members don't want
to offend (Medicare physicians serving seniors, for example).

Such is the way of American policymaking in health care. What we pay for
health care, how much we let the market restrict competition, how much we
continue to support care that we know is excessive, unneeded, potentially harmful, and often not high quality, and who runs into access barriers when they try
to get care are all aspects of health policy that are shaped by many forces: the
president, Congress, drug companies, unions, hospitals, physicians, medical equipment companies, insurance companies, managed care organizations and other
interest groups, federal agencies, state legislatures and state bureaucracies, and

all of us consumers of health care who demand that we get all the care that's available, whether we need it or not.

This book explores how government makes health policy. Most health care in the United States is delivered by the private sector, but because public policy pays for and regulates so much of it, health policy is vitally important. Moreover, private payers for health care tend to mimic the payment approaches of public policy, so public policy's reach extends even further into the private portion of health care policy. For these reasons, and because so much of health care is out-sourced and becomes the income stream of private sector providers, claims pro-cessors, makers of health care products, and others, private interest groups have a huge stake in public policy and find it a good bargain to spend rather lavishly on lobbying and other strategies aimed at influencing public health care policy.

One result of this lobbying for private health care delivery is that public health, which has few dollars to fund its advocacy, tends to be neglected. Public health spending by the federal government for health education to battle sexually trans-mitted and other infectious diseases, reduce smoking, prevent cancer, and do sur-veillance and inspections to mitigate environmental hazards, prevent food-borne illnesses, and promote water safety has been flat for years; public health spending by states has also been dropping, especially in recent years, when economic woes have adversely affected state revenues. The federal government spent only $17.60 per person for disease prevention in 2009 (Levi et al., 2009, 1). Yet health insur-ance premiums for an individual in that year cost more than $8,000, suggesting a huge disparity in spending for health care versus preventive efforts through pub-lic health agencies. This pattern has been long-standing, according to Beitsch, Brooks, Menachemi, and Libbey (2006), who found that public health spending in 2004 and 2005 amounted to barely over 2.3 percent of total health spending.

Despite its complexity and fragmentation (or perhaps because of these fea-tures), few issues have the personal, social, and economic significance of health policy—which is, by the way, responsible for one-seventh of the nation's gross domestic product. And few problems have so persistently demanded public action from presidents, Congresses, legislatures, bureaucracies, courts, and the interest groups that want to influence their decisions. This no doubt reflects the reality that health policy problems are never really solved; rather, they are only managed better (or at times worse).

The nation continues to face a plethora of health policy problems, some new (the obesity epidemic) and some very old (medical errors and patients' safety). A persistent one, getting worse for many rather than better, is access to care. Indeed, in recent decades access to care has become worse at faster rates as more and more employers reduce the scope of their health care coverage or give it up altogether, leaving much of the workforce uninsured. Most Americans enjoy health care that at times, for some conditions, is the best (and most expensive) on the planet, but 45 million or more of us go without health insurance, and nearly as many more have inadequate or intermittent coverage, thanks to our nation's incomplete, uncoordinated, and very expensive health policy approaches. Even more Americans go without coverage, or adequate coverage, of their prescription drugs, although beginning in 2006, elderly people—especially poor elderly people—have some level of coverage under the Medicare Prescription Drug, Improvement and Modernization Act of 2003 (or, in brief, the Medicare Modernization Act, MMA). Mental health coverage, dental coverage, and long-term-care coverage are particularly lacking, even for middle-class Americans. Those who have access to insurance are not always able to get appropriate care within a reasonable time or within a convenient geographic area. Rural and inner-city areas suffer shortages of facilities and specialty medicine.

Mainstream health care for most Americans is now delivered by managed care organizations. Even Medicare beneficiaries, who have generally shunned managed care, have begun to embrace it, although they still lag the rest of the country in their participation.

The Centers for Disease Control and Prevention has as its mission the responsibility for helping Americans curb unhealthy lifestyles and behaviors, but that agency's budget is tiny next to those of the Centers for Medicare and Medicaid Services (CMS) and the National Institutes of Health, which focus on cures rather than prevention. Teen smoking persists as a problem, and low-birth-weight and out-of-wedlock births, while showing some improvement, are problems of epidemic proportion in some subgroups. HIV/AIDS and other infectious agents continue to spread through risky behaviors and lack of adequate progress toward vaccines and cures, often bouncing back after being suppressed as affected populations relax their vigilance with the availability of improved life-sustaining treatment regimens. Again, some improvements have occurred, but there has also been some backsliding—for example with the growing vaccine refusal movement.

No one can be sure that the care he receives will be free of errors, omissions, or excesses. The quality of care delivered in the United States has come under broad attack for high rates of medical errors, inappropriate and ineffective treatments, periodic reports showing little relationship between higher quantities and costs of health care and better health outcomes, and the lack of any systematic mechanism for defining, monitoring, reporting, and working to correct patterns of inadequate care. In general, improvements in technology have come much more slowly to health care administration than to health care delivery. There seems to be little political will to confront the medical care delivery system with a broad demand to heal itself.

Health care is very expensive in the United States. Research into understanding diseases and finding cures has seldom been better publicly funded than it is now, but public and private health care costs continue to rise at alarming rates, especially the cost of prescription drugs. It is not uncommon for drugs to cost twice as much in the United States as in many other industrialized countries, sometimes even more. Many new drugs cost five and ten times as much as older treatments but treat more effectively the conditions of only a small fraction of patients who switch to the newer form. The federal agency that attempts (sometimes unsuccessfully) to protect the public from adverse side effects often requires the testing of new drugs only against a placebo, not against existing treatments.

For these and other reasons, per capita spending for health services vastly exceeds that of any other country. Although most other industrialized countries pay for much more of their citizens' health care publicly, while in the United States we rely more heavily on private sources, health policy choices nonetheless dominate our public budgets, federal and state, even when policymakers try to make other issues their priority. States have always played a major role in health policy, accepting responsibility for basic health and safety laws, innovating in everything from care for the poor to control of prescription drug costs, and paying nearly half of Medicaid costs. Our federal system continues to require a partnership between the federal and state governments when it comes time to implement major reform programs such as the Patient Protection and Affordable Care Act (PPACA). States will play two major roles in breathing life into the health reform law: implementing expansion of the Medicaid program to millions of Americans brought into Medicaid eligibility by the law and implementing the health insurance industry reforms mandated by the law.

Most of the costs of the PPACA Medicaid expansion—estimated to bring perhaps 16 million new enrollees into care—will be paid by the federal government, at least for the first several years of the program's operation. The expansion will take place in 2014. Eligibility will rise then to 133 percent of a poverty-level income, and limitations previously barring childless couples and individuals from receiving care will be removed. States will be charged with finding those who are newly eligible and enrolling them. The federal government will pay 100 percent of costs of the newly eligible through 2016, then 95 percent in 2017, 94 percent in 2018, 93 percent in 2019, and 90 percent in 2020 and beyond.

States already regulate the health industry for small-group and individual insurance. Among new insurance industry rules to be enforced by the states under the PPACA are prohibitions on charging extra for—or denying coverage due to—preexisting conditions, imposing lifetime limits on policies, and charging excessively for old age. States are required to set up insurance exchanges that will solicit insurance policies from private companies and make them available to poor and near-poor individuals and to small businesses that qualify to use them. The exchanges will market the five standardized policies called for in the law, provide the subsidies called for to those who qualify, and provide buyers with help with their purchases. If the states fail to set up their own exchanges by 2014, the federal government will do it in any state that doesn't meet the standard. States were also called upon to set up high-risk pools by 2010 for persons who could not buy insurance due to preexisting conditions. The pools will not be needed after 2014. The federal government took on the role if a state failed to establish a pool that met federal standards. States also have responsibility for coordinating enrollment and standardizing income standards between Medicaid and the exchanges.

Federal health policy harks back to the earliest days of the nation, when the federal government extended its reach up the rivers and into port cities to control infectious disease. Current times have seen an expansion of the federal role (the PPACA's individual and employer mandates), insurance industry reform, and some small efforts to reduce costs. Health savings accounts—a fixed contribution of funds (from employer or government) that the consumer uses tax-free for health care—may come to replace employers' previous commitment to pay for a set of health care benefits. The great benefits of these accounts for employers are that the payments are fixed, predictable, and potentially not adjusted to health care cost inflation, which is almost always higher than general inflation. But the people who choose these savings accounts are likely to be those who enjoy good health status. When they withdraw from the common insurance risk pool, they leave behind a population likely to face higher insurance premiums, because the average risk in the remaining risk pool is now higher.

Proposals for comprehensive national health insurance coverage have been particularly important public policy concerns in decades past. With rare exceptions, these proposals have failed to become policy. Democratic and Republican presidents since Harry Truman have moved onto the national agenda one or more proposals to expand Americans' access to health insurance or improve their coverage. Yet each saw his proposals radically scaled back or rejected. All proposals tend to stumble over the same concerns: the role of the public sector versus the private sector; who will pay the enormous costs; whether the plan will be means-tested, so that those who can pay more do pay more; and the potential burden on employers of the paperwork that tends to be associated with most plans.

Nevertheless, progress does get made. Proposals once regarded as revolutionary and fiercely opposed—an employer mandate, for example, or means-testing Medicare premiums—are now the law of the land.

This book examines the U.S. experience with governing health. It is a political science book about health care policy. As such, it presents health care policy as the product of the U.S. system of government, combining several forces:

—the persistent power of ideological polarization and party politics;
—the dominant need for members of Congress to constantly seek reelection, claim credit, trade votes, and overcome uncertainty in their policy choices;
—the waxing and waning persuasive power of the presidency, promising much, sometimes delivering but more often disappointing;
—the discretion exercised by the bureaucracy in its role as agent of the president, Congress, the courts, its clients, and the public;
—the pervasive and well-financed influence of the burgeoning army of health interests, the coalitions they form, and the strategies they employ to frame issues and shape health policy to their liking;
—the continuing struggle of the states, torn between sovereigns and supplicants in their wish to call on the federal government for more financial support but desperate to control their own health policy destinies; and
—the challenge of effective problem definition, the choice of solutions, and various models of the policy process, all incomplete but each capturing an aspect of the insights we need if we are ever to predict policy outcomes.

The first edition of *Governing Health* grew out of a frustration at the absence of a text written by political scientists for use in health politics classes. Sociologists and economists have authored or contributed to a small number of worthy volumes bringing their own disciplines' perspectives to the topic of health politics and policy, and although they have much to offer, a gap remains. Politics is more than the sociology of institutions or economic self-interest. And health care policy is politics at its richest and fullest. Politics is about power, and the making of health policy is nothing if not the wielding of power. Institutional rules endow some actors with more power than others, differential endowments of other types give some interests more power than others, and the fleeting saliency of the issues themselves sometimes gives one side more bargaining power than another. This book illuminates how the institutions and the policymaking process work to wield power over health policy.

The intended audience is health policy analysts who want to become more adept at gauging the political feasibility of their proposals; health professionals who seek a better understanding of how policy is made and how they might change it; health system managers who are savvy enough to see that in a system in which nearly half the money and most of the paperwork burden come from government, they need to understand how government makes its policies; and political scientists who seek illustrations of how the principles of government work in a policy arena with all the magical ingredients of political conflict: saliency, huge financial stakes, powerful interests, and venues in all the institutions of government. We present a comprehensive synthesis of political science research on the institutions of government and the policy process and an extensive review of the policies that have governed health care for more than a generation.

Part I of the book describes the institutions of government, reflecting the insights of political science research into the interaction of structures and motivations influencing their members. Part II describes the policy process and includes an illustration of how the theories worked to produce the PPACA. The conclusion pulls together the political and policy components of the book.

A central focus is documenting change in the nation's chief political institutions over time. In part I, we begin each chapter with a comparison that shows how different the institution under study looked during various periods when new presidential administrations began their policymaking quests, each one ushering in a new era of public health policy.

—President Lyndon Johnson in 1965 rode the crest of a Democratic wave of power and ideas and a growing consensus that the elderly poor, at least, deserved public health care subsidy. But he stretched the compromise by eliminating means testing from his Medicare proposal.

—President Ronald Reagan in 1981, elected with a mandate to shrink and constrain government-supported health care, welfare, and social services, oversaw the passage of a major Medicare expansion program to cover catastrophic events and costs.

—President Bill Clinton in 1993 quite inexpertly misinterpreted Americans' concerns that their insurance might be canceled as a mandate for employer-subsidized universal coverage. As a result, his congressional supporters were punished at the next election, and the House became dominated by Republicans for the first time in 40 years.

—President Barack Obama in 2009 took health care policy by the horns, but even with a Democratic Congress he was unable to produce the comprehensive, cost-saving health care reform he promised in his campaign. Even when the stars are seemingly in the right alignment, health care reform remains elusive.

Each chapter in part I relates changes in the institutions to these touch points and others, reflecting the conviction that only through a longitudinal view of policy-making can one accurately identify trends and chart the enduring progress of ideas and changes in ideologies and political positions.

Chapter 1 describes the structures and functioning of Congress and the motivations of its members. Its theme is that Congress was intended as, and has continued to be, the dominant branch of government. The chapter begins with a review of the motivations and sources of ideas of the framers, who conferred on the legislative branch enormous powers and many binding constraints. We describe shifts in power of party and institutional leadership relative to committee and subcommittee chairs in the context of their roles and responsibilities and sources of power, including personality and institutional rules. Committees and subcommittees of special importance to health care policy receive the most attention. We discuss conference committees, a central source of policymaking in health care but little understood, and give examples of how they rewrite legislation, often on the fly.

Budgeting, the increasingly dominant task of a deficit-swelling Congress, is closely examined; we step carefully between the concepts that are likely to continue to characterize the process and the changing rules and terms that complicate its understanding. A chapter section devoted to legislative parties addresses the paradox of their uncertain importance in the nation at large but their increasingly powerful role in Congress. Incumbency and its benefits and persistent re-election statistics highlight the discussion of congressional motivations, and this discussion introduces a review of the considerable political science literature on congressional behavior and its evolution. This chapter illustrates the growing importance of partisanship and its implications for strengthening the hand of party leaders.

Chapter 2 examines the presidency, starting with the sources and scope of presidential power and the high-stakes but sibling-like rivalry that characterizes the relationship between the presidency and Congress even in the best of times. Focused as the book is on health care policymaking, the subject of this chapter is the domestic president and how he makes choices about proposals and solutions for domestic problem solving. While his role in setting the agenda and proposing initiatives in his State of the Union addresses and other forums, and his monitoring of the progress of proposed solutions, are closely examined, a theme of the chapter is that there is much truth to the axiom that a president proposes but Congress disposes. The president is much more influential than any of the 535 members who work for or against him, but he is not, in the final analysis, a legislator. We examine the measures of presidential legislative success, although their validity becomes somewhat equivocal when the president's party controls both houses. Clearly he would be less successful if he could not count on the strong support of congressional leaders to add to or subtract from his proposals in whatever ways prove necessary to pull support from the wings of his party, manage the conference committee, and discipline recalcitrant party members.

Bureaucracy nominally reports to the president, too, although few presidents have found effective ways to use it; its direction is left much more to Congress than is suggested by government manuals' organization charts. But when the president and both houses are controlled by the same party, bureaucrats find that they have fewer opportunities to resist their political leaders.

In chapter 3 we describe the zealous huckstering of that diverse congeries of niche groups, coalitions, political action committees, and groundswell participants that engage in lobbying, campaign financing, and grassroots organizing to try to keep things off the public agenda or shape them to their liking when they cannot. A theme of the chapter is that interest groups are extremely influential— and in many instances the controlling influence—in health care policymaking. With their money, organizing skills, and singularity of purpose, they are altogether competent and only too happy to show a legislator the correct path toward constituent service and comfortable reelection margins. Another theme is that interest groups have always been one of the key institutions of government. We do not suggest that groups always or even usually act in the public interest. Much of President Bush's success in passing the MMA and President Obama's with the

PPACA can be attributed to party leaders' willingness to remove from the bill or greatly modify those provisions that key interest groups found offensive— whether or not the public strongly supported those provisions.

We examine how interest groups form and stay together, including the roles of economic self-interest, selective benefits, and entrepreneurs; the dominant role of occupational alliances; and the deliberate or inadvertent role of government itself in sometimes spawning groups. The interest-group world of today is much more complex than that of the 1960s or earlier. It is now characterized by permanent and temporary coalitions that share and complement one another's strengths and resources. Counts show a hugely increased number of interest groups. Their unglamorous daily ardor for monitoring legislation and providing information is the essential ingredient in that magic elixir of influence—access—which must precede their ability to provide a pearl or two of information that may sway a critical decision. We describe the ways in which these groups alter strategies as they move through the many venues of government, as well as the strategies they employ in campaign giving and grassroots campaigning. The link, or lack of it, between the giving of money and casting of votes is examined, but there seems little doubt that, coupled with features of congressional decision making described in chapter 1, the role of interest groups makes health reform all that much harder.

Chapter 4 takes a sympathetic view of public bureaucracy. Bureaucracy here is viewed as a repository of expertise, of detail people who bring the long view to the policy process and stand ready to serve their multiple masters—Congress, the president, the courts, their beneficiary constituents, and their regulatory foes—but who suffer as much when pulled in multiple directions as when they are ignored. The differences between careerists and politicos, the nature of an agency's political environment, and the importance of its mission are highlighted in a comprehensive review of the fascinating literature that describes how bureaucrats function, their relationship to the other branches of government, and the incentives and constraints that govern their behavior.

Both sides of the argument over whether bureaucrats are getting weaker or stronger are advanced, and although we choose neither side as more correct, a rich array of examples from health care policy leaves the clear impression that bureaucrats influence all aspects of the process, especially their own particular province: implementation. There is no question that bureaucracy is more effectively controlled by political leaders whose partisan ideology is shared by the president and leaders of both houses when government is not divided by party. Under such circumstances, it is unlikely that complaints to key committees by bureaucrats who feel pressured to bend to presidential will are likely to result in the launching of congressional investigations to haul a secretary before an unfriendly committee hearing.

A substantial portion of chapter 4 is devoted to regulation and the factors that modulate the degree of success agencies enjoy or suffer in gaining industry compliance. An overarching point is that no matter how green the eyeshades, regulation is political and agency performance is evaluated with a political yardstick. We examine the health agencies, describe their turf, and weigh their political fortunes in the light of past performance and as viewed by important beholders.

Chapter 5 traces the evolution of state governments from the good old days of the good old boys of the 1950s and 1960s through their own awakening and federalism's many redefinitions. The case is easy to make that most states today are modern, savvy, lean, innovative, socially responsible, and politically independent power centers—with huge differences in resources, to be sure, but determined to regain their autonomy and not to lose their identity. They still want all they can get from the federal domestic budget, but they have grown weary of the federal government's presuming that Washington knows better how to spend the money to solve problems.

A theme of the chapter is that while no one was watching, the states reformed their governance and became important players in health care provision and policy. States are innovators in health policy, and many, if not most, ideas about health policy reform offered by the federal government began as state initiatives. One message we want to convey is that the future is likely to see more of the same, especially if the federal government removes some of the barriers it has erected to state innovation. However, states, unlike the federal government, must balance their budgets—leading to programmatic cutbacks rather than expansions in tough economic times. Unfortunately, interest groups have figured out that when state innovation begins to cut into their profits too substantially, they can appeal to Congress to preempt state law by going forward with a federal program.

Institutions are again a central focus in chapter 5, highlighted by a close examination of state-to-state differences and similarities and comparisons with the federal government in the areas of budgets, spending, revenues, and documentation of the rapacious effects of Medicaid and other health spending on states' ability to set their own agendas. We examine the unique state feature known as direct democracy—initiative, referendum, and recall—and consider its benefits and liabilities. Also discussed is the impact of legislative term limits in more than a dozen states, including several of the nation's largest.

Beginning the discussion of the policy process in part II, chapter 6 defines public policy and its evolution. We describe various attempts to categorize public policies and their value in understanding the effect of the type of policy on its politics, and vice versa. We also describe several frameworks of the policy process and provide a compendium of examples of the political ways in which health care problems get defined as part of the effort to widen the scope of conflict and to interest the uninterested so that topics move to the public agenda. Problems do not just emerge; they are carefully nurtured, defined, framed, and often exaggerated to promote a desired policy solution. Ultimately, a decision must be made on whether a problem augurs for a public or a private solution, a choice inevitably tied to the often controversial concern about the role of government. Finally, theories of policy change are presented and analyzed.

Chapter 7 summarizes and critically evaluates the contribution of the 2010 Obama health reform, the Patient Protection and Affordable Care Act, to solving the problems of the American health care system. While the act is a laudable contribution, which really does tackle and fix some serious abuses in the health insurance industry and represents an amazing political success story, sadly it falls quite short of solving many of our most pressing problems—especially escalating health care costs. And assuring high-quality care.

For those comparing the first, second, third, and fourth editions, we offer the following guide to changes:

—Our first priority was to update examples and theory perspectives, keeping older examples only when they were too good to lose and favoring more recent incarnations of theory perspectives over more dated presentations of what may be classic ideas.
—We updated statistics.
—We replaced the third edition's case study of the MMA with a brief treatise on the Obama health reform.
—We updated our prognostications, which, wisely, we had made for the coming 10 years, so that in most cases we were either right or not yet wrong.

PART I / Health Policy and Institutions

CHAPTER ONE

Congress

A Look Back

1965

Democrats seemed to be everywhere when the first roll of the 89th Congress was called on January 4, 1965. So tightly squeezed in were House members that many found it more comfortable to stand at the railing around the back of the chamber. There were 155 more Democrats than Republicans in the House, and 36 more in the Senate, the product of a Democratic landslide victory that would make possible feats of legislative legerdemain seldom seen in the almost always fractious Congress. There was the usual splintering of Democrats, which typically separated Northerner from Southerner and big-city from small-town Democrat, but when sufficient numbers of Democrats stuck together, they could pass almost anything. Their newly elected president, Lyndon B. Johnson, meant to take full advantage of the majority held by his party to tackle a huge legislative agenda: Medicare, Medicaid, maternal and child health programs, health planning, regional medical programs, physician training programs, and programs aimed at specific diseases (including cancer and heart disease)—not to mention civil rights, education, economic opportunity, model cities, urban mass transit, nutritional programs for the poor, and more. Although some of these subjects—civil rights and Medicare, for example—were among the most divisive issues in American politics, this Congress would tackle them all and pass legislation on most of them.

In 1965, John McCormack was the Speaker of the House, and Mike Mansfield the majority leader of the Senate. While both were well-respected and talented legislators, their powers were constrained by the strength of the committees, headed by Southerners. The North-South split was the greatest source of conflict in the Democratic Party. The 1964 Johnson landslide brought 42 new Northern Democrats into the House and forced a change in the balance of party power. The Ways and Means Committee was transformed; a bare majority of curmudgeons had steadfastly refused to allow a payroll tax to finance Medicare. Legislative leaders, urged by the president, took every opportunity to replace them one by one.

Medicare, usually in its broader incarnation called "national health insurance," had been the subject of bitter debates, media fear campaigns, and committee-blocking tactics for some two decades. But with its decisive majority, the 89th Congress would (after considerable bargaining and compromises aimed at splitting interest-group opposition) roll over its opposition. As the final vote on Medicare was being tallied and the outcome became clear, one member of the Republican leadership stormed out of the House center-aisle doors, in exasperation turned to the pages and house doorkeepers gathered there to watch the show, and exploded: "We've got Goldwater to thank for this." He was referring to the fact that the defeat of the 1964 Republican presidential candidate, Barry Goldwater, had been so decisive as to sweep in the large Democratic majority, which could now run roughshod over the shrunken Republican minority.

1981

Contrast the bold, decisive, ideologically unalloyed Democratic juggernaut of 1965 and its massive show of party strength with the Congress of 1981—a time when the seeds of conservatism and antigovernment sentiment, growing in the late 1970s, had flourished to produce a Republican landslide presidential election and the first Republican majority in the Senate in a quarter century. Republicans picked up 34 seats in the House and 12 in the Senate. An oppressed minority so long, they relished their new leadership role in the Senate. Liberal critics said Republicans had been put in charge only because voters were dominated by the "me" generation, yuppies who had lost faith in—or could no longer see themselves benefiting from—public programs. Republicans retorted that liberals had had their chance. Health care reforms would take the shape of reduced spending, prospective budgets, and narrowed eligibility rules for subsidized services. This was nothing short of a sea change in the role of government, made possible by the Republicans' majority in the Senate, a large enough minority in the House to forge a majority with Democrats who strayed from their party's dominant positions, and, for a time, Democrats' fear that the popular Republican president could hurt them in the next election.

But the Democrats had a few resources of their own. They were not so easily split as in the old days, when quarrels over racial policies sent Southerners across the aisle looking for allies. Party leaders were stronger. No longer could they be held hostage by feudal committee chairs who bottled up legislation they didn't favor, thumbing their noses at their party's majority. Leaders had been given their own weapons by a series of reforms in the early 1970s, which were gleefully used by the large first-year class of 1974 elected on the heels of Watergate (named for the site of the attempted burglary of the Democratic National Party Headquarters in 1972, which led two years later to the resignation of President Richard Nixon). The party's leaders now appointed members of the Rules Committee, which set the rules for floor debate on most bills; leaders could refer bills to multiple committees, virtually ensuring that at least one committee would report a bill; and leaders played a crucial role in awarding committee assignments by appointing a majority of the members of the steering and policy committee—the committee that made appointments. Leaders were more aggressive and more willing to use institutional resources to a greater extent than those who had served in previous Congresses (Herrick & Moore, 1993).

One price of clipping the wings of committee chairs, however, was fragmentation. Subcommittees had filled the power vacuum, and, with their own staffing and considerable autonomy, subcommittee chairs and members could become expert in health policy and use their influence to profoundly shape the legislative proposal that went to the full committee (Bowler, 1987). House Energy and Commerce Health Subcommittee chair Henry Waxman embodied this new entrepreneurial subcommittee chair. Accepting the reality that no comprehensive health care program would see the light of day in the near term, he adopted an incrementalist approach: gradual expansion of Medicaid, the federal-state health care program for people who are poor or disabled, to cover more and more near-poor individuals, starting with children and their mothers. This approach worked for eight years. Every year between 1984 and 1991, at least one federal law expanding Medicaid eligibility or services, or both, was enacted, until opposition from state governors finally persuaded the powerful Senate Finance Committee chair to put an end to Medicaid mandates in 1991 (Weissert, 1992).

1993

The Congress faced by President Bill Clinton in 1993 was again different. The 1992 elections had brought in the largest first-year class in the House since 1946: 76 Democrats and 54 Republicans. But these newcomers were not political neophytes. Many had come up through the political ranks, including state legislative stints. Along the way they had lost the patience and humility usually expected of first-year representatives. After five months of toeing the line, they began showing their independence. With 82 more Democrats than Republicans in the

House, the president's hallmark budget and tax package passed with only two votes to spare. Was this the party that would try a year later to overhaul a health system comprising more than one-seventh of the economy, potentially displacing 3.1 million workers?

Leadership had also changed. Though powerful on paper, the current crop of leaders had a more mellow style than their predecessors. Rather than commanding their troops, modern leaders had learned to act as "agents in pursuing the party's legislative agenda" (Rohde, 1991, 35). Their job had become more collegial, so they used the powers granted to them to accomplish goals they held in common with other members of Congress. Rather than raw power, leaders counted on homogeneity of values. Where it existed, leadership could be granted discretion and expect to be followed; where it did not, members would go their own way. Since the late 1970s, Speakers had relied heavily on the party whip organization to enhance morale, build support for party positions, and poll members. Since the 1980s, around 20 percent of Democratic House members had been part of the whip "organization," which met weekly with the leadership to "enhance their two-way communication with members" (93) and make the leadership more effective in advancing its program.

House Speaker Thomas Foley (D-WA) showed his distaste for bare knuckles early in the session. Eleven Democratic subcommittee chairs voted with the Republicans against the administration's budget. Some in the party wanted to "strip" the chairs of their subcommittees, but Speaker Foley demurred, preferring instead to share the task of reprimanding recalcitrants by forcing caucus elections of all subcommittee chairs.

The president had even less power to force compliance with his program. Thanks to independent candidate Ross Perot, President Clinton had been elected with only 43 percent of the popular vote—a smaller margin than any member of either House. He would be of limited use at reelection time. This would become important when members of his party splintered in their support for health care reform: one gaggle demanded complete government takeover of financing while, at the other extreme, another group pressed for everything to be voluntary. In a word, the Democratic Party controlling the House lacked the discipline required to produce a legislative program.

2009

Democrats may have swaggered a bit as they strode through swinging doors to assemble for their first session of the 111th Congress, boasting one of the largest majorities they'd enjoyed in decades and well supported by a newly elected Democratic president. They had held a majority in the House since 2006. In July 2009, nine months after a breathtakingly close November 2008 Minnesota senate election, recount, and subsequent court battle, Sen. Al Franken (D-MN) took his seat, giving the Democrats a 60-vote, veto-proof majority (including two independents). They used it to pass health reform through the Senate without a single Republican vote. But before they could even begin negotiations with the House over differences in their bills (resolution of which could result in the need for a new vote in both houses), Massachusetts upset things by electing a Republican to the seat long held by Sen. Edward Kennedy (D-MA). That left the Democrats with only 59 votes including two independents, not enough to defeat a filibuster against repassing the health reform bill if needed. Six months later, the longest-serving member of the Senate, Democratic stalwart Robert Byrd (D-WVA) died, robbing the Democrats of yet another vote at a critical time in the legislative process.

Yet despite their accordion-like majority, no Congress since 1965 would pass more major Democratic agenda items, including bank and auto company bailouts, economic stimulus packages, health reform, banking reform, major expansion of the troop commitment and funding for the Afghanistan war, and many other reforms. Much of the credit would go to House and Senate leadership, especially Nancy Pelosi (D-CA), the first woman in history to hold the Speaker's gavel in the House. She was widely regarded as one of the toughest and most effective Speakers in the history of the House.

Yet popular opinion of Congress would sink to depths rarely seen in the past, and an anti-incumbent fever would sweep the nation, probably in reaction to the enduring recession, the bank bailouts, and the growing federal debt, surpassing $14 trillion and growing by $1 billion or more each year. The rancor could not help but carry over to Congress. Already partisan, the parties began to see that they shared fewer and fewer policy positions. The Democrats wanted to stimulate the economy and extend unemployment benefits; the Republicans wanted to reduce the deficit and voted to defeat extending benefits to people who had been out of work for more than a year. The Democrats wanted to reform health care and the Republicans did not like expanding the role of government. The Democrats wanted to reform the banking industry; the Republicans opposed them. The Democrats wanted to enact climate change legislation; the Republicans did not. And these were their differences before the grassroots conservative movement called the "Tea Party" began running conservative candidates in Republican primary elections in 2010 and defeating incumbent and party-endorsed Republican candidates. Incumbent Republicans responded by steeling their determination to oppose Democratic proposals of nearly every sort. One exception: on the same day they voted to oppose extension of unemployment benefits for the long-term unemployed, both parties supported legislation to give physicians a 2 percent pay increase under Medicare and to shield them from a scheduled 21 percent cut due to be implemented the next month. No one wanted to rile the doctors or their elderly Medicare patients.

Less than two years later, the Democrats' fortunes would change radically for the worse: they lost the House to the Republicans and watched as the GOP took control of both legislative houses in 26 states and many governorships. Having passed health reform 2010 would be credited as a key factor in the Democrats' defeat.

Powers and Constraints

It's easy to forget that for its first 13 years, the United States operated under the Articles of Confederation, which set up a weak national government and strong states. The experiment failed, and a convention ostensibly called only to modify the Articles of Confederation took the opportunity to rewrite the institutional power structure in significant ways. When the debate ended, a national government had been designed that placed primary power in a legislative body that was split between a popularly elected House of Representatives and an elitist Senate elected by the state legislatures. Congress was further checked by the powers of an energetic executive with veto power and a strong appointed judiciary. Any tendencies central government might have to wield power with a heavy hand would be checked internally by its own structure. In turn, democracy running amok in the states could be restrained by the powers granted to the national government.

The Constitution, like the country it reflects, is far from static, however, and the carefully balanced power relationships of 1789 have been skewed over the years. Thanks in part to some key Supreme Court decisions, the national government is the most important player in federalism. (The Court in the late 1990s rediscovered and reinvigorated federalism by ruling against broad federal power in a number of cases; see, for example, Schram & Weissert, 1999). Congress is the dominant player among the three coequal branches. Such dominance would have suited at least one of the Founding Fathers, James Madison, just fine: "In republican government, the legislative authority necessarily predominates" (quoted in Oleszek, 1989, 1). Two hundred years have proved him correct.

Congressional Structure

The bicameral nature of the congressional structure, carefully designed by the framers, is an important element in national policymaking. Political scientists have studied the effect of bicameralism and concluded that the presence of a second chamber does tend to provide a check on potentially volatile and misled majorities in one house and that bicameralism is central in shaping policy outcomes (Hammond & Miller, 1987; Janiskee, 1995). But most measures don't make it through both houses. Over six recent Congresses, some 43 percent of the major measures passed by the House were not passed by the Senate. During that same period, only 3 percent of major measures were passed by the Senate but not by the House (Dodd & Oppenheimer, 2009).

The institutions and those who serve in them are vastly different. U.S. senators serve six-year terms, are elected statewide (thanks to a 1913 constitutional amendment), and tend to have a broader, more long-term focus than their colleagues on the other side of the Capitol. This allocation of seats leads to some breathtaking representational disparities. The population of California has two senators. A population of the same size, living in 24 small states, has 48 senators. The Senate has 100 members, two from every state regardless of population. The House has 435 members, allocated on a state's relative population. Delegation sizes vary from one member representing each of the Dakotas, Alaska, Montana, Wyoming, Delaware, and Vermont to 53 from California (111th United States Congress, 2010). Since the size of the House membership remains stable, population shifts cause changes in the distribution of members every 10 years, following the census.

In an unusual move, in 2003 the newly Republican Texas legislature redrew congressional districts that had been in place for only one election. The redistricting was the result not of court rulings but rather of the desire of the Republican congressional leadership to increase its margin in the House by drawing lines that would help ensure Republican victories by pitting popular Democratic members against each other. It was clearly a power play, fully acknowledged by House majority leader Tom DeLay from Texas, the mastermind of the plan. He said simply, "I'm the majority leader, and we want more seats" (Riddlesperger, 2005). And he got them. The 2005 Texas congressional delegation added six new

Republicans (increasing from 15 to 21). But in late 2010 DeLay was convicted of money laundering in connection with this very effort; he was found to have channeled corporate contributions to Texas candidates through the national Republican Party in contravention of Texas law barring direct corporate contributions to candidates (Lozano, 2010). The indictment that preceded the conviction, as well as other legal problems, had forced him to resign his speakership and his congressional seat in 2006 (Hulse & Shenon, 2006).

In recent years, the Senate has attracted extremely wealthy people, often without prior political experience, who use their own resources to fund their campaigns. For example, in the 2010 election, Hewlett-Packard chief executive Carly Fiorina spent $5.5 million of her own money to win the California Republican Senate nomination, but she failed to defeat incumbent Barbara Boxer (D-CA) in the general election (York, 2008). But she is far from the first, nor did her lavish spending come even close to setting a record. In the same election cycle, Connecticut Senate candidate Christine O'Donnell (who made herself famous by uttering what many called the quote of the year: "I am not a witch") spent a record for the state of $7.3 million, failed to win, and then became the object of a federal investigation for using some campaign funds to pay for personal expenses. She blamed the investigation on political opponents of her Tea Party–supported campaign.

Six years earlier, Blair Hull spent $28.6 million of his own money in an Illinois U.S. Senate race, only to drop out when reports of spousal abuse emerged. That left the field open for political unknown Barack Obama, then a state senator, to be elected to the Senate (March, 2010).

Self-funded candidates often lose, perhaps for at least two reasons: First, running a company—the way most self-funded candidates get their money—is different from running a campaign; second, and perhaps most important, self-funded candidates typically have not come up through the ranks of politics. In that case they have not run before. When they do, they learn—often too late—that candidates get a lot more scrutiny, and are cut a lot less slack in what's found out, than they may be accustomed to in the business world.

About one in four senators is a millionaire. Few are women, and far fewer are African American or members of other minority groups. The House is more representative, but only in comparison to the Senate. In good years, 10 to 17 percent of representatives may be women, and perhaps another 10 to 15 percent members of a minority group. A total of 260 women have served in Congress, 88 of them in 2011, of whom 73 were House members and 15 were senators (Office of History and Preservation, 2010).

The banner year for election of women to the House remains 1992, when 24 freshman women were elected. In 2007 Rep. Nancy Pelosi (D-CA) became the first female Speaker of the House of Representatives when the Democrats took over the House. She had been elected majority leader of her party five years earlier.

Senators and House members in 2011 were changed little demographically from recent earlier Congresses. In the 112th Congress (2011–12), Senators' average age was 62, about a year younger than the 111th Congress, probably influenced by the 2010 death of the Senate's oldest and longest-serving member, Robert C. Byrd (D-WVA), at 92. He was first elected January 3, 1959, 51 years before his death. (Byrd credited his election to his fiddle, which he played at campaign events large and small throughout his career.) Most members of the 112th Congress had served considerably fewer years than Senator Byrd; the averages were 5.5 years in the House and 12.9 years in the Senate. Senator Byrd was not the longest-serving member of Congress, however. In 2010 Detroit congressman John Dingell (D-MI) had already served even longer than Senator Byrd. Dingell was first elected in 1955 (Manning, 2010).

Newspaper columnist and commentator David Broder (1993) contended that the compromise that made the Senate a smaller and more lordly body than the House had run amok in recent years. A majority of senators come from states that collectively elect only 20 percent of the members of the House, and Senate leaders typically come from smaller states such as Maine, Kansas, Kentucky, Wyoming, West Virginia, Mississippi, and Nevada. In 2009, the chairs of the powerful Appropriations, Finance, and Budget committees were from Hawaii, Montana, and North Dakota. The Senate majority leader for that session was from Nevada, and the minority leader from Kentucky. The leaders of the House tend to come from large and medium-sized states such as Texas, Illinois, Michigan, Washington, Missouri, Georgia, and California. A similar disparate domination of state legislatures by rural legislators in the 1950s made it impossible to pass progressive legislation for cities and suburbs until the U.S. Supreme Court ruled that state legislators had to be apportioned on the basis of population, not geographic area (*Reynolds v. Simms 1964*). Is such a reform possible for the Senate? No: the Constitution precludes amendments that strip away the geographic basis of Senate membership. Perhaps populous states should seek permission to split into two or more states to gain more equitable representation. Or the nation might follow the extreme remedy of one prominent congressional scholar, whose advice regarding the Senate was "Close it down. Put it out of its misery. It's just a bunch of egomaniacs looking around for people to fawn over them."

And no wonder they feel important. Senators have a greater chance of serving on desirable committees, and they achieve chair status more quickly than their House counterparts. Wording of legislation is hammered out in full committees, instead of subcommittees, and the Senate has fewer rules of procedure to restrict members' individuality. Amendments do not have to be germane to the subject of a bill. A senator can put a "hold" on a bill, requesting consultation before a measure is scheduled, and the common use of unanimous consent agreements (similar to rules issued by the House Rules Committee) requires extensive consultation and negotiation. "Holds" on bills can halt the progress of even a widely supported measure. For example, in 2007, following the massacre of 32 students and faculty at Virginia Tech University by a mentally deranged student, there was consensus in Congress to ensure that mentally unstable persons be barred from purchasing guns. A bill to grant funds to states to provide information on persons with criminal backgrounds and dangerous mental illness in a national database quickly passed the House and seemed destined to do the same in the Senate until Oklahoma senator Tom Colburn (R) put a hold on the bill that lasted several months. When the hold was finally lifted at the end of the session, the measure quickly passed and was signed into law. Sen. Richard Shelby (R-AL) made an unusually aggressive use of the hold in 2010: he held all Obama nominations via an unusual "blanket hold" in an effort to pressure the defense department to award two multi-billion-dollar contracts to firms in his state.

One senator can also temporarily halt floor action with a filibuster, which can be stopped only with 60 votes. And senators are no longer shy about using it. Once a rarity, the filibuster has been used with increasing frequency since the 1970s, and its use reached a profound peak in the 110th Congress. After the Democrats took control, a block of 43 Republicans began invoking the filibuster so frequently that cloture motions rose to 139, more than twice the number in the previous Congress (Secretary of the Senate, n.d.). Democrats charged that the GOP was deliberately trying to create a "do nothing Congress" so they could run against it. But frequently the filibuster or threat of it brought about concessions sought by the minority party. Threats of filibuster have become even more frequent than actual filibusters, with some votes for cloture (to end the filibuster) taken before a filibuster actually occurs. Senators may also threaten a filibuster simply to take a stand on an issue they feel strongly about. Targeting one bill to exact concessions on another happens frequently enough that a term has been coined for it: "hostage taking" (Sinclair, 2009, 8). In 2005, the Democrats' use of filibusters on judicial nominations so angered the Republican majority leader that he threatened to abolish the use of the filibuster for judicial nominees. On the eve of the vote for the "nuclear option" to eliminate this use of the filibuster, a compromise was reached, preserving the judicial filibuster for extraordinary circumstances.

Unless a bill has 60 aggressive supporters, a small group can defeat it in the Senate. No wonder that fewer than one-fourth of the bills introduced in a given two-year Senate session pass, compared with more than half of all bills in the middle of the twentieth century. The House passes an even lower percentage (around 15%), but about twice as many bills are introduced in the House as in the Senate—around 5,000 per session in the House (and dropping), compared with fewer than 3,500 in the Senate (also dropping in recent years). House sessions are longer (more days in session) and the number of roll calls is greater than 20 years ago (Mann & Ornstein, 2009).

Many factors go into explaining why Congress may be working harder and producing less. They include divided government, sharp partisan differences, budget constraints, and rules changes such as permitting cosponsorship of bills (which should produce fewer introductions and more passages per introduction, but may not). And increasing complexity of the content of bills is also a factor.

Leadership

Both houses are organized by the political parties. The majority party selects a leader (the Speaker in the House, the majority leader in the Senate), who makes the decisions on scheduling, committee membership, the committees that bills get referred to, membership of "conference committees" to resolve differences in legislation passed by the two houses, and more (see box 1.1 and table 1.1).

Not surprisingly, the strength of party leadership is affected by party unity and the personality of those chosen as leaders. Where party leadership is weak, committee chairs often gain in power. Congressional history is replete with pendulum shifts in the predominant source of power. In the 1890s, the Speakers were so strong as to be dubbed "Czar" Reed and "Boss" Cannon. The Speaker's powers were curbed shortly after the turn of the twentieth century, and for decades the power of committee chairs, and later subcommittee chairs, increased.

Box 1.1 **Party Leadership in the U.S. Congress**

The main leadership positions in the Congress are the Speaker of the House, the House majority and minority leaders, the House majority and minority whips, and the Senate majority and minority leaders.

The House of Representatives

The Speaker of the House is formally elected by the chamber as a whole, though really chosen by majority caucus. The Speaker presides over the House, shapes the agenda by deciding which bills have priority and on which calendar they appear, refers bills to appropriate committees, and designates members of joint and conference committees. The Speaker is the majority party spokesperson in the House, assisted by other party leaders, including

—the majority leader, who formulates that party's legislative program in cooperation with the Speaker and other party leaders, helps steer the program through the chamber, and assists in establishing the legislative schedule;

—the minority leader, who has the top leadership position for the minority party, formulates the party's legislative program in conjunction with other leaders, helps steer the program through the chamber, and serves as the party spokesperson for that chamber; and

—party whips, who assist both the majority and the minority leaders, mobilize party members behind legislative positions that the leadership has decided are in the party's interest, and keep an accurate count of the votes and preferences of members on bills.

The Senate

According to the U.S. Constitution, the vice president of the United States assumes the post of president of the Senate and presides over it. In the vice president's absence, the president pro tempore (a powerless, honorific position) generally presides over the Senate.

The primary leadership duties are performed by the majority leader, who is the spokesperson for the majority party. He schedules floor action, formulates the party's legislative program, schedules bills, works with committee chairs on actions of importance to the party, and directs strategy on the floor. The minority leader is the spokesperson for the minority party, mobilizes support for minority party positions, and directs the minority party's strategy. He does not appoint committee chairs. Until 1995, seniority dominated chair selections. When the Republicans became the majority party, they changed the rules, permitting members to select their chair by secret ballot, regardless of seniority.

The role of Senate whips is similar to that of House whips: aiding party leadership in developing a program, transmitting information to party members, conducting vote counts, and persuading members.

Table 1.1.   Congressional parties and leaders in 1965, 1981, 1993, and 2009

Year and Congress	House of Representatives	Senate
1965, 89th Congress	295 Democrats	68 Democrats
	140 Republicans	32 Republicans
	Speaker:	Majority Leader:
	John McCormack (MA)	Mike Mansfield (MT)
1981, 97th Congress	243 Democrats	46 Democrats
	192 Republicans	53 Republicans
	Speaker: Thomas P. "Tip"	Majority Leader:
	O'Neill (MA)	Howard Baker (TN)
1993, 103rd Congress	258 Democrats	57 Democrats
	176 Republicans	43 Republicans
	Speaker: Thomas Foley (WA)	Majority Leader:
		George Mitchell (ME)
2009, 111th Congress	256 Democrats	55 Democrats
	178 Republicans	41 Republicans
	Speaker: Nancy Pelosi (CA)	Majority Leader: Harry Reid (NV)

Sources: U.S. Senate, 2011a; U.S. House, 2011.
  Note: Excludes independents and vacancies, typically one or two of each per Congress.

Information is important to party leaders—both providing information to rank-and-file members about the party position and obtaining information on the preferences of the rank and file. Information sharing takes place through (1) the activities of the party whips, whose job it is to serve as liaison for the rank and file; (2) the views of party whips who represent different "factions" of the party; and (3) regular caucus meetings (Jones & Hwang, 2005).

However, when Newt Gingrich was Speaker of the House (1995–98), he reminded us how a dedicated and resourceful Speaker can make an enormous difference in both process and policy. Under Gingrich, House rules changed to strengthen the Speaker and to expedite passage of desired legislation. There were changes in informal rules as well, including an increasing role of some interest groups in policy development, manipulation of the media, reliance on task forces rather than committees, and extensive use of political consultants to chart legislative strategies and to gain public support. The Republican Speaker following Gingrich, Dennis Hastert, continued the strong Speaker role, but in a much less public and egocentric manner.

Hastert also used the Speaker's powers on the House floor to good advantage— holding roll-call votes open for long periods of time, calling tough votes at a very late hour to minimize media attention, and keeping certain issues off the floor entirely. He orchestrated efforts to keep Democrats out of committee delibera-tions until a consensus among Republican members was fashioned. And he used the resources of a Republican president to help rein in possible Republican hold-outs (Dodd & Oppenheimer, 2005).

Nonetheless, the Republican leadership did not always win—particularly in the early years of Hastert's leadership, when he lost on several important bills, including a patients'-bill-of-rights measure. To ensure the success of his proposal, he virtually shut down the work of the House health committees and shifted the debate to the House floor—where his own provision withholding the right of patients to sue their self-insured health maintenance organizations (HMOs) went down to defeat (Rogers, 1999).

However, in the early 2000s, the House Republicans were increasingly suc-cessful in getting their way, generally by marshaling every possible Republican vote. Although bipartisanship was initially promoted under the George W. Bush presidency, it was quickly abandoned in the House. The Republican strategy in 2004 was to win 218 votes (of 229) from House Republicans, thus obviating the need for Democratic crossovers. Leadership put pressure on members (threats of loss of committee chairs and earmarked district funds; promises of votes on cherished bills and of funding for a family member's congressional campaign) and bent the rules to get what it wanted. A case in point was the MMA of 2003, a major change in the Medicare program and one that was strongly desired by Congress and the president. In a vote beginning at 3:00 a.m. (unusual in its own right), Republican leaders held the floor open for votes for nearly three hours, until the initial vote of 215–219 became 220–215 (Schickler & Pearson, 2005).

Democrats under Speaker Pelosi began to show more discipline than political commentators typically expected of Democrats. Some thought the new unity was an artifact of the defection of the party's Southern Democratic wing to the Republican Party in the years following adoption of the civil rights laws of the 1960s. Southerners had always forced the party to compromise with conserva-tives, in part because House rules guaranteed these long-serving Southern mem-bers from safe seats advancement to chair key committees under seniority rules. They were independent of leadership, held up liberal legislation including civil rights and Medicare during the 1960s, and often sided with Republicans who shared their conservative views. As they left the party because they viewed its leadership as too liberal, the remaining membership became more homogeneous and more liberal.

But make no mistake: conservative opposition to liberal House leadership persists. Most prominent in recent years has been a coalition of 52 House conservatives (they say "centrists") calling themselves Blue Dogs. By holding sufficient numbers on key committees to block bills, they manage to hold the liberal tendencies of their party in check on many votes, especially including health reform in 2009, when they forced Chairman Waxman and Speaker Pelosi to include more cost control measures in the House bill (Blue Dog Days, 2009).

The name Blue Dogs comes from a painting of a blue dog by Cajun artist George Rodrigue, under which they hold their meetings. Ideologically, their view is that a Yellow Dog Democrat is one who will vote with the party every time. (Originally it was a Southern Democratic voter who would vote for even a Yellow Dog if it was on the ballot as a Democrat.) But a Blue Dog (House member) is said to have a better sense of smell and will bite you if you try to pull him where he doesn't want to go, especially on taxes and federal spending. The coalition formed after the GOP took control of Congress in 1994, when conservative Democrats felt their party had moved too far left. The Blue Dogs vowed to make sure this didn't happen again, but their voice was weakened following the 2010 election, when the voters in the marginal districts that many of them represented replaced Blue Dogs with Republicans.

Regardless of its cause, party unity strengthened the ability of the party majority to impose its will on its members. A sentinel event marking the new unity and new leadership prowess came with the organizing of the 111th Congress, when the Speaker orchestrated removal of the longest-serving member of the House from his chairmanship of the House Energy and Commerce Committee. John Dingell (D-MI) had chaired the committee during Democratically controlled Congresses for nearly three decades, all the while protecting Detroit carmakers from demands for higher fuel efficiency and clean air standards (even though he was also a major champion of health care reform). He was replaced by Rep. Henry Waxman (D-CA), an unrelenting enemy of tobacco companies, an advocate of higher CAFÉ (clean air and fuel efficiency) standards, a Medicaid expert, a leading advocate of nursing home reform, a master of House rules without equal in bill-passing prowess, and a Pelosi ally. Waxman would be much more closely aligned with the policy preferences of Speaker Pelosi, the newly unified Democratic majority, and President Obama.

Waxman used his new chairmanship to quickly coauthor the House Democrats' broad-based attack on global warming, the president's Cap and Trade bill, surprising many with its early passage by the House.

Recognizing Speaker Pelosi's new ability to marshal support and impose discipline, one conservative commentator called her "the strongest speaker in a century" (Fortier, 2008, para. 1). (Indeed, Pelosi was so accomplished a leader that the Republicans decided to make her their 2010 congressional-election-battle "poster child" for runaway liberal government, using advertising to link nearly every Democrat running for reelection anywhere in the nation to the Obama-Pelosi agenda. One northern Florida congressman quipped that he felt at times that he was running in San Francisco rather than Florida. Pelosi's home is in San Francisco.)

On "party votes," or those votes important to party leadership, both Republican and Democratic leaders often expect their members to vote the right way. Failing to do so can lead to future problems. In the past few years, the House Democratic leadership has become tougher—punishing members who do not vote with the party. Asked by a reporter if the White House would punish Democrats who voted against health reform, a senior aide suggested that time of the president and the vice president would be focused on those who had supported the bill. "We're going to have to focus on our friends," he said, implying that opponents would get little help from the White House in their reelection campaigns (Schulman, 2010, para. 2). As it turned out, though, the White House—to their surprise and chagrin—had no such luxury. As the 2010 election neared, they were desperate to keep any Democrat who had any reasonable chance of being elected. The president was happy to travel anywhere he was wanted to support a Democratic candidate.

The trend toward party discipline and polarization between the two parties reached a peak in both houses in the 110th Congress, rising to a level not seen since Reconstruction (McCarty, Poole & Rosenthal, 2006). The impact of this polarization is difficult to quantify, but two scholars found that the impact on productivity was curvilinear. Amid moderate policy conflict, Congress can enact laws on controversial policies. But when the partisan polarization becomes extreme, crafting and enactment of public policy suffers (Dodd & Schraufnagel, 2009).

The strengthening of party leadership is to be expected, say Aldrich and Rohde (2005), when the policy preferences of party members become more homogeneous and the differences in ideology between the parties widen, as seemed to be the case in the 110th, 111th, and 112th Congresses.

Committees

To Woodrow Wilson, writing in 1885 (1913, 79), "Congress in its committee-rooms" was "Congress at work." More than a century later, Wilson is still correct. Standing committees, about 20 in each house, are "the main paths along which Congress moves [and] all lead through the committee system" (Keefe, 1984, 92). They are the "workhorses" of the legislature: considering legislation, holding hearings (often outside Washington), amending legislation, and supporting their product on the House floor. Conference committees are temporary, created to adjust differences between the chambers when the two houses pass different versions of legislation. Conference committees are crucial in resolving remaining issues but also serve as additional venues for lobbyists and others whose proposals failed to pass one or both houses.

Standing committees are those with stated jurisdictions, created by the rules of the House, permanent (unless rules are changed), and responsible for screening, examining, and reporting on the legislation referred to them. Committees are where ideas are debated, deals are cut, and interest groups ply their trade, and in committees partisanship is paramount. The stakes are high in committees, and members know it.

The influence of committees extends beyond Congress itself. They also wield considerable clout over the bureaucracy, conducting oversight or congressional review of the actions of the federal departments, agencies, and commissions and of the programs and policies they administer. When the party in the majority in a chamber is different from the party in the White House and charged with overseeing administrative agencies, the committees turn up the heat. But even a president of their own party does not go unwatched. Cabinet officers say they spend one-third of their time on Capitol Hill testifying before committees and meeting informally with congressional staff. One cabinet secretary serving under Clinton said he was "astonished at the degree to which Congress is present in my daily life and shares at every level" in the direction of his department (Broder & Barr, 1993, 31).

Congressional oversight hearings may also change the behavior of private sector organizations by calling attention to their shortcomings. As chair of the House Government Oversight Committee, Henry Waxman held hearings on steroid use in major league baseball and many other sports. He proposed the Clean Sports Act of 2005. Although it did not pass, baseball responded by implementing strict testing procedures, hoping to head off congressional action and probably contributing to its loss of momentum (Waxman & Green, 2009).

Committee chairs often get their way. However, under the Republicans, the power of committee chairs declined relative to party leadership, since selection was no longer based on seniority and chairs could be deposed or members with less seniority installed as committee chairs—particularly if the lower-seniority members had agreed to be loyal to the party leadership goals.

Committees are not equal in power or popularity among members. House Ways and Means, Senate Finance, House and Senate Appropriations, House and Senate Budget, and House Rules are typically referred to as power or prestige committees. Membership on these committees is competitive and highly prized by legislators who want to make a name for themselves in Congress. Leaders usually get their training there, learning to cut deals, avoid minefields, and work to balance the conflicting pressures of other committees, lobbyists, and the broader house membership.

Policy committees are responsible for authorizing legislation and are organized by subject area. Some policy committees are more attractive than others. Popular House policy committees are Energy and Commerce, Education and the Workforce, and Financial Services. Constituency committees are those that provide electoral benefits to members, including Agriculture, Transportation and Infrastructure, and Veterans' Affairs committees. Committee attractiveness can wax and wane with changing policy priorities and the recent esteem or repute in which a committee is held. During the 1980s, the House Judiciary Committee's popularity plummeted, and in the 1990s, following its embarrassing racially and gender-bias tainted hearings on the Supreme Court nomination of Clarence Thomas, it found itself for a time unable to find enough members to fill all its slots.

Box 1.2 lists the eight committees and six subcommittees that have the most impact on health legislation. Only two are policy committees—the Senate Health, Education, Labor, and Pensions Committee and the House Energy and Commerce Committee—yet these two are extremely important in defining health policy. These committees plus a few others try to carve out a piece of any major health care reform proposal. The House Rules Committee and the leadership must then find a way to put the pieces together.

In recent years, with the rise of party leadership power, the importance of committees has diminished—especially compared with the 1950s and 1960s, when committee chairs could single-handedly stop legislation desired by most of their colleagues and the nation. Party leaders can bypass committees by setting up independent task forces, attaching legislative riders to appropriations bills,

Box 1.2 **Committees and Subcommittees on Health**

Senate Committee on Finance
Subcommittee on Health Care

House Committee on Ways and Means
Subcommittee on Health

Senate Committee on Health, Education, Labor, and Pensions
Subcommittee on Primary Health and Aging

House Energy and Commerce Committee
Subcommittee on Health

Senate Committee on Appropriations
Subcommittee on Labor, Department of Health, Human Services, and Education
   and Related Agencies

House Committee on Appropriations
Subcommittee on Labor, Health, Human Services, Education, Labor,
   and Related Agencies

Senate Committee on the Budget

House Committee on the Budget

having the House Rules Committee bring bills to the floor without committee hearings or markup, or adding provisions to conference committee reports. Nevertheless, the committee chairs are key players in the legislative process, especially for legislation that does not have high party interest. Committee chairs continue to control the staff and name subcommittee chairs. They also oversee individual committee rules and norms, including the level of input from "rank and file" committee members, the power of subcommittees, and even the seating charts for members during hearings.

Theories of Committees

Political scientists have developed three theories to explain congressional organization: gains for trade, or distributive theory; information theory; and partisanship. All have an important element in common: they explain the institution's structure as the result of individuals pursuing their self-interests to solve collective-action problems. All members seek reelection, constituent benefits, and policy outcomes. The actions they take to achieve these individual ends more or less coincidentally serve the collective ends and explain why the institution is structured the way it is.

Gains for Trade

Legislatures can be viewed as a collective of members acting together to allocate public benefits. However, since legislators seek to please their constituents in order to be reelected, they must seek selective benefits for their constituents. To link these selective benefits with collective action, legislators try to capture gains from trade or cooperation. Legislator A agrees to help legislator B by voting for B's bill, in exchange for B's help with A's bill. As long as the help A provides is worth less than the reward she gets from achieving her objectives, there is a net gain. This happy circumstance occurs more often than not, because legislators are heterogeneous in their preferences and priorities. Some care deeply about health policy, while others care little about it but have strong constituent or personal motivations for an interest in agriculture or international trade. Votes on health policy issues can be traded at little cost by the legislator with interests in agriculture in exchange for votes on agricultural issues, at low cost to the giver but high value to the receiver. This heterogeneity of preferences and priorities is an essential element of the gains-for-trade model. But one more element is needed to make the model work: some way to enforce the deals—to make them "stick" over the months of congressional decision making. Because some votes are taken early in the session and others late in the session, legislator B needs a way to guarantee that legislator A does not renege or strike a new, better deal with legislator C. The body needs a way to institutionalize the exchanges so that a large number of decisions can be made efficiently and with the assurance that deals will be honored. Enter committees.

Those who care about health policy self-select onto health committees, for example, while those more concerned with agriculture or other issues choose one of those committees. Each committee is given disproportionate control over its issue by virtue of jurisdiction. Health committees control the agenda by receiving all health-related bills and deciding which ones they will kill and which they will hold hearings on, mark up, and send on to the full chamber. These "institutional endowments" related to agenda-setting authority are a priori because they precede the legislative process (Shepsle & Weingast, 1994). Other endowments are called post hoc because they come after the house has acted (such as the high likelihood of serving on the conference committee or having over-sight responsibility for the agency implementing the law). Together these en-dowments assure the committee that it will have disproportionate influence over policy in its area. This assures members interested in health policy that no one else has much of a chance of breaking the implicit deal these members made when they gave up similar disproportionate influence over other issues such as agriculture. Committee membership seals the deal because all members agree to give the committees disproportionate power over a set of issues within their jurisdiction.

The upside is that everybody gets rewarded by being able to influence the policies of most importance to them. The downside is the potential for moral hazard: raiding the treasury by writing policies that serve committee members' own districts outrageously at the expense of everyone else. To prevent this, more generalist committees such as Ways and Means and Rules were structured by leadership to be more representative of the whole party. Bills giving too many benefits to specialty committee members (health committee members, for ex-ample) will be rejected by the power committees. If not, they may be rejected on the floor. Fearful of such rejection, the specialty committees are well served by not being too selfish in the bills they write.

Information and Expertise

In contrast, the informational approach or theory argues that committees form because of the need of individual members to ensure that the entire legislative body acquires and disseminates information. Information is vital because it re-duces uncertainty. Expertise is essential because it helps members choose poli-cies most likely to accomplish their policy goal and enhances their reelection prospects. Committees generate and provide information and expertise (Kreh-biel, 1992). Committee members who bear the high transaction costs of gather-ing information become experts and share their knowledge, not from altruistic motivations, but because they are rewarded by the organization. Transaction costs are lowered because only members with special interest and perhaps special background join the committees whose jurisdictional property rights give them incentives to become experts in such arcane fields as Medicaid policy. Free riding is discouraged because members' self-interest is served by gaining enough exper-tise and working hard enough on bill drafting to be able to cash in on the dispro-portionate influence that accompanies committee membership: agenda-setting power, bill drafting, hearings, the likelihood of conference committee membership, and oversight of the law's implementation. Committees that include a broad range of ideologies and views best serve the information needs of the body. Leadership, in this view, serves the party's interests by shaping committee membership to represent all the views of the party.

Partisanship

The third model explains congressional structure by focusing on legislative parties: it is the parties that provide the means for cooperation by which gains can be made for trade. Committees are the best way to organize, but committees require oversight and orchestration by party leaders to ensure that legislative efforts benefit party members (Cox & McCubbins, 1993). Leaders serve as the agents of the membership, knowing that if the party is ill served, they will lose their power positions following defeat at the polls. Leaders thus face incentives to protect the membership by making sure committees represent party views; free riders are punished with loss of committee membership; bills not representative of the party preferences don't make it to the floor; and party priorities are helped along by exercise of the leadership's prerogatives, including power to control the calendar, interpret the rules, and make deals with the minority that help the party achieve its policy goals.

Forgette and Scruggs (2005) quantified anecdotal reports that the committee selection system is more partisan than in earlier years. They found that party loyalty, as measured by a member's attendance rate at Republican Party conferences, was a better predictor of Appropriations Committee and Ways and Means Committee assignments after the 1994 Republican takeover of Congress than before that time. They also found that traditional norms of key committee assignment behavior, including restrained partisanship, decayed in the wake of Republican House reforms. "Claimants today recognize that party fundraising and party fidelity on key floor votes are more important now compared to the old-school tactics of regional and state alliances," concluded Forgette and Scruggs (14). "As this trend continues, the committee system will increasingly function as an organizational means for party caucus governance . . . [and] will function less and less as bodies for mediating partisan and ideological conflict, crafting bills that are informed by diverse committee members' policy expertise and compromises."

Balancing Committee Interests

In the gains-for-trade perspective, one result of the passion and district-interest motivations of committee members is that they are not typical of Congress as a whole. Shepsle and Weingast (1984, 345) called committee—and especially subcommittee—members "preference outliers." Not surprisingly, this puts committee and subcommittee members in a difficult position. If they draft legislation to their own liking, it may not be approved by the larger, more general committees through which it may have to pass, or by the whole house. The result: committees are often constrained in their actions by the expected reception on the house floor. They risk rejection if they report bills that deviate substantially from the majority's values. Hence, one of the jobs of an astute representative or senator is to become expert at anticipating chamber reactions (Shepsle & Weingast, 1987; Kiewiet & McCubbins, 1991). Committees that too frequently do not correctly adjust to the prevailing political winds lose power (Fenno, 1973). That some committees are more responsive to outside forces than others is usually explained by the salience or visibility and level of conflict of the issues assigned to them (Price, 1978).

Some committee members are especially vulnerable to self-interested behavior, and this makes clear that an old adage applies to Congress: Money isn't everything, but it can be exchanged for everything. The House Appropriations Committee usually takes the lead on budget actions, and even though its power was reduced in the 1970s with establishment of the Budget Committee and the consolidated budgeting process, it is still a highly desirable committee. It offers opportunities for legislators to "bring home the pork" in the form of appropriations targeted to benefit programs and projects in their home districts.

Writing the Rules

Bills that make it out of Senate committees go directly to the floor, but most major House bills need an additional stop: the House Rules Committee. This committee decides the rules of floor debate for the bill, including time for debate, whether or not amendments will be allowed, the level of detail at which sections of the bill must be voted up or down, and other aspects of the amendment process. Two political scientists compared the House Rules Committee to the "crossroads of the legislative process," where most members must come at one time or another to ask for favored treatment or protection with special rules (Bach & Smith 1988, 12). At one time the Rules Committee was a formidable barrier to a bill's progress. Democrats on the 1965 Rules Committee—over the objections of the Republicans on the committee—allotted only 10 hours to debate the original Medicare bill, permitted no amendments, and required an up or down vote on the entire complex bill rather than allowing section-by-section votes. Disallowed by that rule were votes on amendments that might have passed, such as relating premiums to income. Members who wanted to support the bill but with changes had to vote for it "as is" or go home and explain during reelection campaigns why they voted against a popular bill.

The authority of the Rules Committee has ebbed and flowed. Sometimes it is used by leadership to pull a bill back to leadership's liking after a committee has set out its different preferences. At other times it is used to strike deals that make it possible to get enough support for a bill to assure its passage once it gets to the floor. President Obama's health reform bill would not have garnered enough conservative House Democratic votes in 2009 had a deal not been struck in the Rules Committee that permitted conservative Bart Stupak (D-MI) to offer an amendment aiming to further restrict abortion coverage in the new bill over what was already the law of the land prohibiting federal funding of abortions. The rule permitted the amendment to come to a vote even though leadership knew it would be adopted if that happened and even though Speaker Pelosi (D-CA) favored more liberalized abortion policy. But she needed the support of those conservative members of her party, and this was their price. "This is a small facet of the bill that's very important to a lot of people," Democratic majority leader Steny Hoyer (D-MD) said (Montgomery, 2009b, para. 8).

The committee also can give preference to members in electorally challenging districts by offering them the opportunity to introduce amendments that will be politically advantageous. These members "take credit" for these provisions and get the public spotlight on the House floor and media venues (Lipinski, 2009, 337–60).

Leaders can also use both the committee and existing House rules to block issues that they do not want coming to the floor. For example, to facilitate passage of a $50 billion deficit-reduction package that the leadership wanted in order to placate angry party conservatives, leaders arranged for the Rules Committee to remove from a reconciliation bill a provision that would have raised copayments for Medicaid recipients. The change made the package acceptable to Republican moderates, who without removal of the offensive provision would have opposed the whole package. Conservatives regretted the change but were willing to accept it as the price of moving the bill (Cohn, 2005).

Subcommittees

Since the mid-1970s, subcommittees have played an increasingly important role in congressional decision making, especially in the House. There have been as many as 140 or more subcommittees in each house in some Congresses. The numbers dropped for several years to around 85 in the House and fewer than 70 in the Senate (Ornstein, Mann & Malbin, 2002) and then swelled again in the 111th Congress to 104 House subcommittees (including some task forces and panels) and 77 in the Senate. Appropriations committees in both houses have the most subcommittees, 12 each in the 111th Congress. Homeland Security committees in both houses were next.

The two houses vary in the ways they use subcommittees. The House subcommittees are heavily involved in legislating: holding hearings and marking up bills. Full committees conduct their own markup but generally do not hold additional hearings. Senate subcommittees often hold hearings but frequently do not mark up (or write) bills; markup is usually the province of the full committee. The Senate Health, Education, Labor, and Pensions Committee retains jurisdiction over two dozen major health programs at the full committee level.

In the House, the responsibility for health care policy lies mostly with Energy and Commerce's Health Subcommittee, not the full committee. That subcommittee traditionally sets its own agenda, picks its own battles, and usually wins them. One exception was the major health care reform initiative of the Clinton years. Neither the subcommittee nor the full committee was able to reach consensus on a bill.

The larger clout of House versus Senate subcommittees can be quantified. Smith and Deering (1990) found that 85 percent of measures brought to the House floor were first referred to subcommittees, compared with only 42 percent in the Senate. Sinclair (2005) noted two reasons that the Senate does not use subcommittees to write legislation. First, senators have a larger workload, since they deal with the same issues as the House but with fewer than one-fourth of the members; second, the individualistic nature of the smaller Senate is to give all committee members the opportunity to participate in decision making—thus favoring a committee, rather than a subcommittee, decision-making venue.

Conference Committees

Conference committees are ad hoc congeries of representatives from both houses charged with the responsibility of reaching a compromise version of a bill. Conference committees are older than Congress itself: state legislative bodies used them to resolve differences before the U.S. Constitution was put in place (Oleszek, 2004). Membership in conference committees, dubbed by scholars the "penultimate power" (Shepsle, 1991) or the "third house" of Congress (Oleszek, 2004), is prized because the decisions made in conference are usually final. Conference committee language cannot be amended: the houses must vote the whole bill up or down. Conference committees can rewrite or change the legislation (for example, by choosing to "give up" items passed in a member's own house in favor of the other house's language). Sometimes they add provisions out of whole cloth or delete measures that were included in both House and Senate bills. "It is elementary," said Sen. Mitch McConnell (R-KY), "that if you get a bill to conference, you have wide latitude to produce a bill the majority is comfortable with and the president is comfortable with" (Oleszek, 2004, 270).

Conferees are named by House and Senate leadership based on recommendations from committee chairs, and the conferences are usually dominated by members of the committees that originated the legislation. On major bills, the party leaders often serve on the conference committees themselves. A conference on the 2003 Medicare prescription drug bills had both the Senate and House majority leaders as members (the latter was the lead negotiator for the House). The House and the Senate can adopt motions instructing the conferees, but the conferees can disregard their instructions. Party leaders can—and do—box out members with views they do not support. For example, Sen. John McCain (R-AZ), sponsor of the bill to repeal the Medicare catastrophic coverage program in 1989, was not named to the conference committee reconciling his bill with its House counterpart. Rep. Charles Norwood (R-GA), sponsor of the House-passed patients' rights bill, was not named as a conferee in the 1999–2000 conference committee trying to settle differences between House and Senate bills, because he had rammed the House bill through over the leadership's objections. In fact, only 1 of the 13 House members appointed to that conference committee had actually voted for the final version of the bill the House had passed (Rogers, 1999).

In recent years, the role of the minority party in conference has been minimized. Health reform passed without benefit of a conference committee. Conference committees can be quite large, especially when bills have been considered by more than one committee. In 1971, the average number of House conferees was 8; in 1991, it was 25. The average number of Senate conferees increased from 8 to 12 over that period of time (Oleszek, 2004). Since any agreement must have the majority vote of both houses, such a mismatch in numbers is not problematic. However, sheer mechanics may be difficult. Subconferences sometimes are named to deal with specific issues. On large conference committees, much of the work is done by staffers, who conduct major negotiations on behalf of members on key issues.

Sometimes conference committees bring out "power" issues between the House and the Senate or simply between powerful representatives of those bodies. A case in point was the conference committee for the MMA in 2003. Sen. Charles Grassley (R-IA), chair of the Finance Committee, and Rep. Bill Thomas (R-CA), chair of the Ways and Means Committee, clashed over who would chair the conference committee (both wanted to do it) and later over provisions increasing Medicare payments to rural areas (wanted by Grassley but not by Thomas). At one point Senator Grassley and his staff boycotted the sessions when his issues were not on the agenda (Pear, 2003).

Most Americans do not appreciate the formidable power of conference committees. Few are aware, for example, that the conference committee on the Employee Retirement Income Security Act (ERISA) of 1974 inserted a preemption clause that has proved a major impediment to state-level health care reform. A few House conferees inserted language that preempted state laws relating to "any employee benefit plan" to replace language that prevented states from legislating about subject matter regulated by the act. A second phrase was then added stating that no employee benefit plan shall be deemed an insurance company. The result: state insurance regulation of self-insured or corporate health insurance plans was prohibited. Together, the two provisions—added 10 days before final passage of the law without the knowledge of many health insurers, the Department of Labor, or the state government associations—have withstood efforts in Congress and the courts to make changes and have played a powerful constraining role in state health care innovations (Fox & Schaffer, 1989).

Similarly, a last-minute "surprise" in the 1988 catastrophic health insurance conference bill was a mandate that state Medicaid programs must pay all Medicare premiums, deductibles, and copayments for beneficiaries with income below the federal poverty level (Torres-Gil, 1989). This provision for the "dually eligible" was one of only two major initiatives not repealed the following year. Ironically, dually eligible beneficiaries became major users of the program—accounting for 40 percent of total Medicaid spending in 2007 (KCMU, 2011).

It is not uncommon for bills to languish and often die in conference committee—the fate of the patients' bill of rights noted above. Although the bills were passed by the House and the Senate in October 1999, by August 2000 the conference committee was still stymied over major issues such as which patients should be covered under the new law and whether to allow patients to sue their self-insured HMOs. Since the issue was one of high visibility, there were many efforts to disgorge a bill from the conference. President Clinton met with conferees at the White House to try to resolve issues. The American Association of Health Plans launched a two-week, $200,000 television ad campaign aimed at the conference committee. Both Republicans and Democrats thought the issue was important to the upcoming congressional elections. So, seven months after floor passage, the conferees began a marathon series of meetings that included late-night sessions. As a sign of desperation, a House leader on the issue who had been excluded from the conference committee (Rep. Charlie Norwood) was brought into the conference negotiations in their seventh month (and four months before the election). Republicans wanted a bill passed before the election, because the issue gave Democrats a popular claim to use against them. But the differences were too great, and even with the election just days away, conferees went home with no agreement, leaving the bill to be reintroduced in the next Congress. The bicameral process, said House Ways and Means Committee chair Bill Thomas, is "akin to mating a Chihuahua with a Great Dane" (Oleszek, 2004, 269). No wonder, then, that it is often unsuccessful.

Budgeting, Washington Style

Under the U.S. Constitution, Congress has the "power of the purse," embodied in the language that gives it the power to "lay and collect taxes . . . to pay the debts and provide for the common defense and general welfare of the United States." Congress can also borrow money. The congressional allocation of resources gets to the basic political question of who gets what and who pays. Further, the budget not only represents a document of government operations but also is a statement of government priorities.

The legislative process is defined by two types of bills: authorizations, which establish or continue an agency or program and describe its operations, and appropriations, which provide the funding for the agency or program. The two-part system is designed to separate the policy from fiscal decision making. The process is generally sequential, with the authorization preceding the appropriation. There have traditionally been 13 annual appropriations bills, considered by the 13 appropriations subcommittees in each house. These appropriations are generally specific about the money to be provided and the use to which that money is to be put. Unless a program is funded by appropriations, it ceases to exist. Congress must vote affirmatively to increase the funding level of a program each year; the funding cannot grow automatically (entitlements are an exception).

Traditionally, the appropriations bills were processed and enacted separately—involving 13 different votes. In recent years, however, a new approach has emerged, in which the measures are combined into an omnibus appropriations bill (Taylor, 2004). The 2009 omnibus spending bill totaled $410 billion and covered spending by all agencies except Defense, Homeland Security, and Veterans Affairs (Neal, 2009). It passed in February 2009, about five months behind the congressional budgeting schedule. But that turned out to be a quick pace by comparison to the next year, 2010, when appropriations were done only as a series of continuing resolutions, because no budget bill ever passed. As the last one expired March 4, 2011, Republicans who had taken control of the House demanded cuts of $61 billion from current discretionary spending as a condition for signing another continuing resolution. Senate Democrats and the White House refused. And, as they had in 1995, differing ideologies and partisan objectives threatened to shut the government down for lack of a budget.

Entitlements

Entitlements are guaranteed services that will be provided to all beneficiaries who meet the specified qualifications for the program. Entitlements are funded automatically and do not require appropriations. Entitlement spending makes budget control difficult: there is no overall limit on spending, but rather the spending is determined by the number of eligible beneficiaries, those legally entitled to the program funds. The largest entitlement programs are Social Security, Medicare, and Medicaid. Income Security (a broad category of welfare, retirement, unemployment, Black Lung, nutrition, and related payments) is also large. Smaller but important entitlements include veterans' health care, defense health care, federal employees' health benefits, and a few others. But Medicare, Medicaid, and Social Security dwarf all others, collectively accounting for over 40 percent of all federal spending.

The growth in entitlement spending has eclipsed other domestic spending over the past 20 years. The Congressional Budget Office (CBO) predicts rapid and unsustainable growth in entitlement spending, primarily for Medicare and

Medicaid. Social Security will increase from its 2011 value of less than 5 percent of gross domestic product (GDP) to only about 6 percent by 2035. But Medicare and Medicaid will grow from almost 5 percent of GDP in 2011 to nearly 10 percent in 2035, so that over that period nearly 80 percent of the growth in the three big entitlements will be due to growth in Medicare and Medicaid spending. The increases will be driven by rising health care costs per beneficiary and aging of the population, according to CBO estimates. Medicare was projected by the president's 2012 budget to rise from $6.2 billion in FY 2010 to $8.1 billion in 2020, an increase of more than 30 percent in a decade (OMB, 2011a). See figure 1.1.

Once an entitlement program is enacted, it can escape yearly evaluations. Further, many entitlements are indexed to the cost of living, so payments are increased automatically without congressional action. Entitlements can be curbed only by changing the law that set up the program or the regulations governing its implementation. Other "uncontrollable" elements of the budget are interest on the debt and outlays from prior obligations (largely related to defense spending).

Cutting entitlements is extremely difficult. Entitlements are popular programs—especially to the recipients. Elderly people, a major category of recipients, are well organized and are quick to fight any possible cut in their programs. President George W. Bush ran into a buzz saw when he tried to convert Social Security holdings to private investments. When the stock market crashed two years later, many who had opposed his proposal felt vindicated. As economist

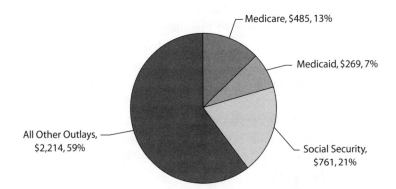

Figure 1.1. Medicare, Medicaid, and Social Security as share of FY 2012 federal budget ($ in billions). *Source:* United States Federal Budget FY 2012, Historical and Summary Tables (OMB, 2011b, 2011d).

Henry Aaron (2009) put it, "It has [been] driven home that Social Security is, and must remain, the bed-rock of retirement income security . . . Private income sources cannot do what social insurance does."

But some analysts and a few politicians have begun to question whether the problem is all entitlements or simply *health care* entitlements. House member Kevin Brady (R-TX) observed: "A good Medicare solution is more difficult than the war on terrorism, education, Social Security and homeland security combined" (Roth, 2005).

Brookings Institution health and retirement policy expert Aaron (2009) agrees: "Growth of total health care spending is not an entitlement problem . . . It is a health care financing and organization problem." While Aaron's argument is compelling and is correct about the importance of health care costs in aggravating the entitlement problem, there is no denying that the plethora of subsidy programs directing funds to individuals—most of them as entitlements—is growing at an alarming rate and consuming much of the federal budget. Payments to individuals nearly doubled from 2000 to 2010 and are projected to fall just short of $3 trillion by 2016, accounting for almost two-thirds (65.7%) of the total budget (U.S. Government Printing Office, 2011).

Republican House Budget Committee chair Paul Ryan (R-WI) decided he would try to take on the entitlement problem in his proposed 2012 budget (Tully, 2011). He recommended capping the government's contribution to Medicare and block-granting Medicaid. While his budget passed the House (with no Democratic votes), Democrats were quick to target vulnerable House members who voted for his bill with ads charging that they had supported the Ryan plan to abolish Medicare as we know it (Yadron, 2011).

The Congressional Budget Process

For the country's first 150 years, there was a surplus of funds; and federal spending, with the exception of military pay, equipment, and supplies, was relatively low. But in the 1930s, the federal budget began to grow as the government assumed new domestic responsibilities, including regulating business and providing for people who were temporarily or permanently disadvantaged. Presidential control over the budgetary process dates back to 1939, when the Bureau of the Budget (BoB) was made part of the executive office. In 1970, the BoB became the Office of Management and Budget (OMB) and its responsibilities expanded (see chapter 2). The presidential budgetary power peaked in the early

1970s, when President Nixon aggressively "impounded," or refused to spend, funds appropriated by Congress for programs he did not support. The Congressional Budget and Impoundment Act of 1974 (Public Law 93-344) was passed in part as a response to congressional unhappiness over this increased presidential role. It was also enacted as a way to improve congressional control over the federal budget, thus allowing Congress to set fiscal policy and make choices among programs (Ellwood & Thurber, 1977). The law set up the House and Senate Budget committees and the Congressional Budget Office. It also mandated a concurrent budget resolution setting forth aggregate federal spending, which serves as a fiscal blueprint to guide the actions of authorizing, appropriating, and taxing committees. Finally, it established the process known as reconciliation, designed to bring existing law into conformity with the budget plans.

The budget process has evolved since it was set up, with the focus changing from the process of priority setting, to controlling the size of the federal budget and federal budget deficits, to controlling domestic spending. In the early 1980s, it became clear that something was needed to control government spending and reduce the burgeoning deficit. Although it had taken more than 200 years for the debt to get to $1 trillion, it took only four more years to get to $2 trillion and little more to pass $5 trillion. It passed $10 trillion in the final months of President George W. Bush's second term. Two years into President Obama's first term the debt had passed $14 trillion.

One mechanism Congress sometimes uses to try to reduce yearly shortfalls of revenues compared to spending (called deficits) is "Paygo," an agreement among members of the majority party that they will offer no new spending without paying for it through either new taxes or cuts in other programs. Democrats used it when they had the majority in Congress during the Clinton administration. Republicans did not adopt it during their control. Democrats adopted it again when they took Congress back in 2006, and then Republicans embraced it in 2011 when they took back the majority, but they agreed to apply it to everything except tax cuts.

The *New York Times* did an analysis of what brought about the reversal of fortune from surpluses in 1998 through 2001 to deficits starting in 2002 and continuing for the foreseeable future (Leonhardt, 2009). They pointed to five factors:

- 37 percent of the swing from surplus to deficit is due to the business cycle reversal: decreasing revenues and increasing unemployment and other automatic payouts;

- 33 percent is due to legislation signed by President George W. Bush, including tax cuts and the Medicare prescription drug law;
- 20 percent comes from President Barack Obama's decisions to continue President Bush's policies, including the Iraq war, tax cuts, and Wall Street bailouts;
- 7 percent comes from President Obama's Stimulus Plan, directed at reviving the economy, in the first months of his term; and,
- 3 percent comes from President Obama's plans for health care reform, education, energy, and other reforms.

The Reconciliation Process

As it has evolved over the years, the budget process has weakened the power of authorizing committees and given more power to party leaders. Authorizing committees rarely have the opportunity to launch new programs but rather must work hard to protect established programs from budget cuts. The Appropriations committees—once viewed as the "cardinals" of the appropriations process—now have control over only about one-third of federal spending. This is because so much spending is in the form of entitlements, not subject to appropriations. Further, the party leaders and Budget committees often make key decisions about what programs to fund and how much to alter entitlement programs to produce savings or increase the amount of spending they will require to cover new benefits or newly eligible beneficiaries.

Beginning in the early 1980s, the reconciliation bill, a compilation of legislative committee recommendations implementing the budget resolution, began to be used as a vehicle to enact new provisions and programs and otherwise change policy. Its attractiveness was clear. Measures could become law with minimal attention and no hearings and would likely sail through both houses, which were eager to vote to reduce the deficit. Importantly, reconciliation bills cannot be filibustered in the Senate and permit actions to be taken in tandem that arguably would never survive separately.

Most major changes in Medicare and Medicaid over the past 20 years have been in the reconciliation bill—with the rare exceptions of the 2003 Medicare Modernization Act, which made substantial changes by adding drug coverage, and the 2010 Patient Protection and Affordable Care Act, which made more limited changes in Medicare than did the MMA.

While consideration in reconciliation bills is given special treatment, rules have been made along the way—particularly in the Senate—to curb excesses in the reconciliation process. For example, reconciliation provisions cannot contain non-revenue-related items and cannot incur revenue loss beyond 10 years; but these provisions can be waived by a three-fifths vote of the Senate (Oleszek, 2004).

This process became highly relevant in the 2009–10 legislative planning for the Obama health reform plan. Liberal Democrats pressed the White House and Senate leaders to use the reconciliation process to pass health reform. That way they could include many provisions, such as a public plan option, that would be sure to invoke a Republican filibuster if the bill was considered outside reconciliation. Only 51 votes would be needed to pass the bill, so even if conservative Democrats defected, the bill could pass. Furthermore, reconciliation rules limit debate to 30 hours, so there was no chance of talking the bill to death. But reconciliation has many limitations. Provisions that don't affect the federal budget can be struck on a point of order, so individual mandates to buy insurance, employer mandates to offer it, and limitations on insurance companies' excluding patients with preexisting conditions could all be struck. The bill would also have to save money: $1 billion within five years to show net deficit reduction. "Many of the advocates of major health reform would be quite disappointed with what came out of the use of reconciliation," Sen. Kent Conrad (D-ND), a Senate Finance Committee member and an opponent of reconciliation, told the *Washington Post* (Murray & Montgomery, 2009, para. 22). That is, many of the most important provisions in the reform bill would have been struck out on a point of order because they represented policy change rather than budget reductions. The result was a compromise that permitted the House to accept the Senate version of the bill, obviating the need for a conference by putting into two reconciliation bills some language that had the legal effect of amending the Senate reform bill. Both of the reconciliation bills were passed with simple majorities.

"Pork" in the Budgeting Process

Pork is the fanciful appellation given to projects garnered from Congress by a member for her district. "Bringing home the bacon" means being successful in winning projects that send federal money back home. While pork is often contained in appropriations bills, it finds its way into other bills as well. For example, the global warming reduction bill that passed the House of Representatives early in President Obama's first year may have hit new records for including giveaways needed to garner votes. Small change to the tune of $50 million went for hurricane research in Florida, while rural and farm state members drew down billions to support their constituents' agricultural and forestry businesses. Utilities were the biggest winners, capturing both free pollution permits and promises to let them keep burning coal, but also billions in research money to help them develop carbon recapture technologies (Broder, 2009). Republicans had done much the same when they were in charge. The House-passed MMA of 2003 contained numerous elements called "rifle shots" for their narrowly targeted effects. In a high-profile bill such as health reform or climate change, these components can help build support for the bill and provide interest groups with a mechanism for passage of provisions that might not make it alone.

Appropriations committee and subcommittee chairs and members are often the primary purveyors of pork. The subcommittee chairs in charge of veterans' spending will often see veterans' hospitals built in their districts, while defense plants and contracts often go disproportionately to the districts of Defense Committee and subcommittee chairs. But those districts do not get all the veterans' hospitals or defense plants. Self-interest must be balanced with the public interest if committee power is to be maintained. When it is egregiously abused, chairs may be replaced when the next Congress is formed, or a committee's jurisdiction may be narrowed or shared with another committee, or an entire committee may be abolished by the next Congress, or the house membership may gather the simple majority of votes for a discharge petition, forcing a committee to give up a bill so that it can be considered by the whole house. Likewise, contracts for some expensive military procurement projects are sometimes deliberately spread among many members' districts to assure widespread, enduring support for the airplane, ship, helicopter, or other expensive piece of equipment being designed and built over a period of years.

Appropriations committees, especially in the House, have become more partisan in recent years. Before the mid-1990s, decisions by these committees were based on consensus, and bipartisanship was the norm. Former House Speaker Newt Gingrich recognized that appropriations were crucial to his vision and to the Republican agenda, so the type of member appointed to the committee was changed—from someone willing to work across the aisle to someone closely tied with the leadership agenda. Appointees are now more party-loyal and more electorally challenged than in earlier years, when members of the committee were chosen largely from "safe" districts as a way of ensuring longtime members with appropriations expertise (Gordon, 2005, 278). Today's members are increasingly from marginal districts (where both parties are well represented in the electorate) and can use their position to help solidify their importance to their district.

Another change has been the increase in riders—or legislative language in appropriations bills. Exceptions to allow riders can be made by the House Rules Committee, largely controlled by party leaders. Thus, more and more appropriations bills now carry substantive riders (Aldrich, Perry & Rohde, 2009).

Finally, there are earmarks, provisions slipped into a bill that direct specific funds to specific projects in a specific member's district. Earmarks passed the 10,000 mark in 2009 but fell back slightly to 9,413 in 2010, according to Taxpayers for Common Sense, which noted that the more than $16 billion appropriated by this selective method of funding represented about 2 percent of all congressional appropriations in 2010 (Kane, 2010).

The problem was not simply the increasing amounts being earmarked but also the way they were added—often in the middle of the night in a conference committee report, without the knowledge of other committee members. One example was a California road project in a highways appropriations bill that ballooned from $30 million in the original proposal to $750 million when it came to the final vote (Abrahms, 2006). The most famous earmark in recent years went to Alaska in 2005, connecting very small towns to Anchorage and dubbed by critics "bridges to nowhere." Following that embarrassing controversy, Congress made some improvements in earmarking rules, but none of them would have prevented the bridges to nowhere.

Earmarking attracts much media ink and talk, frequent promises of reform, and little actual improvement. The fiscal year 2009 budget bill included $7.7 billion for 8,570 earmarked projects. For Ohio, they included $95,000 for "cataloging and preservation activities" at the Columbus Museum of Art and $122,871 sent to the Greater Toledo Arts Commission to support local artists with marketing help and for two gallery events. Requests came both from Ohio House members and the state's senators. Sen. Sherrod Brown (D-OH) said that he succeeds in garnering federal money for only about 2 percent of the 1,500 requests for earmarks that he gets from constituents each year. He claimed that he seeks funds for only those that create jobs and help economic development in Ohio. Sen. George Voinovich (R-OH) was less defensive in his explanation of earmark support, saying through a spokeswoman that he was "elected to represent Ohioans" and supports "common-sense" earmarks rather than leaving project choices "to somebody who's never been in Ohio, let alone never been out of Washington, D.C." But bureaucratic agency heads complain that earmarks trample their authority and curb their ability to allocate funds according to national plans and priorities (Eaton & Koff, 2009).

To address this specific problem, House rules were adopted by the Democrats at the beginning of the 110th Congress and continued in the 111th requiring that earmarks be publicly disclosed by the earmarking committees. Taxpayers for Common Sense, a nonprofit group opposed to earmarks, now compiles a database of all earmarks by starting with the committee reports and then adding other earmarks they find on their own. Their methods include searching members' websites and other sources for earmark disclosures, member by member. Thus, in their reporting they also include categories for "unknown" sponsor, because in some cases no name is associated with what is clearly an earmark in a bill. They follow the rule that "what looks like an earmark, talks like an earmark" is probably an earmark, including items tucked into legislation but not counted by the committees, or included in an agency's appropriation bill as part of the president's budget but not actually requested by the president (instead, requested by a committee member). These reporting practices make the estimate of total earmarks made by Taxpayers for Common Sense about twice as high as the total reported by congressional committees (Taxpayers for Common Sense, 2010).

Reform is not easily accomplished. With the rules on earmarks tightening, members have resorted to a different strategy, which came to be called "lettermarks" or "phonemarks." Members call or write to agency heads urging them to direct funds appropriated for a particular type of project to the member's district (Nixon, 2010, paras. 7–8). Efforts by presidents to restrict agency response to these demands are not always successful, perhaps in light of the fact that the member making the demand often wields influence over the agency's budget.

Legislative Parties

Few people argue with the statement that political parties in the United States are fairly weak. Crossover voting, split tickets, and the growth in the number of voters calling themselves independent provide evidence that voters can no longer be considered stalwart partisans. Direct primaries, growth in political action committees (PACs), and the increased role of the media in campaigns have contributed to a weakened position of parties in recruiting candidates and in funding and guiding their campaigns. The party in government—the role of the political party in organizing and overseeing legislative action—was once characterized as weak (Burns, 1984; Schlesinger, 1966; Scott & Hrebenar, 1979). However, more recent observers have argued that congressional parties have become stronger as members are more ideologically similar and party leaders are increasingly active in shaping public policy.

There is evidence that parties have an important role in defining and shaping the legislative product. Parties help facilitate communication among members of a particular house, members of the other house, the president, and the states. Legislative parties provide a place to air issues, collect support, and broker compromise. Importantly, the legislative party reduces information overload by providing cues to members (especially important to new members). Finally, the legislative party facilitates the identification of issues that differentiate it from the other party. Most members' daily activities are much more dominated by party activities than they were in the 1970s, when committee work occupied most of their time.

Party leadership picks its battles, staking out positions on the bills most important to the party ideology and to future elections. These "party" bills or issues are the ones that party leaders expect their members to support. On highly visible and salient bills, the party leadership usually expects cooperation from its members. If they do not get that support, some retribution may result. "The hyperpartisanship has been getting more hyper with every passing year," Sen. Joe Lieberman (I-CN) told the *National Journal*. "It's almost like the Serbs and the Bosnians. They go back to the 11th century about who started what first," added Sen. Tom Harkin (D-IA) (Cohen & Friel, 2010).

Party leaders can also play an important role in "framing" issues to appeal to voters "back home." One example of such framing occurred when Senate Republicans stopped pushing the "Patients First Act of 2003" and in its place began talking about the "Healthy Mothers and Healthy Babies Access to Care Act." Both bills were actually tort reform measures designed to cap the size of awards in medical malpractice court cases. The second bill, which targeted only obstetricians and gynecologists, was cast as a measure to improve women's access to care. "This is about women," said Sen. Judd Gregg (R-NH), sponsor of the bill. The renaming and retargeting of the tort reform bill in 2004 may well have been part of a Republican effort to lessen, if not eliminate, the advantage Democrats usually have among women (Martinez & Carey, 2004).

Rick Wilson (1992) described three problems inherent in the congressional structure that political parties can help solve: problems of coordination, collective action, and collective choice. Parties and leaders can be focal points to coordinate individual members following sometimes similar, sometimes dissimilar, interests. They can bind individual members to collectively desired goals that without parties would not be articulated or achieved. They can provide needed stability and force the compromise necessary to prevent domination by individual members representing widely differing district interests. In short, parties can transform the actions of 535 independent agents in the House into a workable, more focused institution that has the opportunity to act in the public interest.

Increased Party Loyalty

A crucial factor in parties' effectiveness is how homogeneous they are. Do they speak with one voice or many divergent voices? For years, the parties, particularly the Democratic Party, have fallen at the divergent end of the spectrum. In recent years, first the Republicans and then the Democrats have become more homogeneous and are voting more in line with their party.

Party unity scores, the percentage of votes on which a majority of Democrats opposed a majority of Republicans, are a measure of conflict or interparty disagreement. In 2010 a majority of voting House Democrats opposed the majority of voting Republicans on 89 percent of the votes. House Republicans opposed the majority of Democrats on 88 percent of the votes. The 2010 freshman class helped: through April 2010 they voted 96 percent of the time with their party on party unity votes. Senate unity votes show a similar trend toward more party voting, especially for the Republicans (CQ Weekly, 2011, 37). These high scores reflected determined partisanship. In a January 2011 online update to their book on party polarization, McCarty, Poole, and Rosenthal (2011) reported, "Polarization in the House and Senate is now at the highest level since the end of Reconstruction."

While these unity scores are useful, especially in their ability to mark trends, they are not without critics. Political scientists have developed other measures to quantify partisan pressure (Ansolabehere, Snyder & Stewart, 2001; Binder, Lawrence & Maltzman, 1999; Snyder & Groseclose, 2000), but it is difficult to separate out the party influence from the ideological proclivity of the member of Congress and the preferences of her constituents. What seems to be clear is that party influence is greatest on procedural issues—such as votes on rules—that are key to shaping the legislation but are not as transparent to voters. Nevertheless, most observers agree that allegiance to party is strong in the modern Congress and that differences between the parties are notable. One reason often cited is the loss of many members in the middle or moderate stream of both parties.

Increasing party unity can also be attributed to other factors, including the increasing homogeneity of the voting population, the effects of legislative reforms that strengthen the role of party leaders, and the personalities and persuasiveness of party leadership. In fact, an argument can also be made that voters' disdain for electoral party loyalty might well lead to strengthened parties in the House and the Senate, because "candidates need all the help they can get; they are finding that the best place to get it is from their fellow partisans" (Schlesinger, 1985, 1168). Rohde (1991, 170) argued that the two are related in that members of Congress are linked to their party through their constituency. Where these party constituencies are similar across the country, the positions taken by their representatives become more similar.

At the same time that parties are becoming more homogeneous, the conflict between the parties is growing. This has led to more acrimony in committees and on the floor and to stronger party organizations.

Today's parties have been characterized as legislative cartels, which use procedural powers—including naming committee members, using the legislative calendar, and spawning favorable rules—to produce outcomes favorable to the party (Cox & McCubbins, 2002). These cartels work best in a majority party that has near-complete control over the procedural powers, particularly in the House.

Political scientists and media organizations bemoan the polarization in Congress. Binder, Mann, and Reynolds (2008) refer to Congress's "venomous" partisan atmosphere, where members are often encouraged to obstruct the legislative process on nonsubstantive grounds to garner support for their partisan base. Such political grandstanding reduces the likelihood of thoughtful deliberation and stymies passage of measures their own constituents may support.

There is evidence that partisan differences in the House and the Senate— more so than differences between the parties of Congress and the president— increase legislative "gridlock," with a low percentage of legislative output produced in proportion to the policy agenda (Binder, 1999). Partisan differences also have resulted in increased bickering and finger-pointing. When the health reform bill passed the Senate in 2010, using the reconciliation process to avoid a GOP filibuster, Republican senators were so angry that they refused to participate in further legislative business, effectively shutting the Senate down by invoking a rule that stops committee action two hours after the opening session and again at 2:00 p.m. unless unanimous consent is granted to continue later in the day (as it typically is). Hearings were shut down by both the Judiciary and the Armed Services committees amid acrimonious criticisms of the GOP tactic by Democrats: "For a second straight day, Republicans are using tricks to shut down several key Senate committees. So let me get this straight: in retaliation for our efforts to have an up-or-down vote to improve health care reform, Republicans are blocking an Armed Services committee hearing to discuss critical national security issues among other committee meetings? These political games and obstruction have to stop—the American people expect and deserve better," said a spokesman for Majority Leader Harry Reid (D-NV) (Grim, 2010).

Funding Congressional Elections

Particularly in the House, party leadership has become very active in raising campaign funds. Of course, congressional campaign support has a long history. Rep. Lyndon Johnson of Texas was among the first to see the value to the party of actively seeking funding for congressional candidates. However, even his enthusiastic and persuasive efforts pale compared with today's campaign juggernaut.

In 2010, the average Senate candidate spent $2.4 million on her campaign, and the average House candidate spent nearly $587,000. Members seeking reelection spent more than their challengers. The average amount of money raised by Senate incumbents was $11.2 million, compared with less than $1 million by their challengers. Similar differentials were found in the House, where incumbents raised more than $1.5 million, compared with a bit over a quarter million, on average, raised by challengers. Perhaps most interesting is that for open seats, which one might expect to engender the most money, less money was raised in both the House and Senate. On average, open seats in the House saw $437,000 raised, and in the Senate $2.8 million, in the 2010 election (Center for Responsive Politics, 2011f).

But none of these totals tells the whole story of campaign spending. Unassociated with the candidate's own campaign spending are moneys spent by outside groups. One type of group is called 527 committees, named after the section of the Internal Revenue Service (IRS) code that authorizes their tax-exempt status. They can raise and spend unlimited amounts of money so long as they spend it on issues rather than to *directly* support or oppose a candidate. But many are clearly partisan and work in ways that flatter or condemn a particular candidate or party. Most famously, the self-styled Swift Boat Veterans ran ads challenging 2004 presidential candidate John Kerry's wartime service, despite his well-supported valorous service record. Big-spending 527s in the 2010 election cycle included American Solutions for Winning the Future, $28 million (this is a group created by former GOP House Speaker Newt Gingrich [R-GA]); the Service Employees International Union (SEIU), $15 million; Citizens United (a Tea Party–style conservative group that successfully led a Supreme Court challenge to limits on campaign spending by corporations and unions; see chapter 3), $9.2 million; and Emily's List, $9 million. These topped a list that included many others (Center for Responsive Politics, 2011d).

Parties and party-related groups are also big spenders on congressional campaigns, including both the national parties themselves and their House and Senate campaign committees. Other spending comes from nonprofit groups authorized to be tax free by IRS code section 501(c). These groups are not primarily engaged in political action but may spend a modest share of their budget on elections and campaigning. Their donors are permitted to remain anonymous. Finally, PACs representing businesses, industries, labor unions, or ideological interests such as the environment or opposition to regulation are groups organized for the express purpose of raising money to spend on behalf of their favored candidates. Physicians have a PAC, as do hospitals, pharmaceuticals, nursing homes, and even individual members of the House and Senate. Statistics available for the 2008 election cycle show that the average Senate winner received over $2 million from PAC contributions, while the average House winner received about $609,000 (Center for Responsive Politics, 2011g). (See chapter 3 for details on PACs.)

All together, outside groups of various kinds were big spenders during the 2010 election cycle, spending more than $489 million (excluding party committees), according to the Center for Responsive Politics. Prior to the 2010 election cycle, liberal outside groups tended to outspend conservative outside groups, but the ratio reversed in 2010, with liberal outside groups spending barely half what conservative groups spent, excluding party committees (Center for Responsive Politics, 2010e).

Legislative Behavior

Fenno's research (1973) on congressional motivations found that members of Congress strive to meet three goals: reelection, influence within the house, and good public policy. Individuals differ in how much importance they place on each. Someone secure in her district may prefer to try to gain influence or promote her idea of good policy. Mayhew (1974) argued that of the three goals, reelection underlies everything else. It keeps members accountable, and without reelection the other goals mean nothing. Members can, if they choose, focus on producing particularized benefits to their districts in the form of casework and federal funding for projects ("pork"). Or they can take the high road: trying to help enact good public policy that produces collective or generalized benefits. They can choose committee membership that best meets their electoral needs, either a constituency-responsive, reelection-oriented committee (Agriculture or Resources, say), a policy committee (International Relations or Energy and Commerce), or a power committee (Appropriations, Rules, or Ways and Means).

For most, reelection is their proximate goal, in Mayhew's terms (1987), a goal that must be achieved over and over to make everything else possible. Incumbency helps make that happen. Incumbents are overwhelmingly reelected, with margins that have increased markedly in most elections in recent decades. From the mid-1960s through the early 1990s and beyond, members were rarely defeated, and changes were usually instigated only by retirement—reminiscent perhaps of Robert Audrey's dictum "Where there's death, there's hope." In the mid-1960s, reelection rates in the House were nearly 90 percent. A downturn in the early 1990s, which was probably due to redistricting, anti-incumbent feelings, and fewer contested seats, saw the rates drop back to the high 80s (Ornstein, Mann & Malbin, 2002). By 2004, the House reelection rate peaked at 98 percent. But 2010 was a "wave" election, turning out incumbent Democrats in almost unprecedented numbers. Some thought it was because they had passed health reform, but others blamed the high unemployment rate. But even in this "wave" election, the House reelection rate for 2010 fell only to 85 percent.

The Senate has at times been somewhat more volatile but still a pretty safe place to work, with typical reelection rates in the 80th and 90th percentile. But in 2010 it dropped to 84 percent, which was, however, not nearly its low of 55 percent in 1980 (Center for Responsive Politics, 2011a).

This many losses represent a departure from the typical election, in which not only incumbents but their party prevails. That is, when a member departs, her seat is most often filled by a candidate from the same party. Political scientists refer to this situation as "uncompetitive" seats: districts in which one party or the other will almost certainly win. In 2008 only 46 seats in the House and 9 in the Senate were won by less than 10 percent. The average winning margins were 67 percent in the House and 60 percent in the Senate. Most political analysts consider 60 percent the marker for a safe (uncompetitive) seat.

Nonetheless, evidence abounds that even incumbents with seemingly healthy electoral situations remain worried about reelection and continue to support their districts' interests. But their district can still move out from under them. Arlen Specter (R-PA) is a case in point. First elected to the U.S. Senate in 1964 as a Republican, he was one of a group of centrists who over the years saw their ranks thinned election after election as more and more Republican constituencies became more conservative. Despite trying to move in directions that would keep his voters happy, in 2009, realizing that he could not win a Republican primary, he switched to the Democratic party, only to be defeated in the Democratic primary in 2010. Even House Speakers and Senate majority leaders have been tossed out when voters perceived them as having moved away from hometown values or priorities.

The fear of electoral loss helps keep members accountable and assures that they will carry out the duties associated with reelection: advertising, credit claiming, and position taking. Advertising promotes name recognition and plants an image of personal qualities without the distraction of policy content. Credit claiming paints the member as personally responsible for some desirable policy or program, such as individual casework assistance and bringing specific benefits (pork) to the district. Federal agencies announcing grants phone the good news simultaneously to each member of Congress representing the area, so each can claim credit. Position taking can range from votes on issues to speeches on the floor or press releases on the member's website. As Mayhew (1987, 23) put it, "The position itself is a political commodity."

Incumbents win in part because they handle constituency issues exceedingly well. They have mastered the art of using the federal bureaucracy to make them look good on pork barreling, casework, and leaning on agencies on their constituents' behalf. Compared with lawmaking, these tasks are a cakewalk. They make constituents happy, they are mostly done by the staff, and they are rarely controversial.

Agency oversight—another task in a member's job description—is even less fun and noticed by very few. Not surprisingly, it often is overlooked, except in dramatic cases or those with photogenic causes. Political scientists call the process "fire alarm" oversight, whereby Congress generally ignores day-to-day oversight until there is a fire, when it brings out the fire trucks: highly televised hearings accompanied (often) by heavily exaggerated accusations about violations of the public trust (McCubbins & Schwartz, 1984). Hold an oversight hearing on the evils of smoking, with a teenage movie star talking about her personal convictions on not smoking, and the session has to be moved to the Caucus Room to hold the crowd and network television crews. Similarly, taking an agency head to task for excessive spending or an unflattering evaluation, or grilling the head of an oil company for its slow progress in cleaning up an oil spill often proves appealing—especially to those of the congressional party opposite the party in the White House. Much of this oversight is carried out by staff. When the cameras leave, so do the legislators.

Good oversight involves long hours of work by well-trained staff. It also requires interest from members of Congress on issues that might not make the network news or Sunday morning talk shows. "Oversight is very tedious work," said Lee Hamilton, former House member from Indiana. "It takes a lot of preparation, and it tends to be very complicated. Members are very busy now and they just don't make oversight that high a priority" (Nather, 2004, 1192).

The 110th Congress conducted 844 committee oversight hearings, compared to 521 in the 109th Congress (Mann & Ornstein, 2009, 66). Enthusiasm picks up when there is divided government (when the president is of one party and Congress is controlled by the other). Congress then takes the opportunity to deliver what are often partisan jabs at the president, demanding reports and testimony from agency heads, setting short deadlines for detailed reports, and trying to show that poor policies and decisions are emanating from the White House, leading the agencies astray.

But some members relish the oversight role and use it to create demand for legislation that they want to see passed. Rep. Henry Waxman (D-CA) was a master of this tactic, first as chairman of the Health Subcommittee of House Energy and Commerce, later as ranking minority member, and finally as chairman of the House Committee on Oversight and Government Reform after the Democratic takeover of the House in 2007. Whether chairing or serving in the minority, Waxman was able to muster committee support to hold hearings on such disparate issues as AIDS, orphan drugs, clean air, tobacco marketing tactics, food supplements, steroids in major league baseball, Iraq military trainees' progress, nuclear plant safety, and many other topics (Waxman & Green, 2009).

Revealed Preferences and Intensities

Congressional decision making is not easily dissected. Members take into account various influences, including district preferences, interest groups' requests, demands from party leadership, individual members' preferences, and the characteristics of the issue on the table. Some commentators have suggested that how members vote is not as important as where they put their resources and focus their energy. Back in the (what now seem to be) lazy days of the mid-1970s, a political scientist decided that time was "a House member's scarcest and most precious political resource" (Fenno, 1978). Today's member of Congress is even more stretched—sandwiching committee introductions, votes, and constituent responses into the few minutes when she is not feeding the persistently yawning jaws of the campaign coffer or questing for 30 more seconds of media coverage.

Deciding How to Vote

Reelection takes top billing in deciding how to vote. Members do a type of personal-impact assessment to answer two questions: how will this decision enhance my chances for reelection, and how might it be used against me by opponents?

Sometimes the answer may be to vote yes and no: no to add a provision to a bill, yes to report the bill to committee, no on a rule permitting no amendments, yes to crippling amendments if the member wants to kill the bill, yes to recommit the bill to committee, yes to substitute another bill, no to a motion to cut off a filibuster, yes on a vote to postpone the final vote, no on a voice vote to pass the bill, but yes on a final roll-call vote that may be reported back home. The complicated nature of congressional votes came out in the 2004 presidential campaign when the Democratic candidate John Kerry, a longtime senator, had to explain his votes for and against the same issue. While congressional scholars might have understood, few others were persuaded that his actions were rational and principled.

Arnold (1990) argued that members will vote in ways that reflect both current and "potential" preferences of constituents. They anticipate what the voters will think, how they will interpret an issue and an action, and respond accordingly. Constituents are not equally informed; only a few can be called "attentives": those who have opinions about a particular policy, know what Congress is doing, and communicate those opinions to their legislator. Interest groups affected by the policy are part of this attentive public. "Inattentives" have no preferences and no knowledge of congressional activity. According to Arnold (84), to make a decision, a legislator needs to

—identify all the attentive and inattentive publics who might care about a policy issue;
—estimate the direction and intensity of their preferences;
—estimate the probability that potential preferences will be transformed into real preferences;
—weight all these preferences according to the size of the attentive and inattentive publics; and
—give special weight to the preferences of consistent supporters.

Conflict can lead to different decision-making strategies. Kingdon (1977) believed that a member would implicitly ask whether there was any controversy in the issue. If no controversy, the legislator would vote with the consensus in her "environment" of party members, ideological companions, predispositions, and constituency. But in the face of controversy, Kingdon believed, she would subdivide the environment into those actors most critical to her: constituency, party leadership, and fellow members. When these three conflicted, she would most likely vote with her constituency. But the reality is that on many issues, the constituency is uninterested or uninformed. This means the choice is between party and policy goals.

The saliency or visibility of the issue in the press and with the public also plays a key role. On highly salient issues, the constituent role is the dominant decision-making criterion. For low-saliency, complex issues of little broad public concern, policy or party considerations are more important. Policy content is also important. Health issues tend to be viewed in an ideological manner, affected by the framing of the problem.

Finally, personalization is important to congressional decision making—what Browne (1993, 22) called the "I Know a Man Theory." Browne's example is a former Senate Budget Committee staffer who said when the time came to make a decision, a member of the committee would say something like: "On the contrary, I know a man from Illinois . . ."; language would then be drafted to avoid that man's problems. A variation of this—the "I Know a Woman Theory"—played out in a turnaround of Sen. Trent Lott's views on drug reimportation. He became an advocate after his 90-year-old mother turned to him one night and asked why she paid so much more for her drugs than Canadians did (Schuler, 2004).

Although legislators prize their own decision-making prowess, they are also affected by the positions of respected colleagues, and, to get their own bills passed, they need to be owed some favors, bargaining and exchanging votes with these colleagues. Bargaining includes more than just vote trading, which also goes on. It can include compromising to accept a $1.5 billion appropriation rather than the $2 billion the member might have preferred. Bargaining is constrained by the size principle: the bargainer will bargain only as much as necessary to produce a minimum winning coalition, and no more. When Olympia Snowe (R-ME), Susan Collins (R-ME), and Arlen Specter (R-PA) agreed to support the Senate's version of President Obama's 2009 economic stimulus plan, passage was assured, promising a crucial one-vote margin. Winning those votes had cost Democrats in several ways, including a last-minute agreement to trim an additional

$100 million from a bill that many Democrats thought was already too small. At that point, the search for other GOP votes stopped because a one-vote margin was all that Majority Leader Harry Reid (D-NV) needed to pass the bill (Associated Press, 2009).

While members are generally consistent on votes related to similar issues, sometimes they change their mind. As Meinke (2005) found, members do reverse their positions on important issues, especially when control of the White House shifts, the member's electoral security is high, and the member is subject to cross-pressuring among goals.

Congress at its worst may also be Congress as a collective body. Clearly it seems to suffer from the classic "tragedy of the commons" problem. Members are looking out for themselves and their interests, not the best solution for Congress or the country as a whole. Davidson and Oleszek (1994) referred to this situation as the conflict between the two Congresses: the Congress of individual wills, or guardian of constituent interests, and the Congress of collective decisions. Arnold (1990, 142) argued that legislators will rise above their district's concerns and vote for general benefits over particularized ones under certain circumstances:

—if the general costs or benefits are salient to a large number of citizens;
—if these general effects can be easily traced, permitting credit taking; and
—if the costs to the district are small.

Participation

Looking over the committee list for the 112th Congress, one can easily see that House members in the majority (Republicans in the 112th) serve on two or three committees, while minority members (Democrats in the 112th) serve on only one (Official Alphabetical List, 2011).

Members of a key committee, such as Ways and Means and Appropriations, serve on only that committee. The total number of committee assignments is determined in large part by the size of the party's membership in the House. When one party holds a sizable majority, as in the 112th, minority members get few assignments.

Most members will serve on at least one informal congressional caucus, and a large number serve in party or other leadership positions. Members must answer mail and e-mails, spend time in their district, meet with visitors to their office, attend committee sessions, and go to the floor for quorum calls, votes, and the occasional floor debate, and they must raise money for the next election. There are well over 1,500 recorded votes per session (Ornstein, Mann & Malbin, 2002). Each trip from their office to the House floor and back is likely to take more than a half hour, interrupting whatever they are doing when the bells ring calling them to the floor. They need time for staff briefings, caucus sessions, and chats with colleagues. They also travel home frequently to meet constituents and sometimes travel abroad for investigations or junkets. They go to receptions held by lobbyists and to the annual meetings of groups such as unions or the Chamber of Commerce, who often meet in Washington, D.C., because they want their representatives and senators to drop by their meeting for a meet and greet. Members simply cannot do everything.

How, then, do they choose where to invest their limited time and energy? Hall's work (1996) on participation deals with individual decisions and the impact those decisions have on the collective body. Members devote what Hall dubbed their "intensity" to measures important to a small number of attentive groups or people in their district, to measures in which the member has a personal interest from experience or background, or to those in which the president has a strong interest. While much of this is played out in subcommittees, even there, the intensity of members varies. On subcommittees, participation is highly selective, with small subsets of members dominating the results. Different subsets dominate on different bills. Few issues elicit involvement by more than a small group of members. Hall concluded that the typical game is played by the few, not by the many. Once again an old saw proves true: The world is run by those who show up.

Caucuses promoting various issues and concerns are also popular and can be used to forge bipartisan relationships. Caucuses range from geographic to ideological, bringing together those of the same gender or race or those who share a concern for a cause. Many represent interests of foreign countries (Congressional Caucus on Bulgaria), others business or leisure interests (Congressional Motorcycle Caucus), and still others represent categories harder to define (Congressional Prayer Caucus) (Committee on House Administration, 2009). Health causes are very popular, making up around one-fifth of the total in a 2009 count. One of the most effective health caucuses of recent years was the Diabetes Caucus, which was key in passing at least 10 pieces of legislation in a single recent Congress, including expanding Medicare coverage for diabetes, speeding up Food and Drug Administration approval of a noninvasive blood glucose meter, establishing a Diabetes Research Working Group to advise the National Institutes of

Health on diabetes, and securing major increases in funding for juvenile diabetes research. The caucus is large (more than 200 members) and has powerful members who are leaders of both parties. It used a variety of techniques to focus attention on the problem of diabetes; among them were organizing diabetes screenings on Capitol Hill for members and staff, press events, and sending group letters to administration officials and congressional leaders. The group also used a carefully crafted message, arguing that diabetes-related spending could help produce budgetary savings by reducing the huge burden the disease places on the nation (Burgin, 2003). In contrast, many, probably most, caucuses never meet, do most of their information exchanges by e-mail, or actually do little or nothing. Caucuses are handled differently in the Senate, where they must be officially sanctioned by legislation. The only one to meet that standard is the Senate Caucus on International Narcotics Control (U.S. Senate, 2011b).

Institutional Constraints and Gridlock

Political science research has shed light on the role of institutions (including bicameralism, the Senate filibuster, and the presidential veto) in voting decisions and in gridlock, the position where no action is taken. Krehbiel (1998) argued that the possibility of a Senate filibuster and the possibility of a House override are "pivotal" points in predicting legislative productivity. Martin (2001) documented how the presence of a second chamber and the Supreme Court constrain House and Senate roll-call votes—often leading members to adopt a less-than-optimal policy that has more likelihood of acceptance in the other chamber or the Supreme Court. Martin did not find that the president constrains behavior—this is a result, he thinks, of the fact that the presidential effect may appear earlier in the policy process. In an experimental study, Bottom and colleagues (2000) also found the importance of bicameralism. They concluded that, much as James Madison hoped, bicameralism helps provide stability, in this case a reduced variance in policy outcomes.

Gridlock, or difficulty in enacting legislation, is not new in Congress. In fact, some political scientists argue that the Founding Fathers wanted to make law production ponderous and difficult. Others point out that the early leaders also wanted to design a government capable of responding to national crises and problems (Binder, 2003). This tension between action and deliberation has been present in the system since its original design. Recent research has tried to better understand why gridlock occurs and what its consequences are. One influential scholar (Mayhew, 1991) found that, contrary to the common wisdom, there is little evidence that a divided government produces gridlock (or that a unity government produces significantly higher levels of lawmaking). More recent research has countered Mayhew, showing that both intrabranch and intraparty conflict (but not interbranch rivalries) are important predictors of gridlock (Binder, 2003). Binder also found that while gridlock seems to have a negative effect on the reputation of Congress as an institution, it does not significantly affect members' electoral fortunes, thus limiting legislators' incentive to overcome any impasses.

The Congressional Enterprise

Current and former congressional staff and the congressional campaign workers who help develop and operate a political policy organization headed by the member of Congress have been called the congressional enterprise (Salisbury & Shepsle, 1981). The turnover of congressional staff is so high that an alumni network can be the largest element of the enterprise. Staffers move to executive branch agencies with their bosses, then on to lobbying firms to reap the large financial benefits from their connections. Campaign staffs exist, unnoticed, as ongoing organizations, funded by PAC moneys and other campaign contributions. Yet they may play an important role in defining the policy persona of the member and, especially in the House, provide ongoing political advice.

The revolving door of staff from the Hill to lobbying firms, perhaps to the White House or executive branch, provides a close-knit network of like-minded persons that can easily share information and work together. As one Republican lobbyist put it, "It is the hallmark of a very savvy member of Congress to see the departure of staff as an asset and not a detriment. They are building contacts and networks to the good of both sides. Tom [DeLay] has done that as well as anyone" (Justice, 2005, A11).

In recent years, the congressional enterprise has become increasingly active in placing aides in lobbying firms and associations in Washington. Under the G. W. Bush administration, an operation known as the K Street Project was designed to oust Democrats from trade associations and replace them with Republicans, often those who had worked for House members. Then House majority leader Tom DeLay (D-TX) placed more than a dozen of his top aides in crucial lobbying and trade association jobs. While these efforts largely took place below the radar screen, one effort in 2002 by Rep. Michael Oxley (R-OH) failed when the press learned that one of his staffers notified a trade group whose legislative interests fell within Representative Oxley's Committee on Financial Services that if it fired its Democratic lobbyist, the chair might go easy on investigating practices in its industry (Drew, 2005).

A 2005 scandal involving a Republican lobbyist active in the K Street Project—Jack Abramoff—turned the endeavor into a liability when former Republican staffers and congressional family members were shown to have benefited financially from their connections. Democrats were helped by the scandal, which many thought contributed to their takeover of Congress in 2007. Thus, shortly after taking the Speaker's gavel, House Speaker Nancy Pelosi (D-CA) vowed to sever the link between lobbyists and lawmakers.

While little evidence accumulated that such a severing ever took place, President Obama did issue executive orders soon after taking office that endeavored to curtail the "revolving door" problem of public officials departing to join lobbying firms, and to restrict lobbyists' gifts to public officials (Eisen, 2009). Yet there is little doubt that K Street and other lobbyists still wield enormous influence on Congress, and while the "revolving door" may have slowed from the executive branch, congressional staffers continue to be highly attractive job candidates for lobbying firms eager to gain access to key committee chairs and congressional leaders.

Congressional Staff

One of the reasons members of Congress can follow an entrepreneurial path is that they are well staffed, with both committee staff and personal staff, the latter of which is split between Washington, D.C., and the member's home district. (Senators may have multiple offices in their home state.) No one would expect the modern Congress to operate without an efficient and capable staff, although until the twentieth century Congress did just that. As Congress began to take on more and more tasks and responsibilities through more committees and subcommittees, it began to hire more staff, especially following World War II and again in the late 1960s and early 1970s as Congress decentralized and worked to free itself from dependence on the executive branch for research and analysis. Congressional committee staff doubled, then tripled, from the 1950s through the 1980s, then dropped significantly under the GOP after 1994. Nonetheless, a typical senator in the 110th Congress could count 62 staff, about 27 of them working outside Washington, D.C., and had a staff budget in excess of $3 million, nearly

50 times as large as that of a senator from the same state in the 1950s (Ornstein, Mann & Malbin, 2008).

Personal Staff

Personal staffs are the link between the member of Congress and the district. They keep the legislator in touch and, when the opportunity arises, make the pitch that she is working hard on constituents' behalf. Some do casework, that is, helping constituents solve problems with bureaucratic red tape. Others become expert on issues that the member may find boring but that are of concern to constituents. They also offer expert advice on issues in which the member wants to "specialize." Personal staffs work with committee staffs on issues of concern to their bosses in roughly two stages. The first is a monitoring mode, in which personal staffers spend (relatively little) time keeping up with major issues likely to come before the committee. The second is a more active "cramming" mode, gathering information and getting help from committee staff and other sources so they can help the member prepare for deliberations.

As demands on members of Congress have grown, personal staffs have had to assume a greater role in policymaking. Staffers consult and engage in initial negotiations with each other and then with their bosses to resolve conflicts. Staffers are expected to come up with new ideas, provide support for desired positions, draft language for proposed laws and press releases, and give advice on political issues. They are also the surveillance crew for legislators on the lookout for issues that will garner media and public attention, whether or not there is a viable solution. Not atypical was the experience of one personal staffer who was given the dates that the member of Congress planned trips home. She was told to come up with a major policy proposal and draft bill for him to unveil at a press conference on each return visit. She did, he did, and one of her ideas—a proposal to remove the requirement for a three-day hospital stay before a person became eligible for Medicare home health care—became law.

Some people worry about these developments. Perhaps congressional staffs play too important a role in policymaking, particularly since staffers tend to be young, smart, eager, yet generally inexperienced. "If people only knew how important decisions are really made, with exhausted staffers in their twenties sitting around a table at two in the morning, they would be very upset," confided one health staffer of a U.S. senator, referring to negotiations in a budget reconciliation package. The story is repeated again and again.

Committee Staff

Committee staffers are, on average, older and more experienced than personal staffers. They also stay longer in their jobs. Compared with personal staffers, they are "the people who really know what's going on" (Whiteman, 1987, 223). Whiteman found that on health committees, a small inner core of one committee staffer and perhaps two or three personal staff members who were very knowledgeable on issues dominated things. Staffers outside the core were better informed in the Senate than in the House.

Staffs, of course, tend to reflect the personalities, styles, and political desires of their bosses, although David Price (1971, 325) identified some staffers as policy entrepreneurs who served as independent sources of policy initiation, reflecting "an interest more lively, in some cases, than that of their bosses." Henry Waxman (D-CA), for example, surrounded himself with long-serving staff who were experts in health issues, especially Medicaid. Working with their boss, they often looked for and found ways to push a liberal health reform agenda, typically a small piece at a time, an approach for which Waxman was famous.

Some observers worry that the staffs are running the place. "There are many senators who felt that all they were doing is running around and responding to the staff . . . It has gotten to the point where the senators never actually sit down and exchange ideas and learn from the experience of others and listen," said Sen. Ernest Hollings (D-SC). "Sometimes when the members do talk, they find that they agree; it was the staff who disagreed" (Smith, 1988, 282). Staffs are key in translating general congressional desires into legislative mandates. While the 1995 curbs in committee staffs were intended to help counter this trend toward staff dominance, it is noteworthy that the cuts were not extended to personal staff—the source of major growth. Cynics might point out that it is personal, not committee, staffs that are most closely associated with the reelection of members, clearly an important concern for members of both parties.

Congressional Staff Agencies

Congressional staff agencies—what Martha Derthick (1990) called the congressional generalist staff—have grown, though not recently. From a small start in the 1940s, the Congressional Research Service (CRS) 2009 Annual Report showed that it was staffed by nearly 700 employees—still tiny by Washington standards (CRS, 2010). The CRS is not very visible to the public or even to most policymakers, but it serves an important policy role in congressional decision making. Part of the Library of Congress, the CRS answers questions, provides information, and synthesizes research that is later used in a variety of congressional committee reports and members' speeches.

The Government Accountability Office (GAO) evaluates the effectiveness of government programs and operations and makes recommendations for improvements. It also alerts policymakers and the public to emerging problems. In the 1970s, the agency changed from a "green eyeshade" agency dominated by accountants to an aggressive policy analysis shop staffed by lawyers, social scientists, and policy analysts. Financial audits are still part of the GAO's mandate—but a small part, making up only about 15 percent of the agency's workload. In 2004, this change in focus was formalized in its change of name from the General Accounting Office to the Government Accountability Office (Walker, 2004).

The GAO conducts research requested by congressional committees or subcommittees or mandated by public laws or committee reports. It also undertakes research under its own authority, although a congressional request is typically the preferred source of initiation. The GAO claims that it returns in government savings about $114 for every dollar spent on its support: $58.1 billion in financial savings in 2008, plus 1,400 nonfinancial benefits (GAO, 2009). Over one four-year period of study, more than 80 percent of its recommendations were implemented (2005).

During just a three-month period in 2009, the GAO issued health-related reports on

—approaches for controlling prescription drug costs;
—Food and Drug Administration (FDA) shortcomings in medical device review and oversight;
—holes in pandemic protections for federal workers;
—theft of supplies and equipment from the Indian Health Service;
—how the site of breast and cancer screening can affect Medicaid eligibility of women in various states; and
—continued crowding and long wait times in emergency rooms.

Of course, health is just one of its many, many topics. One of its reports on another topic caused uproar in Congress: the GAO showed that it could carry bomb parts past building security guards in many supposedly secure federal buildings (GAO, 2009).

Between 1995 and 2000, Congress (under the GOP, which felt that the GAO had gotten too cozy with Democratic members) reduced the GAO's staff by 39 percent, to 3,200 employees, and it still had that same number in 2010—down substantially from its heyday of 5,204 employees in 1988. Nonetheless, its 2011 budget request noted that in the past year it had written reports for every single one of the House and Senate standing committees as well as for 70 percent of their subcommittees. The agency maintains 11 offices around the country, although about two-thirds of its workforce is located in Washington, D.C.

The Congressional Budget Office is quite small, with only 230 employees in 2009, 70 percent of whom held advanced degrees in economics or public policy. The CBO was established in 1974 to provide Congress with the institutional capacity to establish and enforce budgetary priorities, coordinate actions on spending and revenue legislation, and develop budgetary and economic information independent of the executive branch. The CBO helps the Budget committees with the congressional budget resolution and budget enforcement, including tracking spending and revenue legislation in a "scorekeeping" system (CBO, n.d.). It provides Congress with cost estimates for every single bill reported by a congressional committee, as well as estimates of the costs to state and local governments of federal mandates and laws, and forecasts of economic trends and spending levels. The CBO "mark," or how much money the agency thinks a proposed law will cost, is essential in determining the feasibility of a provision.

Given the importance of health to the budget, the CBO provides major reports on timely health-related issues, and the CBO staff testifies frequently on the Hill. In one 90-day period in 2009, CBO health reports bore the following titles: "Effects of Changes to the Health Insurance System on Labor Markets"; "Likely Effects of Substantially Expanding Eligibility for Medicaid"; "Health Care Reform and the Federal Budget"; "Questions about Health Care Industry Stakeholders' Proposals"; "Preliminary Analysis of Major Provisions Related to Health Insurance Coverage under the Affordable Health Choices Act"; "The Effects of Proposals to Increase Cost Sharing in TRICARE"; "The Budgetary Treatment of Proposals to Change the Nation's Health Insurance System"; and "Information on Options for the Medicare Advantage Program's Benchmarks for Federal Payments." The CBO and its estimates invariably cause turmoil for one or the other side, or both sides, of major debates involving national health insurance or reforms that have broad effects through Medicare or Medicaid.

In the debate over the Obama effort to reform health insurance, the CBO entered the fray with an estimate of $150 billion in savings over 10 years from a "public health plan option" (a government-sponsored health plan that would compete with private plans—an idea hated by insurance companies and Republicans). For supporters it was good news of potential savings. But critics called the savings small change, considering that the total 10-year cost of health reform would be close to $1 trillion.

Another group that advises Congress, the Medicare Payment Advisory Commission (MedPAC) operates below the public's radar screen but is well known to insiders—particularly to health care providers. The MedPAC, established in 1997 and staffed by only about three dozen people, including administrative and clerical staff, makes extensive use of payment data analysis to provide advice to Congress on issues affecting the Medicare program, including yearly recommendations on payment update amounts. The MedPAC is also charged with analyzing access to care, quality of care, and other issues affecting Medicare.

The MedPAC issues two reports with recommendations to Congress each year. Its June 2010 report revisited and revised a set of recommendations that it had made in the past: reform payment policy to stop rewarding volume and pay instead for performance. Commissioners urged Congress to give the Department of Health and Human Services (HHS) secretary more flexibility in testing new payment approaches, suggested ways to improve graduate medical education subsidies and workforce policies, suggested changes in policy affecting physicians' provision of ancillary services in their offices, and ways of improving Medicare and Medicaid coordination for patients eligible for both programs (Aligning Incentives, 2010).

At a more practical level, the MedPAC gives Congress political cover for some of the tough choices it must make if health care costs are to be controlled. Members of Congress simply point to the commission's recommendations and say they had no choice.

Building on the usefulness of the MedPAC model, the PPACA authorized another advisory board, the Independent Payment Advisory Board, which some wags described informally as "MedPAC on steroids." The legislation directs the secretary of HHS to implement the board's recommendations to "reduce the per capita rate of growth in Medicare spending" (Davis & Newman, 2010, 1).

The board's recommendations are to be given special "fast track" consideration in both the House and the Senate. Because its mandate is to slow the rate of growth, not expenditures, total health care spending will continue to rise despite its policy recommendations. Nonetheless, the CBO estimated that it would result in $15.5 billion in reduced Medicare spending between 2015 and 2019 (Davis & Newman, 2010, 1). If it is successful in its efforts to reduce Medicare growth, its recommendations might be voluntarily adopted by private insurance companies and potentially lead to additional spending curbs. As might be expected, various health care provider groups quickly mounted efforts to limit the board's power to reduce their incomes.

Entrepreneurship and Congress

Although in recent years party leadership has tightened its grip on members of Congress, and even the minority party leadership is stronger than it was a decade or so ago, it would be wrong not to recognize that individual members are still masters of their own fate on most issues. Members can use modern technology to help assure their reelection, employ staffs who cater to constituents' needs and help the member become expert in desired areas and knowledgeable in many others, and avail themselves of a fairly compliant press corps to get their message across to interest groups, constituents, and colleagues. Several scholars have dubbed modern members of Congress "policy entrepreneurs," who can use staff resources, the media, and technology to promote issues and themselves (Loomis, 1988; Parker, 1989; Shepsle & Weingast, 1984).

Wawro (2000) called activities to achieve a member's policy goals "legislative entrepreneurship" and specifically examined whether legislative entrepreneurship benefits a member in her reelection or in PAC contributions. He found little evidence of such a link. However, entrepreneurs are more likely to advance to committee and party leadership positions.

But tell that to Democratic senator Mary Landrieu (LA) or Sen. Ben Nelson (NB). As the final Senate vote on health reform neared, member after member made demands for special concessions. Senator Landrieu asked for and got $300 million in Medicaid relief for her state after weeks of hints that she would oppose the health care reform bill, and then she voted to support it. Conservatives called her a prostitute. While she said that her vote was not exchanged for the deal, she would nonetheless do the deal again on behalf of her state (Mary Landrieu Defends, 2010). Senator Nelson's deal was so good that it brought scorn on both him and his party. He won federal subsidies that would reduce the cost of the bill's Medicaid expansion for his state to zero, permanently. Critics called the deal "The Cornhusker Kickback." As word spread and reaction became fiercely negative, he was eventually forced to ask that it be vacated in favor of a more generous Medicaid subsidy for all states (Ben Nelson's Medicaid Deal, 2009). Indeed, the award created such negative reaction that some felt certain that distaste for the deal-making it represented contributed to the Democrats' loss of the seat held for decades by liberal Democrat Ted Kennedy (MA). The loss cost the Democrats their filibuster-proof majority and nearly scuttled the reconciliation of the Senate's health care reform bill with the House version. Even Nebraskans criticized Nelson for what Tea Party members perceived as sleazy Washington deal-making with the public's money.

Congress and the Press

The press plays a crucial role in the packaging of the modern member of Congress. Media representatives are extremely responsive to the actions and reactions of the member and provide her with almost universally positive coverage. Reporters representing local newspapers, particularly those in small or medium-size cities, are generally uncritical and unwilling to examine issues in depth: whatever the legislator says must be true. Local television stations are similarly happy to have video feeds from their district members, even videos produced by the party's own camera crew, often featuring the legislator's press secretary asking the "probing" questions. For members of Congress primarily concerned with re-election, local coverage is more important than national exposure.

The national press, a harder "sell" for many members of Congress, can also be useful if the member is more concerned about influence in Congress or national public policy (or running for national office at a later date). The plethora of talk shows, C-Span, and YouTube have brought the names and faces of once-unknown legislators into living rooms across the country and into those of their colleagues. Members can use the media to enhance the importance of and improve public knowledge about favored issues and perhaps persuade viewers to support their position. National media coverage can also serve to inform colleagues, the White House, and top-level bureaucrats and can help build winning coalitions.

This media-oriented environment not only has affected the behavior of members of Congress already elected; but it has also attracted a new kind of member— one who is photogenic and fast on her feet. Television personalities, movie stars, and sports heroes have successfully used the media and their experience with it to win primaries and seats in Congress.

Jacobson (1987) concluded that the media, taken together, have not done much to damage members of Congress but that they have damaged the institution of Congress, at least a little. When a president is called a liar by noted commentators such as conservative Rush Limbaugh or liberal Keith Olbermann, and when promotional ads for talk shows state matter-of-factly that Congress is corrupt, one has to ask whether civil discourse is being encouraged. The confrontational style encouraged by the media may stir the fires of a cynical and dissatisfied public viewing audience. Some of the foul-mouthed characterizations of public officials or legislative proposals found on YouTube probably don't raise anyone's esteem either. But those who want to can find quite informative videos on the same website, ranging from presidential speeches to hearings where cabinet officials, bailed-out corporate executives, and embattled oil company CEOs are playing out the democratic process, live, in color, and unedited.

Public Opinion

It is important to keep in mind that the reason the press is valuable to members of Congress is that it helps link the member with the public. Public opinion clearly matters to individual legislators, party leadership, and other policy participants. Social networking is a very useful way for members to gauge public opinion in their districts about issues on which they have not yet taken a position. One congressman used Facebook to solicit questions that he should ask BP Oil and Transoceanic CEOs. Members also try to sway public opinion, turning to mass mailings, newsletters, e-mails, social networking, press appearances, and other means—including personal contacts, robocalls, and orchestrated campaigns. Public opinion is important, particularly as related to the government's role in policy. DeGregorio (2000) stated flatly that for major policy initiatives, it is essential to have mass public opinion on your side. And Binder's 2003 study of gridlock found empirically that the greater the level of public support for government action, the lower the level of policy gridlock.

President Obama clearly had this kind of political insight in mind when he decided that the best strategy for getting health reform passed, despite losing his filibuster-proof majority in November 2009, was to go on the campaign trail and sell the health reform bill that had just passed two houses in slightly different forms but still needed to be reconciled. He also used the process to strike back at the insurance industry, which had decided to vigorously oppose the reform. This process of softening up opposition, beating back opponents' arguments (with a summit where he personally refuted every Republican participant's argument against the bill), and building support for the insurance reforms in the bill at his stump speeches turned defeat into victory and allowed the reform bill to work its way through a reconciliation process that put a consolidated version on his desk for signature.

However, when it came to raising the debt ceiling in 2011 so that the country would not default on its bonds and thereby drive up interest rates, public opinion was clearly divided. Everyone wanted the debt and annual deficits reduced, and even Democrats were willing to endure spending cuts in favored programs to do it. But Republicans wanted to take much of the cutback amounts from Medicare through a "premium support" proposal (so that Medicare would no longer be an open-ended entitlement) designed by House Budget Committee chair Paul Ryan (R-WI), and they opposed any new taxes (Kaiser Health News Staff, 2011). Democrats wanted much more tailored cuts in Medicare, and they wanted to raise new revenues through eliminating tax loopholes, especially those favoring large corporations. Republicans walked out of talks over the taxation issue (Cowan & Sullivan, 2011).

But as the debate dragged on, ironically, the day before the walkout, a Rasmussen poll on June 22, 2011, showed that likely voters weren't happy with their Congress. Only 8 percent approved of the way it was running the government (Just 8% Approve, 2011).

Congress and the Courts

An important balance of power for Congress occupies a lovely building across the park—the U.S. Supreme Court. The Court's relationship with Congress is somewhat cyclical, with some Courts serving to curb congressional actions and others allowing much more leeway. The current Court appears to have moved ideologically to the right, at least according to one analysis (Liptak, 2009, 2010b; Landes & Posner, 2008), and in the opinion of one Supreme Court justice, it has been moving that way for many years. The study reviewed Court decisions in divided cases on ideologically charged issues like criminal procedure, civil rights, and the First Amendment. It found that conservative judges on the 2008 Court voted more consistently than their predecessors on the conservative side of the issue. Earlier conservatives split their votes more frequently. The study concluded, "Four of the five most conservative justices to serve on the Court since 1937, of a total of 43, are on the court right now" (Liptak, 2009; see also Landes & Posner, 2008). Many argue, however, that despite its movement toward the right, the court remains well to the left of the nation's public on issues like individual rights, school prayer, criminal procedures, and abortion (Liptak, 2009).

Congress has limited options to change the Supreme Court (except, of course, that the Senate approves its new members). It has a more direct role in other federal courts and has actively taken on a rather unusual oversight role. One example is a 2003 law limiting federal judges' ability to hand down sentences lighter than those recommended in federal sentencing guidelines for crimes against children and sex crimes. The law requires the Justice Department to inform Congress whenever a judge hands down a sentence more lenient than the federal guidelines, except in cases where the defendant provides substantial assistance to authorities. Another example is the efforts of the House Judiciary Committee to investigate the sentencing habits of specific federal judges viewed as too "soft." Other measures have been introduced to limit the purview of federal courts over such issues as constitutional challenges to the Pledge of Allegiance and the 1996 law against gay marriage. As one scholar put it, "There used to be what we called a reverence for the courts in Congress. Now judges aren't so sure they're safe" (Perine, 2004, 2153).

Conclusion

Despite the tendency to send incumbents back to the House and the Senate, Americans are also willing to express their dissatisfaction with their officials and their government. Few voters respect the job Congress does for them. Presidents seem to consolidate more power with each new administration. But perhaps the biggest cloud on the horizon, one that worries both political scientists and practitioners alike, is the increasing partisanship that is evident in the halls of Congress. In their book *The Broken Branch*, Mann and Ornstein (2006, 59–60) cited a culture of corruption, the demise of debate, and the rise of a destructive form of partisanship. Certainly the long-held Democratic control over Congress promulgated many abuses of power, and the Republicans did not often get their way. But Republicans in the minority did not have their rights quite so blatantly abused: they were not physically excluded from conference committees, and they weren't denied opportunities to review legislation or participate in its drafting. Democrats sometimes suffered these and other indignities during the years ending with the Republicans' defeat in 2006. Democrats, when they took over again in 2007, then adopted some of these abusive techniques, such as bringing massive legislation to the floor at the last minute.

Discourse among members has become increasingly shrill and immoderate— often flowing from a set of talking points produced by party leaders. Even in the Senate, the last bastion of civility and moderation, leaders of the two parties no longer talk regularly, and they even personally campaign against each other. And little such consultation and moderation is in play in the modern House of Representatives. President Obama sought in his initial months in office to encourage bipartisanship, and Democrats, who had come to control both houses, made supportive claims. But voting continued to be split along partisan lines, and much of the rhetoric exchanged on Sunday talk shows and in evening news clips remained highly partisan. Much of the health care debate seemed to break along partisan ideological lines. Debate over the health reform bill seemed to particularly poison the political discourse, especially with the emergence of the Tea Party movement, which saw health reform as the quintessence of big-government intrusion.

Along with heightened partisanship have come entrenched ideological positions—often with punishment meted out to party members who do not toe the ideological line. Although some moderate Republicans have wielded their power, such examples are few, and the number of moderates of both parties elected to office is lessening.

Ideology has long played a role in congressional action in health, often in positions relating to the role of government versus the market. Conservatives seek a smaller role for government and generally protect the role of the market to solve problems; liberals want government protections. Perhaps the biggest sticking point in the 2010 debate over health care reform was whether or not to include a public plan option in the reform package. Private insurers and Republicans were rock solid in their opposition, seeing it as a major expansion of government with potential to drive out private insurance. As a consequence, they hated it with a visceral reaction that would broach no compromise. Liberals, especially the Service Employees International Union, took a similarly impassioned stance in favor of it, despite the likelihood that it would have had very little effect on the industry, since the proposal was to limit access to the public option to those who had been uninsured for at least six months.

The other major sticking point, also ideological, was public funding for insurance that would cover abortion. Debate over nuances of language relating to abortion have tied up budgets and legislation in Congress for more than 30 years and show no signs of producing a compromise other than an unstated one that seems to be "count on a battle over language each time a major piece of legislation comes up that touches on the issue; expect both sides to push for improvement in policy every time they can; and expect the weaker side to push for return to the status quo ante prevailing before this current debate began."

The Congress that has emerged in the twenty-first century looks different in crucial ways from earlier ones, but also in important ways it looks similar.

Partisanship, ideology, strength of party leadership, and presidential leadership and cooperation with Congress, as well as public support, vary across decades and across Congresses. Because health is a major issue across decades and Congresses, it provides an excellent case for understanding the evolving and ever-changing power structure that guides national policy.

CHAPTER TWO

The Presidency

A Look Back

1965

On July 27, 1965, President Lyndon B. Johnson and his cabinet, assembled for their twentieth cabinet meeting, congratulated themselves heartily. The Medicare bill had just come out of the House-Senate conference committee and final passage was hours away. The voting rights bill was following close behind it, in conference, with agreement expected within the week. The landmark Elementary and Secondary Education Act had become law in April, and the War on Poverty was a year old. In all, 36 major pieces of legislation had been signed into law by the time of that twentieth cabinet meeting; 26 others were moving through the House or the Senate.

Tom Wicker, writing in August 1965, said, "They are rolling the bills out of Congress these days the way Detroit turns super-sleek, souped-up autos off the assembly line" (Johnson, 1971, 323). The president was an activist, had been elected with 61 percent of the popular vote, and was working with a heavily Democratic Congress (68% in both the House and the Senate). Johnson had strong public support. Although in the fall of 1965 he sensed "a shift in the winds," or a fading of public support for change (reflected in some congressional calls for a slowing down of legislative action), he pushed forward, largely through the work of 10 task forces, each on a critical area of policy.

By the end of the year, major laws had been enacted dealing with issues ranging from higher education to the formation of the Department of Housing and Urban Development (HUD), from law enforcement assistance to workforce training. Of these laws, seven were in health (Medicare; a heart, cancer, and stroke program; mental health; health professions; medical libraries; child health; and community health services) and four dealt with the environment (clean air, water pollution control, a water resources council, and water desalting). But at the top of the list was Medicare, what Johnson and others considered the premier issue of that year, perhaps of his term.

In 1964, President Johnson was very disappointed when Medicare failed to pass the House after its success in the Senate, and in 1965 he was determined that the Ways and Means Committee should not bottle up the measure again. He worked closely with House leaders, encouraging them to change the composition of the Ways and Means Committee to reflect the Democratic majority in the House, thus adding two crucial seats. He asked the leadership to designate Medicare HR 1 and S 1 (the first bill introduced in both House and Senate), symbolizing its importance. He highlighted the great consequence of Medicare in his State of the Union message on January 4 and in a special message on health. When consulted on a compromise proposed by the Ways and Means chair, Johnson (1971, 216) enthusiastically supported any reasonable move "to get this bill now." He met personally with House and Senate leaders following the favorable recommendation of the bill by the House Ways and Means Committee. When the bill passed the Senate, Johnson called it a "great day for America."

1981

The situation facing President Ronald Reagan in his first year after election was not as rosy as that enjoyed by Lyndon Johnson 16 years earlier. Reagan's winning margin was substantial (nearly 10 percentage points over incumbent Jimmy Carter's), but he faced a Democratic majority in the House and had only a slim (53–47) Republican majority in the Senate. Nevertheless, Reagan, like Johnson, moved quickly. In his first nine months in office, he helped push through major domestic budget and tax cuts and a massive defense buildup. One of his greatest achievements was passage of the entire administration budget and program reform package in the Omnibus Reconciliation Act of 1981, a legislative coup because it allowed consideration of a large number of important measures in one vote rather than as dozens of bills. Included in this measure was the consolidation of 21 health programs into four block grants: primary care; maternal and child health; preventive health and health services; and alcohol, drug abuse, and mental health. The consolidation included a reduction of 21 percent in federal dollars for the programs, compared to the previous year's funding (Feder et al., 1982).

By the fall of 1981, the congressional tide had turned. Congress was less enthusiastic about the administration's cuts and approved only half of those proposed. By February 1982, even the Republican-dominated Senate Budget

Committee rejected the administration's budget, which was defeated 21-0 two months later (Salamon & Abramson, 1984). Yet in those early months, some argue, the long-standing principles governing social welfare policy in the United States were questioned, if not revised. The administration thought public welfare should focus only on those unquestionably unable to care for themselves. For those people who were more marginally disabled or less needy, the approach was to reduce or eliminate benefits and encourage them to work or seek help in the private, not the public, sector. In health, President Reagan's philosophy encouraged less government and had the effect of promoting the idea of market competition and the provision of services by the private sector. Ideas spawned during this period would continue to influence Republican and to some extent Democratic health policy thinking for decades.

1993

The political climate surrounding Bill Clinton as the newly elected president was inauspicious. He had been the governor of a small state and had limited Washington experience. Elected with only 43 percent of the vote, he clearly lacked any "mandate." He had what one writer called the "worst first week of any President since William Henry Harrison who caught pneumonia while delivering a long Inaugural speech and died a month later" (Blumenthal, 1994, 36). There were problems with nominees for attorney general and enormous opposition to changes in the policy on gays in the military. Yet the Congress Clinton faced was seemingly sympathetic, with substantial Democratic majorities in the House and the Senate. This president was enthusiastic and diligent in his efforts to court the Democratic members of Congress in his first year of office, making trips to Capitol Hill and inviting members individually and in groups to accompany him jogging, to ride in Air Force One, or to attend meals or movie screenings, to the point where "few on the Hill . . . managed to escape a talk with Clinton" (38). Early successes included a difficult budget vote (passing by two votes in the House, one in the Senate), ratification of the North American Free Trade Agreement (NAFTA), legislation on family and medical leave, the earned income tax credit, and national service legislation. In his first year, his presidential success rating as measured by the *Congressional Quarterly* was 86 percent—the highest for a president in his first year since Lyndon Johnson's 88 percent in 1964 (Ornstein, Mann & Malbin, 2002). (The score reflects presidential victories on votes on which the president takes a position. It combines major and insignificant bills and reflects the position of the president at the time of the vote.)

Like Lyndon Johnson, Bill Clinton worked Congress to promote his health care agenda, but unlike Johnson, he also used television, in what has become known as the town meeting format, in which citizens ask questions of the president in an informal setting. After a highly publicized appearance before a joint session of Congress in September 1993, the real "selling" of the program began. Hillary Rodham Clinton made five televised congressional appearances and had interviews with five network reporters. The president answered questions about his health care proposal for two and a half hours on a popular network news show, conducted a town meeting in California, invited two dozen newspaper reporters to lunch, and allowed 55 radio talk show hosts to broadcast live from the White House lawn (Kelly, 1993).

But Clinton faced many more obstacles and had fewer resources than did Johnson. Both were Democratic presidents dealing with a Democratic Congress, but the nature of the relationship was starkly different. The member of Congress of 1994 was largely an independent enterprise and could raise her own money and strike her own "deals." Another "plum" from the Johnson era and before—presidential support and appearances in congressional campaigns—was of little use: Clinton's public support reached a low of 37 percent before the midterm elections, and there were relatively few calls for campaign appearances. Party leaders had less power than those of the 1960s and were unable to deliver votes or coerce many votes from party members. With the advent of the Congressional Budget Office, the president's own numbers—on the cost of health care reform, for example—were questioned and discounted in favor of those of the less partisan CBO.

The interest-group world into which President Clinton's health agenda was thrust also varied enormously from that of the mid-1960s. In 1993, numerous interest groups used strategies to mobilize their members and sway public opinion that only one or two powerful groups could have mustered in Johnson's time. Clinton's "bully pulpit" was shared, at least in part, by the fictional characters Harry and Louise, developed by the health insurance industry and wildly successful in framing the public debate on health care reform. Interestingly, Harry and Louise apparently made their biggest initial impact on Washington, D.C., rather than on the people back home. When the Clintons began to refute and parody the ads, they gave the ads additional legitimacy and standing (Clymer, Pear & Toner, 1994).

Finally, President Clinton faced budgetary constraints unlike those confronting any other previous modern president. In the summer of his first year in office, Congress imposed strict spending limits, freezing discretionary spending at the previous year's levels with no allowance for inflation. Under the agreement, any new spending had to be accompanied by offsetting spending cuts or revenue increases or both. To make up for inflation and add money for priority initiatives, such as health care, Clinton was forced to cut back on hundreds of programs. It was a far cry from the days of earlier presidential power. Bill Clinton, the president with an activist agenda topped by health care reform as the defining element, was relegated to near-observer status in the spring and summer of 1994, when the legislative drafting set about in earnest.

2009

"Black Man Given Nation's Worst Job" headlined the online newsletter the *Onion*, in its day-after-the-election issue (Black Man, 2008). A funny headline but, remarkably, not far from the truth. More than any president since Franklin Delano Roosevelt, Barack Obama, the nation's first black president, faced a list of problems that would make an optimist cry. After more than a decade of high prosperity, high salaries, high employment, high home prices, loose credit, soaring stock prices, and unlimited consumer spending, the bottom had fallen out of everything. Jobs were drying up at increasingly rapid rates, the stock market had lost one-third of its value, housing prices were dropping back to levels of six years earlier—before they started to boom—and foreclosures were forcing thousands of Americans from their homes as the value of their houses descended below their mortgages. Home sales had stopped all over the country, putting the brakes on labor mobility, so that many could not afford to move to a distant job even if they could find one. As home sales ceased, so did the business of those who supplied those sales, from construction workers to the restaurants they frequented.

The financial system was on the brink of collapse. The American auto industry was literally going bankrupt, could not find buyers for either their cars or their companies, had already shed thousands of jobs, and threatened to completely collapse without a huge federal cash bailout—on top of much larger bailouts already given to the nation's largest banks and investment and insurance companies. The federal deficit had already reached $1 trillion the previous October and would exceed $2 trillion in the next fiscal year.

Our troops were fighting two major wars, and our country was held in low esteem throughout the world, especially in the Middle East. At home our immigrant population had been angered at our patchwork and arbitrary policy toward undocumented aliens. Arizona and other border states were threatening to take the law into their own hands if the federal government did not curb illegal immigration across their borders.

The United States had long been shown to be the world's worst contributor to global warming but had done little to curb its excesses. We were falling behind Japan and other countries in developments and application of broadband and wireless services and in implementation of electronic records systems. Our schools were again recording startlingly high school dropout rates. And our power grid, bridges, and highways were falling apart.

On top of all this, Medicare was rapidly approaching bankruptcy as costs rose and revenues did not. And the problem would worsen as payroll taxes fell with falling payrolls. States were scrambling to meet their share of Medicaid, whose rolls were growing with expanding unemployment. Social Security would also go bankrupt, though more slowly, unless politically fearsome fixes were put in place, almost certainly involving reduced benefits, increased revenues, and delayed age-of-eligibility. Most pressing of all was the health care system: it cost more than two and one half times the average cost of other industrialized nations' systems, was growing each year in its share of the GDP, and by such measures as infant mortality, life expectancy, and access to care was delivering some of the worst value for the money, when ranked with all other industrialized nations.

In short, our health care, our economy, our infrastructure, and to some extent our national psyche was in tatters. And if the new president was going to have to rely on Congress to partner with him in addressing this distressing list of calamities, he would have to do it facing one of the most fiercely partisan, polarized, antagonistic political milieus in generations.

President Obama promised to fix everything—the financial system, jobs, and health care reform before all else—and do it in a bipartisan way. He also promised not to raise taxes on the middle class. No doubt he was happy to have won the presidency, but he had to be asking himself what he had gotten into.

Yet by the end of his first year, he would expand health insurance for children, bail out the car companies, extend unemployment benefits, stimulate the economy with a massive spending bill, rescue the financial industry, try to help the housing industry, issue executive orders to restore the primacy of science in medical research decisions, expand military resources in Afghanistan, and, most remarkably, pass major health reform through both houses of Congress. He would still face major hurdles in reconciling the two versions of the health reform bill, even as his popularity had begun to wane, but he would look back on a year of substantial accomplishment. Yet, he faced much more to do, quite likely with diminishing congressional support as the midterm elections neared.

Presidential Power, Symbolism, and Roles

The presidency is the institution of executive power in the United States; the president is the person who exercises that power for a limited period of time. Many young boys and girls (and their parents) may aspire to be president, but few will achieve it, and those few will be closely watched, examined, and analyzed. Yet, as Charles Jones (1994, 281) pointed out, the U.S. presidency "carries a burden of lofty expectations that are simply not warranted by the political or constitutional basis of the office." The president, analysts say, is one institutional player among many in the crafting of national public policy.

One of the primary policymaking roles of the president is to put items on the agenda. When a measure is introduced in Congress, his role shifts to one of monitoring and encouragement. The president's margin of victory, his popularity with the public, and the dominance of his party in Congress make up what is known as political capital, an important factor in the president's ability to persuade Congress to adopt his programs. Presidents like to "go public," or take their case to the American people, in the hope that constituents will then pressure their members of Congress to support the president's policy. In 1994, going public was not a successful route for President Clinton and his health care reform initiative, since strong interest groups also invested in advertising to inform the public on issues not to the president's liking. Like Congress, the presidency is much affected by public opinion and the press. The press coverage of presidents is massive; it can be helpful or harmful. The president is responsible for overseeing the executive branch, a task that many presidents do not like but some try to use to their advantage. Finally, presidents appoint members of the Supreme Court and other judicial posts, subject to Senate advice and consent. The president's most significant role in health policy has traditionally been in putting health issues on the national agenda and urging public support for their adoption by Congress.

Presidential Power

The Founding Fathers were leery of giving presidents too much control; their experience with kings and their henchmen had convinced the founders that control vested in one individual was a bad idea. Yet they were also fearful of the "impetuous vortex" of the legislative branch and wanted to prevent "legislative usurpations" as well (Publius, [1787–88] 1961, 309). So they set up a system of balanced powers, with three branches of government, each providing a check to any overzealousness of the others. Since ratification of the Constitution, the struggle between Congress and the president over control has waged almost continually. Some presidents have exercised strong leadership and others have acquiesced to a more dominant Congress.

The president personally embodies most of the power of the executive branch (unlike Congress and the judiciary, where power is highly decentralized and dispersed). This gives the president power because he can act more quickly than other branches and can be the center of press coverage, thus focusing the attention of the entire nation on a particular matter. The president is the only person (except for the vice president) elected to represent the nation as a whole, and thus he has a national constituency. The president represents all the people and is the personification of the national interest. In the development of policy, presidential concerns for the broad national interest can conflict with more specialized congressional concerns focused on the costs and benefits of policies to members' local constituencies.

Another way to look at the president is as the representative of the 200 million or so Americans who are not directly represented by lobbies of some sort. This was the role President Lyndon Johnson described when he explained to a group of Southern senators why, as president, he was proposing major civil rights and other "liberal" issues that he had not supported as a senator. He said, "I'm president now—president of all the people" (Thomas 1999, 37). President Clinton seemed to be appealing to all the people when he said in August 1994 that his White House was really "the home office of the American Association for Ordinary Citizens" (Wines 1994, A9). Later, looking back at his presidency, he had the same view: "I've tried to make my government the government of the people of Watts as well as the people of Beverly Hills," he told a predominantly African American crowd of enthusiastic Democratic supporters in Watts, California, as he stumped for candidate Al Gore in the final days before the 2000 presidential election. "Four more years," his listeners responded, indicating that in their view he had succeeded and, if they had their way, the Constitution would be changed to let him keep up the good work (NPR, 2000).

Presidents are a symbol for the country as a whole, and people sleep better when a president they trust is watching over the country (Kernell, Spelich & Wildavsky, 1975). Journalists focus Washington coverage on the White House, and scholars highlight the power and leadership of the office of the president. Presidents themselves encourage their identification with the nation and the national interest in their speeches and addresses (Hinckley, 1990). In his emotional speech on resigning from the presidency, Richard Nixon drew on this bond, which he called "a personal sense of kinship with each and every American" (Price, 1977, 348). President George W. Bush frequently talked about "the people's business." Yet a president soon learns that promoting unity in the face of the pluralism of the U.S. political system is extremely difficult. Much is expected— often too much. Brownlow (1949) noted that whatever else a president newly arrived in the White House might look forward to, he would be wise to realize from the first moment that he is certain to disappoint many of his constituents, who collectively compose the nation. As George W. Bush (2004, 2072) put it in his speech accepting the Republican nomination in 2004, "One thing I have learned about the presidency is that whatever shortcomings you have, people are going to notice them; and whatever strengths you have, you're going to need them." President-elect Obama quickly recognized the challenges he faced: "We've got a lot of problems," he told *60 Minutes*. "The challenges are enormous, and they are multiple, and there are times during the course of a given day where you think, where do I start?" (Obama Interview, 2008).

Presidential Roles

The president is clearly the most visible government official in the land. Television seems to cover his every move—even stops at fast-food restaurants while jogging, helicopter trips to a forest getaway, and attendance at church worship, parents' funerals, and parent-teacher meetings. The formal speeches, press conferences, and state dinners are well covered by the press and closely followed by many others. Yet the presidency is more than a photo opportunity or dress-up dinner. The president must lead. But how? And in what direction?

Cronin and Genovese (1998) described seven functions of the presidency: recruitment of leadership, crisis management, symbolic and morale-building leadership, priority setting and program design, legislative and political coalition building, program implementation and evaluation, and oversight of government routines and establishment of an early-warning system for future problem areas. The first function facing presidents is selection of leadership. President George W. Bush launched his administration flanked by many old hands brought back to Washington from the days of the first Bush administration or the Gerald Ford administration. His cabinet did not have to spend the first days and months figuring out where to park and how to run their office, as is typical for newcomers to the capital. The experience of these officials was helpful when the president confronted crisis management early in his presidency with the events surrounding 9/11 and when the press and Congress made demands on the new administration. President Bush, like his predecessors, was not very concerned about oversight and early-warning systems for future problem areas. Presidents are, of course, politicians interested in promoting their policies, building their party, and leaving a legacy. President Obama repeatedly stressed that he wanted to move forward, not look back, especially when Democratic colleagues urged his administration to mount an investigation of his predecessor's possible violations of law based upon the Bush doctrine of the "unitary presidency." This doctrine presumed possession by the White House of all powers of the executive agencies. It took the view that actions taken in the pursuit of national security were essentially legal if the president did them and that they were generally unreviewable by the other branches. The Supreme Court eventually disagreed.

While presidents are viewed by the public as the epitome of power in the United States, political scientists have debated whether the president is in fact a leader or a clerk (Neustadt, 1960). Those who subscribe to the clerk mode argue that understanding the presidency is a matter of understanding the institution of the presidency, in which presidential behavior is fully (or mostly) subsumed under the institutional setting, dimensions, and constraints. The president has little individual leeway under this model; rather, any president in the same institutional setting would do pretty much the same thing. The counterargument, the president-centered approach (Gilmour, 2002), is that the president is a leader and imposes his own will on those institutional constraints and opportunities. As in many such debates, the truth may lie between the two models or have a few components of each. The president has institutional constraints but can choose to push those constraints to the limit or live with them. George W. Bush tended to push and generally succeeded in protecting private documents, initiating policies through executive orders, and limiting congressional inquiries. President Obama during his campaign vowed to reverse such secrecy but once in office found that he wanted to embrace some Bush executive privilege prerogatives while reversing others.

A president has to deal with two distinct policy domains: domestic affairs and foreign and defense policy (Wildavsky, 1966). Of the two, the president has more control over (and perhaps more success with) the second. He must deal extensively with Congress on domestic issues, and convincing legislators can be tough indeed. Presidential time and attention are often devoted to mustering congressional support rather than determining the desired policy. In foreign and defense policy, the reverse is often true: "selling" the plan is not the hard part; coming up with the best policy choice seems to be much tougher. The public knows little about foreign policy or defense and tends to trust the president on his proposals. Voters generally like a president to be decisive in foreign affairs; support for the president, as measured by polls, often rises after presidential action to deal with a difficult foreign issue. Also, the interest groups opposing presidential actions in foreign policy are relatively weak.

In domestic policy, especially economic issues, the public is more informed and is more likely to object to presidential preferences when interest groups are active. And the preferences of the president and Congress may differ more markedly on domestic than on foreign policy issues (Rohde, 1990). Indeed, for many years, members of both congressional parties frequently announced that they honored the principle that "politics stops at the water's edge." Although the growth of free trade has eroded this bipartisanship principle by mixing foreign and domestic issues concerning exported jobs and imported workers, human rights concerns, and other matters, when the nation is engaged in a foreign-policy crisis, there is still a tendency to rally behind the president and save the second-guessing till the dust settles. The country's bipartisan response to the 9/11 terrorist attacks is a case in point; there was initially very little second-guessing from Congress, the press, or the citizenry. The benefit of the doubt is less likely to be given in domestic policy, where frequently the opposition party deliberately tries to differentiate itself from the president's policy choices and members of his own party may feel pulled away from their leadership by constituents, policy, or interest-group pressures.

Our focus here is on the domestic presidency, the one in which the president has major roles in setting the policy agenda, persuading Congress and the public to support the proposed policies, and overseeing the implementation of the policies once enacted.

Setting the Agenda

For the president, unlike members of Congress, reelection is not viewed as the raison d'être of decision making. Presidents also want their policies to be adopted, they want the policies they put in place to last, and they want to feel they helped solve the problems facing the country (Ceaser, 1988). But for the first-term president, reelection is an ever present concern. In *The Agenda*, Woodward (1994) reported that reelection concerns came up in the first term of the Clinton presidency over issues such as NAFTA and a freeze on Social Security cost-of-living increases and their likely effects on key states such as Florida and California in the 1996 election. The closer to an election, the more likely the president is to be concerned with reelection. Other presidential goals are historical achievement, power, and the ability to solve the country's problems. George W. Bush recognized the importance of agenda in his 2000 campaign biography: "The first challenge of leadership . . . is to outline a clear vision and agenda" (Greenstein, 2004, 197).

If President Obama lacked anything in his agenda, it was not a clear vision (or an imposing list): "We are facing an array of challenges on a scale unseen in our time. We are waging two wars. We are battling a deep recession. And our economy—and our nation itself—is endangered by festering problems we have kicked down the road for far too long: spiraling health care costs; inadequate schools; and a dependence on foreign oil," he told his first Fourth of July audience as president in 2009 (Obama Cites His Agenda, 2009, 1).

When a president decides an issue is a national concern—whether it's health care reform, drug abuse, energy conservation, or Social Security—that issue is propelled to the top of the nation's policy agenda. Typically, presidents use the prestige and prominence of their office to focus national attention on the desired policies. As Davidson (1984, 371) noted, "Framing agendas is what the presidency is all about." Presidents communicate their agendas through State of the Union addresses and other major speeches, television addresses and televised news conferences, and the release of special reports and analyses. They use highly visible cabinet members to spread the word and highlight key issues across the country. To affect policy they must convince Congress, and the president has little trouble getting members' attention. Kingdon (1995, 23) quoted a lobbyist as saying that "when a president sends up a bill [to Congress], it takes first place in the queue. All other bills take second place."

President Clinton was committed to health care reform in the early years of his presidency and used the State of the Union and a special address to Congress to make his case. President George W. Bush was less concerned with health but nonetheless did speak about his concerns about access and costs of health care and offer some proposals for Congress during his first term. In his State of the Union address in 2003, President Bush called for Medicare reform, including improved access for seniors to preventive medicine and new drugs. He also called for more choice in the Medicare program. He got all of one and much of the other in the 2003 MMA. However, it is noteworthy that he did not succeed with other health issues he placed on the agenda, including a patients' bill of rights (2002), tax credits for uninsured or lower-income Americans (2002, 2004, 2005), association plans in which small businesses could work together without constraints of state law to negotiate for lower insurance rates (2004, 2005), malpractice reform (2003, 2004, 2004), expanded health savings accounts (2004, 2005), and technological improvements (2004, 2005) (State of the Union, 2005).

According to Light (1991), presidents choose issues to minimize political costs and maximize political benefits. One way to do this is to alternate the promotion of broad policy redirection and noncontroversial incremental change. Indeed, not all presidential agenda items are bold steps. Mark Peterson (1990) found that of the presidential initiatives he examined, only 12 percent involved large new programs. Most of the proposals (58 percent) were best categorized as small changes to existing programs.

Presidents can choose certain issues for strategic, political gain. For example, Torres-Gil (1989) argued that part of the rationale behind President Reagan's decision to put catastrophic health insurance on the agenda was a careful determination that the Republicans needed an issue that would demonstrate their compassion and family orientation. Torres-Gil noted that the "compassion agenda" came on the heels of the Iran-Contra hearings and a loss of party control in the Senate, at a time when the president needed to regain public support. Similarly, the push for Medicare prescription drugs in 2003 was seen as a way to undercut the Democrats' domestic policy positions in the 2004 congressional and presidential campaigns. President Obama's agenda seemed less strategic than genuinely targeted at what he regarded as the nation's most paramount and urgent problems. The fact that his priorities were generally shared by Democrats and liberal-leaning independents probably did not hurt him politically, however.

Although the president cannot introduce legislation, he can and does provide draft legislation or legislative guidance for translating his agenda into legislative language. A leader of the president's party or another prominent party member usually introduces the president's proposal. The president is also responsible for the presidential budget proposal, submitted to Congress in January before the fiscal year begins, which often sets the baseline for further discussions. Congressional budget reforms adopted in the mid-1970s dramatically affected the president's budget-making power, providing Congress with the staff and procedures to formulate its own budgets and allowing it to declare the president's proposed budgets DOA—dead on arrival. However, the president can use the budget process to his advantage as well. President George W. Bush urged Congress to set caps on domestic spending, and President Clinton worked closely with Congress on the 1997 reconciliation measure.

In 1995–96, Congress learned the power of the presidency in the budget process the hard way. Republican leaders refused to compromise with President Clinton over their plan to balance the budget in seven years through major cuts in virtually every area of government spending while also providing a sizable tax cut. Clinton twice vetoed the temporary spending authority for the federal government, and federal offices were shut down. The shutdown was a public relations nightmare for the Republicans, whom the public blamed by a margin of two to one (Quirk & Cunion, 2000). The impasse was resolved, of course, but with considerable loss of face by the Republicans. As Sen. John McCain (R-AZ) said of the experience, "I have to give President Clinton credit. He played us like a violin" (As Elections Loom, 1997).

The president must make three decisions concerning his agenda: the problems to be addressed, the solutions that seem most appropriate, and the relative priorities (Light, 1991). The decision calculus for the three differs markedly. Light argued that the evaluation of which problems to address is based on which are most likely to be politically beneficial to the president—generally these are problems that have been around for a long time rather than newly identified problems. The evaluation of solution options relies on costs; solutions that involve high costs—either budgetary or political—will likely not be proposed. The search for alternatives is important yet very difficult, particularly with the budgetary and political constraints of recent years.

Light (1991) advised presidents to adopt a "satisficing" approach, choosing the first alternative that meets the policy needs rather than continuing the search for a "better" solution. The Clinton administration sought to change the U.S. health care system dramatically—after extensive study by some 500 experts for nearly six months. A year later, the task force process and the product were roundly criticized and were credited, at least in part, with the failure of the Clinton health care plan. Clearly he would have been better advised to follow the recommendation of Light (1991) and others to adopt and amend proposals already before Congress rather than embarking on a new policy path.

President Obama sought to avoid the Clinton stumble. He offered a broad outline for health care reform but left it to Congress to write a detailed bill, planning to enter the fray later in the process (Babington, 2009).

Nonetheless, presidents are not the only agenda setters. Although the agenda-setting role for presidents is important, the agenda is full of nonpresidential initiatives as well. Studying the sources of agenda topics in speeches, hearings, and media—measured in inches of type and minutes of talk—between 1986 and 1994, Edwards and Wood (1999) found that presidents mostly react to events and are generally unable to overcome inertia, world events, and an already full congressional agenda of leftover issues. Only in the area of health did President Clinton seem to be the dominant agenda setter, and even that dominance disappears if the weeks following introduction of the Clinton national health insurance proposal are omitted from the study sample.

Presidential priorities are crucial. The president often chooses to put his prestige behind one or two issues prominent in his campaign and ideologically important to him. As Sullivan (1991, 715) expressed it, the lesson is one of "concentrate or lose." Edwards and Wood (1999, 342) expanded on this: "Under special circumstances, presidents may concentrate their resources and move issues onto the agendas of other institutions and focus issue attention, especially when the issue is a major administration initiative. Under these circumstances, presidents operate as issue entrepreneurs, essentially creating attention where little existed before."

The targeting of priorities is necessary because resources, especially time and energy for both the president and Congress, are scarce and need to be directed to those programs with highest support—usually only one or two key issues. President Carter discovered the value of prioritized issues in 1978, when he began sending to Congress a variety of programs with little guidance on the relative standing of each—with minimal success. President Reagan learned from the Carter experience and was clear about his priorities: cutting government spending, reducing taxes, and increasing defense spending. President Clinton came in with two top priorities: health care and economic stimulus. He had difficulties with both, but especially health care reform. He promised he would introduce his plan in the first 100 days, but it was actually nine months into his term before he gave a major speech to Congress outlining the goals of his plan. And it was another two months before the legislative proposal itself was presented. In the meantime, he dealt with numerous issues not high on his priority list, including gays in the military and Haitian immigration policy, which used up valuable time and effort. But putting items on the agenda and getting them passed are very different; the second is much harder. President Obama left no doubt about his priorities, but he left many wondering if he could possibly enact any of them if he continued to insist on so many of them.

Monitoring and Encouragement

Once the president has put the item on the agenda and offered a preferred solution, it is up to Congress to act. At that point, presidents operate "at the margin" of coalition building in Congress: they must rely on congressional party leadership for support, and their legislative options are essentially limited to exploiting rather than creating opportunities for leadership (Bond & Fleisher, 1990; Edwards, 1989). Presidential skills have less to do with changing votes than with getting the right issues on the floor (Schull, 1989), and presidents prefer to influence the design of legislation rather than the votes on it.

The president's proposals can be dismissed, ignored, substituted for those more acceptable to Congress, compromised, or (sometimes) adopted in full. Most presidents recognize that the probability of success is improved with their active monitoring and encouragement. Presidents can help mobilize public support and assist in the coalition formation necessary to guide the bill successfully through both houses of Congress. They can use their office to encourage legislators "leaning" in their direction or fully in their camp. They can use their prestige and visibility to counter strong opposing interest groups by alerting the public to the groups' tactics.

Personal appeals, on the telephone or in person, can be persuasive, although not conclusive. Harry Truman summed up his role as sitting all day "trying to persuade people to do things they ought to have sense enough to do without my persuading them . . . That's all the powers of the president amount to." Such persuasion includes inducing people "to believe that what he wants of them is what their own appraisal of their own responsibilities requires them to do in their own self interest, not his" (Neustadt, 1960, 10).

In the 1994 congressional consideration of health care reform, President Clinton was asked by congressional leaders to stay out of the first round of decisions and refrain from public comment on what was going on. The White House activity directed at Congress in the spring and summer of 1994 was confined largely to providing expertise when asked and inviting pivotal members of Congress to the White House for special attention and persuasion (Kosterlitz, 1994). Yet by summer, the president was visibly concerned about the slow congressional pace and began meeting with key congressional leaders and stepping up his public appearances and those of the first lady and prominent cabinet members.

President Obama had the opposite experience in his 2009 health reform effort. As the president traveled abroad, members of Congress and commentators began to question whether health care reform could be done in the current year, especially since the president appeared to some to have taken his eye off the ball. President Obama quickly disabused the doubters immediately after returning from his travels: "The naysayers and the cynics still doubt that we can do this. But it wasn't too long ago that those same naysayers doubted that we'd be able to make real progress on health care reform. And thanks to the work of key committees in Congress, we are now closer to the goal of health reform than we have ever been," he said.

He was referring to passage of a health reform bill by the Senate Health, Education, Labor, and Pensions (HELP) Committee the day before. He did not mention that the legislation had passed on a strictly partisan vote or that the HELP Committee was not much of a test, given that it had passed national health insurance reform legislation as early as 1982, only to see it die in the Senate Finance Committee, which would have had to find ways to pay for it. But he had gotten the hint that more involvement was required of him, and his remarks were intended to show that he was, indeed, in the game.

Hands-On Negotiations

Sometimes presidents become much more than monitors and cheerleaders. They can be intensely involved in the day-to-day negotiations on major legislation. These bargaining sessions, sometimes called summits, include chairs of the Budget, Ways and Means, and Finance committees, party leaders, and the president. A case in point was the Balanced Budget Act of 1997, a measure that made major changes in Medicare and Medicaid policies. From the release of his budget in February of that year, President Clinton played an active role, informing Republican leaders of his budget in advance and calling for two reconciliation bills—one to balance the budget and one with tax amendments. When congressional action was stalled, the president would invite congressional leaders to meet with him at the White House to reach agreement. President Clinton was also actively involved in the conference committee, sending letters and statements, calling strategy meetings, and providing staff for day-to-day drafting tasks. Negotiations were not the usual House-versus-Senate ones, but rather the Republican Congress versus the president, and the final solution reflected these actors—with both sides giving and taking until they found common ground (Smith, 2002).

President Obama incurred the wrath of Senate Finance Committee chair Max Baucus (D-MT) when from the White House he immediately rejected a critical element of the Finance Committee's health care reform financing strategy: taxing health benefits above some threshold value. "Basically the president is not helping," Baucus said. "He does not want the exclusion, and that's making it difficult" (Montgomery 2009a, 2).

The President's Relationship with Congress

In the early days of his presidency, George W. Bush was asked how he would deal with Congress. "A dictatorship would be a heck of a lot easier, there's no question about it," he joked (Crawford, 2005). On a more serious note, Lyndon Johnson once said, "There is only one way to deal with Congress, and that is continuously, incessantly, and without interruption" (Kearns, 1976, 226). Indeed, Johnson understood the workings of Congress and was able to work with it very successfully. His successors have had a more difficult time.

Woodward's 1994 chronicle of the first year of Clinton's presidency frequently illustrates the presidential preoccupation and frustration with Congress—a Congress where both houses were controlled by his party. On the budget deficit and economic stimulus package of 1993, the president was involved daily, counting voters, making calls to key members, sitting in on strategy sessions with congressional leaders. At one point, Hillary Clinton claimed her husband had become "mechanic-in-chief"—put in a position of "tinkering" with policy rather than leading the charge to a higher vision (Woodward, 1994, 255). Yet President Clinton managed to squeeze out success with the closest of votes on several issues important to him, including his economic plan and NAFTA. Clinton expressed his frustration by using the analogy of the nation as a ship: "I can steer it but a storm can still come up and sink it. And the people that are supposed to be rowing can refuse to row" (330).

Clinton learned early that sometimes capitulation to members of Congress is necessary to move legislation. When the votes are close, the president even has to persuade members of his own party. Sometimes the price he must pay is fairly low: a round of golf, mention of an issue in the State of the Union address, fund-raising help, or a job for a longtime aide. Sometimes it is higher, such as arranging an appointment to chair a high-profile commission or acceding to a demand on a preferred policy. In one case, Sen. Herbert Kohl (D-WI), in a crucial 1994 vote on the gas tax, set the ceiling on a gas tax increase as the price for his vote. He got it.

Some researchers believe there are swings in dominance between the White House and Congress such that in some years the president is more powerful, and in other years Congress is. Others see the system as much more stable and coopera-tive, what Mark Peterson (1990) described as tandem institutions both contribut-ing to national decision making. Indeed, as Davidson (1984) noted, cooperation between Congress and the president is at least as common as conflict, although we hear more about the latter. The president's relationship with Congress is far from static, varying with the president's political capital, outside influences, and the nature of the policy proposed. One thing that can affect the relationship is scandal or low popularity, making it easier for members to vote against the presi-dent. As one presidential aide put it, "When the president's popularity is low it's advantageous and even fun to kick him around" (quoted in Collier 1995, 6).

The president's influence is greatest when some recent event shows that cur-rent policy is no longer acceptable and presidential leadership can help forge the alliances in Congress necessary to come up with a new solution (Miller, 1993). The president plays a much less important role in issues that are not salient and on which Congress has already reached agreement.

Presidential styles in working with Congress vary greatly. While Bill Clinton was often accused of "policy wonkism," or involvement in details of policy, his successor, George W. Bush, preferred a different style: setting forth broad param-eters of his vision and leaving much of the detail work to Congress. And blessed with a Republican Congress and leadership closely attuned to his views, Bush was extremely successful. When he failed to achieve the desired vote in one house, he was often able to recover in conference committees closely controlled by Repub-lican leaders (Schatz, 2004). One example of Bush's policy leadership style was his approach to the signature health law passed during his first term, the MMA. Bush's overall goals for the program were outlined in the document "Framework to Modernize and Improve Medicare," which was released in March 2003. The framework included some specific suggestions, including allowing private health plans to provide additional prescription drug benefits, but it had few details about how the overall program would work. It stuck by the $400 billion price tag first mentioned in the State of the Union address a few months earlier, but it did not include detail on how that money would be allocated.

This hands-off style is one that many members of Congress prefer. For example, veteran senator Charles Grassley said, "Those of us who have been working on Medicare and prescription drugs for the last two or three years, we feel like we know how to do it. So what we finally talked the president into back in probably February or March, was, 'We ain't going to wait for a bill, we're going to go ahead'" (Krane, 2003, 22). This more general approach contrasts sharply with the Clinton administration's production of a 1,342-page proposal to Congress on reforming the health care system—an approach, it might be noted, that did not result in a bill that passed any committee in either house.

Yet, even with a Republican majority in Congress, in summer 2003 some intraparty opposition arose over the MMA, particularly from rural-state senators, including the chair of the Finance Committee. Some conservatives were concerned about the costs of creating a new entitlement program without adequate changes in the program itself. By June, the president was meeting with conservatives and rural solons about their concerns (Toner & Pear, 2003). In an effort to influence a close House floor vote, Vice President Richard B. Cheney visited the House to meet with members and sent a signal that the White House strongly wanted a bill. President Bush strongly supported the measure, even though it did not contain his preferred provision relating to better drug benefits for Medicare patients willing to join private plans (Goldstein & Dewar, 2003). Importantly, the bill did pass—and the president took full credit. Late in his first term, some Republicans complained that they were not included in discussions on key policy, but the dissent was muted in part by the importance of the upcoming presidential and congressional elections.

With Republicans already solidly opposed to the Democrats' health reform proposals, President Obama ran into similar Democratic intraparty dissent, especially among House Blue Dogs (fiscally conservative Democrats), who expressed major concern about the expected costs of their party's health care bill under consideration in the House Commerce Committee: "We cannot support the current bill," said Blue Dog representative Mike Ross (D-AR); "Last time I checked it took 7 Democrats to stop a bill in Energy and Commerce." He was suggesting that the bill would die in committee unless Blue Dog concerns were addressed (Soraghan, 2009, para. 3).

Political Capital and Midterm Elections

Political capital is the strength of a president's popularity and of his party in Congress, along with his electoral margin. Political capital is important because it affects Congress's receptivity to the president's proposals. Presidential popularity, reflected in public approval polls, is a crucial component of political capital, since presidents who can arouse and mobilize the public are apt to "greatly lessen" their problems in Congress (Sullivan, 1987, 300). Rivers and Rose (1985) estimated that a 1 percent increase in the president's popularity leads to a 1 percent increase in his legislative approval rate. Even legislative sponsors can be persuaded by public opinion influenced by the president (MacKuen & Mouw, 1992). Similarly, potential opponents may think twice about voting against a measure supported by a particularly popular president. The president's popularity is especially important when he is of the party of the congressional majority. The components that make up the political capital of presidents beginning with Lyndon Johnson are shown in table 2.1.

The strength of the president's party in Congress is an important component of political capital. Thomas Jefferson is purported to have said that "great innovations should not be forced on slender majorities" (Light, 1991, 106). Indeed, Lyndon Johnson's successes of 1965, including the passage of Medicare, must be attributed mainly to the election of a large number of liberal Northern Democrats in November 1964. There were 295 Democrats in the House in 1965—a level not met in the decades since. The amount by which presidents lead or trail congressional candidates of their party can be important as well. If individual members drew more votes in their district than did the president, the perceived political value of the president to those members is reduced. Mark Peterson (1990) found that when the opposition controlled Congress, the proposals of presidents who had smaller winning margins than their party's House candidates had difficulty finding a consensus, and public fights over the proposals were common. Although Bill Clinton did not face a House controlled by the opposition party in his first two years, he was in the unenviable position of having trailed every member of the House and one-third of the Senate at the polls in November 1992. And in the fight over health care, consensus was slow in coming and public fights, even among members of his own party, were frequent.

A second important component is public approval, which is often extremely volatile. Lyndon Johnson enjoyed strong public approval in the first year following

Table 2.1.   Presidential political capital, 1965–2011

President	Year	Senate seats held by president's party	House seats held by president's party	Public approval (%)	Percentage of popular vote
Johnson	1965	68	295	80	61.1
	1967	64	248	46	—
Nixon	1969	42	192	59	43.4
	1971	44	180	51	—
	1973	42	192	65	60.7
Ford	1975	37	144	39	—
Carter	1977	61	292	66	50.1
	1979	58	277	43	—
Reagan	1981	53	192	60	50.7
	1983	54	167	38	—
	1985	53	182	62	58.8
	1987	45	177	48	—
Bush, G. H. W.	1989	45	175	51	53.4
	1991	44	167	58	—
Clinton	1993	57	258	58	43.0
	1995	47	204	47	—
	1997	45	207	58	49.2
	1999	45	211	63	—
Bush, G. W.	2001	49	220	57	47.9
	2003	51	228	63	—
	2005	55	232	52	51.3
Obama	2009	55	256	67	52.9
	2010	58	256	50	—
	2011	51	242	48	—

Sources: Light, 1991, table 1, p. 32; updated using Ornstein, Mann & Malbin, 2002; House Clerk's Office; U.S. Senate Historical Office.

Note: First approval rating of the year from the Gallup Opinion Index.

his election but saw it nearly halved by his last year. Presidents Reagan, George H. W. Bush, and Clinton saw major changes in their approval as well. Figure 2.1 shows the volatility in public support during the first term of George W. Bush. His approval ratings spiked shortly after the 9/11 attacks in 2001, then showed a small spike in May 2003, shortly after he declared the end of major combat operations in the Iraq War, and a smaller spike shortly before the 2004 election; after that they began to fall again. Generally, however, the pattern is one of declining popularity. Ironically, as Light (1991) noted, the cycle of decreasing

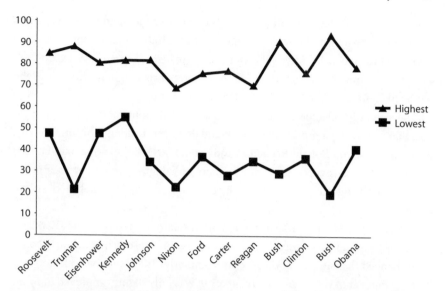

Figure 2.1. President approval ratings, as percentages, highest and lowest scores, Roosevelt to Obama. *Source:* Authors' graphic from "Presidential Approval Highs and Lows," Roper Data Center, Cable News Network, *USA Today,* CNN/USA Today/Gallup Poll No. 2000-20: Microsoft/Parents/'Socially Responsible' [computer file], 1st Roper Center for Public Opinion Research version, produced by Gallup Organization, Lincoln, NE, 2000. Distributor: The Roper Center, University of Connecticut, Storrs, CT, 2001.

presidential approval coincides with a cycle of increasing effectiveness as the president learns about the office, makes mistakes, and learns from those mistakes. Indeed, Sullivan (1991), while confirming the reality of declining support for the president as his popularity declines, also finds that presidents gain some influence due to congressional successes. Presidents might be well served to wait on their big issues until they have established a track record of success on smaller ones. Unfortunately, Sullivan's data suggest that declines due to lost popularity seem to be larger than gains due to successes.

Interestingly, President Clinton maintained relatively high popularity throughout the years of investigation for his alleged sexual harassment and lying under oath. Even during his removal trial in the Senate in January 1999, his approval ratings were no lower than 60 percent (in contrast, Ronald Reagan in his last year had only 48 percent approval). In Clinton's case, the public disliked the person of the president but liked his policies—or the booming economy they enjoyed during his terms of office. In polls taken over 1998 and 1999, two-thirds of respondents repeatedly said they did not like Clinton as a person, but more than 60 percent consistently said they liked his policies (Sonner & Wilcox, 1999). President Obama seemed to be having the opposite problem in his first term: the public liked him but not his policies (Dickerson, 2009).

The size of his electoral victory is also a factor in political capital, to the extent that it provides a president with a mandate to act. Lyndon Johnson, Richard Nixon in 1972, and Ronald Reagan in 1984 could (and did) claim a mandate for change that Congress recognized. Members of Congress are sometimes reluctant to face the wrath of an electorate by opposing the implementation of such a mandate.

But some presidents don't have much of an electoral mandate. John Kennedy squeaked by in 1960; a change in one state, or even a large city like Chicago, could have changed the outcome of the election. Similarly, Bill Clinton was elected by a scant 43 percent of voters in 1992; the margin was only slightly improved in 1996, at 49 percent (table 2.1). George W. Bush became president without a plurality of the popular vote in 2000 and with a small majority in 2004. Yet his administration expressly ignored this lack of mandate. Barack Obama had a strong mandate in 2009 and for a very brief time in early 2010 an all-but-veto-proof majority in the Senate between his sizable Democratic majority and two independents.

Political scientists have examined the linkage between approval and policy success. The assumption is that high approval leads to more success with Congress, since high approval levels either (1) affect or alter citizen approval or (2) reflect public preferences about the president's agenda. There is some evidence that high presidential approval is a significant determinant of policy success in Congress, especially when the issue is complex and salient (characteristics that define many health policy issues) (Canes-Wrone & de Marchi, 2002).

Presidents tend to think of themselves as being strongest politically in the earliest months of their tenure and to act accordingly. Lyndon Johnson (1971, 323) was especially concerned in the early days following his election that he should "use his strength while it still existed," pointing out that the popularity of other presidents had diminished, and then their problems with Congress increased very quickly. Edwin Meese, a key Reagan aide, told a reporter that the White House knew that if it wanted to get the radical changes it proposed through Congress, it had to do so in the early months of the administration. "We're fighting the clock," he said. "We think about that all the time" (Kernell 1984, 256). Indeed, by the fall of the first year of the Reagan administration, the presidential victories declined abruptly, and the following spring even the Senate Republicans on the Budget Committee voted against the president's budget (Salamon & Abramson, 1984). However, some political scientists believe the value of "hitting the ground running" has been overestimated. Sullivan (1991), for example, argued that quick action is secondary to the value of a focused presidential agenda.

As if to follow Sullivan's advice, George W. Bush was very focused during his first term. "The president doesn't like to lose," said one observer. White House officials are "very attuned to which bills and legislation they should let Congress write and which ones they should write" (Schatz, 2004, 2900). The president was very active on the issues he cared most deeply about, such as tax cuts and education policy, while "staying on the edges of many debates, even some of the ones on which he eventually [took] a decisive position" (2903).

The midterm elections, at the end of the president's second year, when one-third of the Senate and all seats in the House are up for election, are an important outside influence affecting the relations between the president and Congress. As election day nears, members may shy away from controversial issues and may prefer to provide visible programs to their districts. After the election, the president may be worse off, because midterm elections generally go against the incumbent's party, regardless of his efforts or popularity. In the 1994 health care reform debates in Congress, the approach of midterm elections was a crucial outside influence. The Republicans wanted to delay a vote until the new Congress was seated in January 1995, hoping they would have greater numbers, perhaps even a majority, in one or both houses. (They were right: they took over both houses in 1995.) The Democrats wanted to make health care a campaign issue, ideally taking credit for the passage of a laudatory bill or, alternatively, taking the opportunity to blame the Republicans for any failure to do so. Yet health was markedly absent from most campaign debates. And, most significantly, Sen. Harris Wofford (D-PA), whose election to an abbreviated term in 1991 was credited with alerting politicians to the public's concern about health care and catapulting health care to the top of the national agenda, lost in November 1994. Some thought his defeat symbolized the coming dormancy of comprehensive health care reform in Washington.

Presidential Persuasion

The "power to persuade" is one of the most important aspects of the presidency. One foremost presidential scholar, Richard Neustadt (1990), argued that presidents get what they want through persuasion, not through command or institutional authority. Kernell (1991, 90) called the president "doubtless the Washington community's most prominent and active dealmaker," who can provide the "much-needed coordination in assembling coalitions across a broad institutional landscape."

Consultation with Congress is important. The likelihood of meaningful consultation between the president and Congress is greatly enhanced when the issues involved are salient and when the president wants a solution, the White House cannot solve the problem alone, and prominent figures on the Hill want to reach an agreement or the president wants to work with Congress on a solution (Peterson, 1990).

Bargaining, whereby a legislator agrees to vote with the president in exchange for presidential support for her pet issue, is extremely common and an important weapon in the presidential arsenal. The president must bargain even with those who agree with him, because most members have interests of their own beyond policy objectives, and their votes cannot be guaranteed (Edwards, 1980). Bill Clinton was accused of "giving away the store" for crucial votes on the 1993 budget bill and NAFTA. Other presidents have been similarly accused. Ronald Reagan angered party leaders when he offered not to campaign personally against Southern Democrats who supported him and gave them policy concessions beneficial to their constituents (Salamon & Abramson, 1984). Coercion, or arm-twisting, is generally the last resort, and then it is used only on particularly important votes (Edwards, 1980).

Compromise is obviously an important factor in the relations between the president and Congress, but compromise can be difficult for a president whose every move makes national news. In the spring of 1994, for example, Bill Clinton was criticized for compromising too much to make his health care reform plan pleasing to a variety of people. When he seemed to be wavering in his support for universal coverage—or at least its definition—he was criticized for retreating or backsliding and was forced to reiterate his full support for coverage of all Americans. Interestingly, Ronald Reagan was criticized for the opposite behavior—not compromising enough, what Salamon and Abramson (1984, 59) called "ideological intransigence." Senate majority leader George Mitchell (D-ME) described the situation in 1994 as one in which Clinton would be criticized for whatever he did. If he took an inflexible position or refused to compromise, he would be attacked for not knowing the ways of Capitol Hill or not having the experience to win. If he participated and made the necessary compromises to get the plan approved, he would be attacked for being willing to give in. "You can't escape criticism in the process," Mitchell said (Woodward, 1994, 183).

The personality component of the presidency can be of great importance on some issues but may be overstated. Some presidents (Clinton and Johnson) seemed to enjoy meeting with and attempting to persuade members of Congress; others (Nixon and Carter) preferred a hands-off approach, with minimal personal interaction. President Reagan was widely viewed as an excellent communicator whose informal, friendly style was disarming and charming to members of both parties. Barber (1985) characterized four types of presidential personalities, based on the level of energy and enthusiasm the president brought to the job and his positive or negative views about himself in relation to that activity. Reagan would be classified as passive positive, Clinton and George W. Bush as active positive, Eisenhower as passive negative, and Nixon as active negative. It would be hard to think of Obama as anything but active and positive. Indeed, critics often asked if he was too active with too broad an agenda, too many speeches and too many interviews. His campaign slogan told the rest of the story: "Yes we can." And if that wasn't enough, he classified himself when talking about health care reform: "I actually am optimistic," he told the NBC *Today* show (Herszenhorn & Pear, 2009a).

Vetoes and Threatened Vetoes

Another presidential "tool" is the veto, a disapproval that requires a two-thirds vote in both houses to overturn. Unlike 43 state governors, the president of the United States does not have a line-item veto: he is forced to veto an entire law rather than just offensive parts of it. In 1996, Congress enacted a law allowing the president a type of line-item veto in which he could cancel specific items of spending or specific tax breaks (but only when the budget was in a deficit). Two years later the Supreme Court overturned the law, saying it was incompatible with Article 1 of the Constitution. Within that short period, Clinton vetoed 82 items, including 38 in a military construction appropriations bill (Aberbach, 2000).

While presidential vetoes are most likely when Congress passes legislation that is objectionable to the president, some presidents are more likely than others to veto bills. Gerald Ford, the only unelected president who assumed office without serving as an elected vice president (he was appointed vice president when Spiro Agnew resigned), had no electoral margin of any kind and faced a heavily Democratic Congress. He used the veto more than any other modern president, vetoing

37 bills in the 94th Congress (1975–76), compared with Reagan's 15 vetoes in the 97th Congress (1981–82) and Carter's 12 in the 96th Congress (1979–80).

Typically, the presidential veto has served more as a threat than a reality, although presidents facing a Congress controlled by the opposite party and those with declining public popularity are particularly likely to use the veto (Rohde and Simon, 1985). A veto override is relatively difficult to achieve. For example, George H. W. Bush vetoed 46 bills in four years and was overridden only once (Ornstein, Mann & Malbin, 2002). His son George W. Bush did not veto any bills in his entire first term—the first president to avoid the veto over a four-year period since John Quincy Adams (Cochran, 2004).

The president's threat of a veto, particularly one issued early in the policy process, greatly increases his stake in the policy outcome and clearly articulates his priorities. Such a threat means that the president has thrown down the gauntlet (especially to the opposition party), that unless certain policies are enacted (or omitted), he is willing to sacrifice the entire policy package. It also provides "comfort and cover" to members of Congress inclined to follow the president but wanting assurances that he will back them up (Priest & Broder, 1994). President Reagan "drew the line in the dirt" on tax cuts in 1981. President George H. W. Bush uttered a "no new taxes" pledge. President Clinton, in his speech to a joint session of Congress introducing his health care reform proposal, used the threat of a veto to attempt to prove his intractability on universal coverage. Although he offered to compromise on other aspects of the proposal—managed competition, health care networks, and global budgets, to name a few—he continued to demand that universal coverage be in the legislative package or the package would be vetoed. President Obama wanted health care expanded, the deficit reduced, and the military reshaped for what the Defense Department calls "asymmetric warfare"—war between the Superpower United States and stateless fighters using improvised devices and other low-tech weaponry. Helpful to achieve all these goals would be deletion from his budget of funds for the purchase of more F-22 fighter jets. The jet was designed in the 1980s to fight Soviet fighters in air-to-air combat, no longer considered a priority. He threatened a veto if the Senate did not reject an amendment adding the purchase to the budget. The use of the veto reminds Congress that the president can be a powerful constraint, especially since successful override votes are difficult to muster. Franklin Roosevelt was known to ask his supporters for something he could veto as a reminder to Congress that this form of policy enforcement could and would be applied (Spitzer, 1983).

Executive Orders

Presidents have one way to make policy without congressional approval: they can issue executive orders, which have the force of law and establish requirements for the agencies and departments under the president's direct authority and supervision. Presidents have great leeway in executive orders; the only constraint is that they must have the statutory or constitutional authority to support their actions. Since the late 1970s, presidents have relied less on statutory authority and more on their constitutional powers when justifying their executive orders. Executive orders can be especially attractive to presidents facing a Congress controlled by the opposite party. For example, in his first year in office (with a Democratic Congress), President Clinton issued 27 executive orders; in the first few months of 1998, with a Republican Congress, he issued 102 (Aberbach, 2000). But another analysis, of executive orders between 1936 and 1999, found little evidence that the party of Congress was a significant factor in the number of executive orders issued. Only twice has Congress overruled an executive order—most recently in 1998 when Congress prohibited expenditure of federal funds to carry out implementation of an executive order on federalism (Mayer, 2001).

The assumption is that what presidents cannot get through Congress they implement through executive orders. President Clinton was straightforward about this when he said in a July 2000 radio address that if Congress did not act, he would use his own authority to create a home heating oil reserve to help avoid shortages in the Northeast (Lacy, 2000). He issued several orders in his last days in office, including one requiring Medicare to cover the costs of clinical trials for testing the value of new drugs and procedures intended for use by beneficiaries who are elderly and disabled (Pear, 2000a)—a change long sought by beneficiaries, many of whom have chronic illnesses. Before this order, Medicare did not cover experimental drugs and procedures. Another order required plans offering health insurance to the federal government's 9 million employees to provide mental health parity—equally generous coverage of mental health services and physical health services. Supporters hoped the order would inspire private employers to adopt similar standards (Goode, 2001). Although Congress passed the mental health parity act in 1996, the act's many loopholes allowed plans to continue to limit mental health coverage. President George W. Bush used executive orders frequently, many of them associated with homeland security and the war in Iraq. His first executive order established a White House Office of Faith-Based and Community Initiatives. As with other presidents, health was not a major focus for executive orders in the George W. Bush White House.

In one count, domestic policy (not including civil service, public lands, and labor policy) accounted for less than 4 percent of executive orders between 1936 and 1999 (Mayer, 2001). Nevertheless, it is important to recognize the importance of executive orders as a policy tool available to the president. With the stroke of a pen, the president can issue a directive that has the force of law (although, if it conflicts with a statute, the statute will prevail). Presidents have used the executive order to establish or abolish executive branch agencies, determine how legislation is implemented, launch dramatic civil rights policies, determine how national security information will be handled, and set up dozens, if not hundreds, of commissions and advisory bodies.

Possibly the most interesting saga of executive orders has concerned abortion. In January 2001, the newly elected president used an executive order to ban federal aid to international organizations that promote or perform abortion as a way to implement family planning, reversing an executive order that President Bill Clinton had issued in his first month of his presidency, January 1993. Clinton's executive order reversed the ban imposed by the Reagan administration and maintained by the administration of President George H. W. Bush (Pal & Weaver, 2003). President George W. Bush also banned the use of federal funds for stem cell research using any newly created cell lines. Critics argued that existing cell lines were contaminated with mouse genes and that the Bush ban permitted other countries—especially the United Kingdom—to surpass our progress in stem cell research. Many feel that such research promises cures to Alzheimer's disease and other catastrophic conditions. But some religious groups regard the destruction of embryos, which is involved in producing the cell lines, as tantamount to abortion. President Obama said that reversal of the Bush executive order would advance research and vowed to "make scientific decisions based on facts, not ideology." He joined signing of the stem cell order with a companion memo to the White House Office of Science and Technology Policy, instructing it to "develop a strategy for restoring scientific integrity to government decision-making" (Stolberg 2009).

Institutional Constraints

Historically, among the institutional constraints on presidential action are the decentralized nature of congressional policymaking, the expansion of interest groups and policy networks, and the reduced importance of political parties in the past 30 years. A modern president cannot work with a few key committee chairs and party leaders and a few dominant interest groups; rather, he must deal with a spate of individuals and groups, all of whom have their own particular interests. As Jimmy Carter (1982, 80) put it, "Each member had to be wooed and won individually. It was every member for himself, and the devil take the hindmost!" Further, the underlying consensus animating the national majority politically and philosophically is different from that which animates the majority party of the legislature (Marini, 1992). In a time of weak party discipline, ideology, not partisanship, is key.

In Light's view (1984, 217), presidents must now "pay more for domestic programs." And the cost is high. Joseph Califano (1994, 41), White House staffer and secretary of Health, Education, and Welfare (HEW) in the Carter administration, noted that President Clinton's willingness to compromise on most things in his health care package reflected the dominance of Congress and the recognition that he would have to sign whatever it sent to him and "declare victory." In Lyndon Johnson's time, wrote Califano, the president had some leverage over Congress with campaign contributions, patronage jobs, and assistance in writing bills. Today, Congress needs little help in those areas. In fact, as Light (1984, 207) noted, the president often does not get "star billing" for his domestic agenda; the presidential aura has lessened because of increased competition among the other policy initiators, more resources for such initiation, and less reverence for the wisdom of presidential planning.

President George W. Bush benefited not only from Republican majorities in both houses but also from strong party leadership. While the Republican Party in Congress was far from homogeneous, it nevertheless understood the importance of staying in the majority and working with the White House to do so. President Bush trusted the House and Senate party leaders to hold their party members in line and deliver the vote on important legislation. They were able to do so by taking advantage of rule changes and curtailing the independence of committee chairs (see chapter 1). In return, the congressional party benefited from a popular president who campaigned enthusiastically for members, helped raise money for the party, and articulated a strong ideological position shared by many in the party.

President Obama for a few months appeared to have a similarly supportive congressional party in both houses, but as the recession lagged on, unemployment went well beyond his worst predictions, housing foreclosures peaked, and his health bill began to bog down over cost cutting and financing disagreements, the two wings of his party began to pull in different directions: liberals wanting taxes on the rich to pay for health care expansions, Blue Dogs wanting more cuts to avoid extra spending and tax increases. As his poll numbers dropped, particularly those associated with support for health care reform, his problems with Congress seemed to grow and sharpen.

Presidential Successes

The president generally has an easier time when Congress is controlled by members of his own party: his legislative success scores do not drop below 75 percent (Ornstein, Mann & Malbin, 2002, 198). Ronald Reagan was successful an average of 62 percent of the time over his eight years in office. Richard Nixon's average success rate in office was 67 percent; Gerald Ford's, 58 percent. Lyndon Johnson's, in contrast, was 83 percent. When Bill Clinton had a Democratic House and Senate to work with, his success rate was 86 percent; when the Republicans took over both houses in 1995, it dropped to a low of 36 percent. Over his two terms, George W. Bush had an average success rate of 82 percent—the highest of any president since Lyndon Johnson (Schatz, 2004).

The success rates shown in table 2.2, compiled by *Congressional Quarterly*, are used frequently by presidential researchers and the press. However, these ratings probably overstate presidents' successes, for several reasons. First, the scores are

Table 2.2.   Presidential victories in Congress

President	Year elected (or assumed office)	Percentage of bills supported by the president that were enacted		
		Highest	Lowest	Mean
Johnson	1963	93.1 (1965)	74.5 (1968)	82.6
Nixon	1968	76.9 (1970)	50.6 (1973)	67.2
Ford	1974	61.0 (1975)	53.8 (1976)	57.6
Carter	1976	78.3 (1978)	75.1 (1980)	76.4
Reagan	1980	82.3 (1981)	43.5 (1987)	61.9
Bush, G. H. W.	1988	62.6 (1989)	43.0 (1992)	51.6
Clinton	1992	86.4 (1993; 1994)	36.2 (1995)	61.4
Bush, G. W.	2000	87.8 (2002)	72.6 (2004)	81.5
Obama	2009	96.7 (2009)	85.8 (2010)	91.3

Sources: Ornstein, Mann & Malbin, 2002; *CQ Weekly,* Jan. 3, 2011, 18.

based on issues on which the president took a clear-cut position, and they treat seminal legislation and more trivial pursuits equally. Second, the *Congressional Quarterly* score considers the president's position at the time of the vote, not his position much earlier when the item was first placed on the agenda. Finally, roll-call measures such as this understate the complexity of the policy process, in which the president is only one of many actors. Making "victories" attributable to the efforts of one player can be somewhat suspect.

In a more in-depth look at a sample of some 300 presidential proposals of five presidents (Eisenhower through Reagan), Mark Peterson (1990) found that about 54 percent of the proposals between 1953 and 1984 were passed in some form; more than one-third passed exactly as introduced. However, presidential success varied with the nature and scope of the proposal. Presidential proposals involving new and costly comprehensive policy initiatives often engendered opposition, and they were defeated outright 40 percent of the time. An analysis of 20 health policies in the final two years of the Carter administration and the first two years of the Reagan administration found that half were initiated by the White House, but only 12.5 percent of those proposals were enacted (Heinz et al., 1993).

Divided Government

A president facing at least one house controlled by the opposite party has to use a different strategy from the president blessed with a Congress led by his own party. Traditionally, presidents facing a unified Congress often rely on informal party mechanisms to achieve their goals. When facing a divided Congress or one controlled by members of the other party, the president must resort to the veto (or the threat of the veto) and support from the public. Yet both strategies are somewhat risky. Clearly the president cannot veto every bill he does not like; he must pick those that arouse public interest or strong public opinion. Similarly, the president cannot take every issue to the public.

One reason that relations between the president and Congress are especially dicey when government is divided is that opposition politicians often gain electoral advantage by frustrating the president. According to Kernell (1991), the main business of an opposition Congress is to prepare for the next election. Members of the minority party will tend not to bargain in good faith—it is not in their best interest. Perhaps the best recent example demonstrating the accuracy of this observation came amid the first signs of difficulty for President Obama's health care reform effort. Rather than pressing for specific policy changes to make the bill more acceptable to the GOP, Republican senator Jim DeMint (R-SC) characterized the issue conflict as a political opportunity: "If we're able to stop Obama on this, then it will be his Waterloo—it will break him" (Editorial, 2009; Smith, 2009a).

Interestingly, President Clinton had a Democratic Congress in his first year yet encountered difficulties (from his own party and the opposition) not unlike those of a president in a divided government. The Republican leadership talked about "sitting at the table" but spent more time carping at the Democrats' health care plan and forming coalitions with conservative Democrats to defeat key portions of the proposal. In the remaining years of his two terms, Clinton faced an opposition Congress, and his tactics changed as expected. He had fewer meetings with members, was less visible to the public, and offered little in the way of legislative initiatives.

In his second term, Clinton played obstructionist politics, reverting to fighting Republican initiatives rather than launching his own. He also compromised with the Republican leadership, often to the point of alienating some members of his own party. In fact, the president tried to distance himself from both congressional Democrats and Republicans in his second election campaign, adopting a centrist strategy between traditional Democrats and Republicans.

Going Public

Closely tied to presidential success in Congress is the desire of the public at large. Lincoln once commented on the strength of public approval: "Public sentiment is everything. With public sentiment, nothing can fail; without it nothing can succeed" (Collier, 1995, 1). Presidents often make direct appeals to the public, urging constituents to put pressure on their elected officials, in a manner Collier called "merchandising." Ronald Reagan often tried "to go over the heads" of members of Congress to mobilize public opinion behind a desired policy. Although this tactic is not new—Woodrow Wilson used it in an attempt to engender public support for the League of Nations—it has been used increasingly in the past two decades, thanks to advances in technology that allow interactive communications from a variety of sources and direct, targeted satellite feeds to television stations across the country. From Franklin Roosevelt's fireside chats to Bill Clinton's town meetings, the purpose is the same: to mobilize public support and build coalitions. As Miller (1993, 314) put it, "The president's most powerful weapon . . . is a public aroused on a specific issue." Public support can be important in building coalitions. It can help convince members of Congress that it is safe to support the president. This is especially important for members of the opposition party.

Presidents and their advisers fully understand the role of strong public support. Kernell (1984) recounted the desires of Reagan and his staff to take advantage of the president's popularity after the assassination attempt in 1981. They decided to push the president's desired budget cuts in a televised joint session of Congress, the first major appearance of President Reagan since the shooting. The broad public support helped; the budget passed, nearly intact. The problem with such an appeal is that the public is typically fickle and will often provide only fleeting support. It is also susceptible to messages from other interested parties and can easily grow bored with a subject. Jeffrey Cohen (1994) found that presidential attention to economic, foreign, and civil rights policy led to increased public concern with these policies. But presidential leadership effects decay within a year (except in the area of foreign policy). To keep the item on the public agenda, a president must repeatedly rally the public.

Presidents also use sympathetic interest groups to help arouse public support. Since Richard Nixon, presidents have established an Office of Public Liaison that mobilizes interest-group allies. In Clinton's health care reform strategy, core natural allies included senior citizens' associations, consumer groups, unions, liberal health care provider organizations, religious associations, and several organizations representing women, children, and minorities. As it turned out, Clinton did not get this base of support. Only one-quarter of the Democratic target group was in favor of the plan (Peterson, 2000). President Nixon also fully understood the importance of developing a message and making certain it got out. According to speech writer David Gergen, Nixon would repeatedly say, "About the time you are writing a line that you have written so often that you want to throw up, that is the first time the American people will hear it" (Gergen quoted in Kelly, 1993, 68).

Presidents can help define public opinion by framing issues in appealing ways. One example from the presidency of George W. Bush concerns his opposition in 2005 to a measure that would permit the importation of prescription drugs from Canada and allow the government to negotiate drug prices. While Democrats viewed the measure as giving seniors more access, the president saw the measure as a threat to the 2003 Medicare law and said, "Any attempt to limit the choices of our seniors and to take away their prescription-drug coverage under Medicare will meet my veto." His press secretary reiterated the "straw man" approach: "He's not going to let anybody take away what we have provided to you" (quoted in Loven, 2005).

A president's access to the media and strong allegiance to the national interest make the public approach appealing. A crucial challenge to the president comes in seeking to shape opinion. The Clinton administration recognized the importance of public opinion and established a "war room" that served to put the best "spin" on information such as the CBO's cost estimates for the Clinton plan and congressional pronouncements such as New York senator Daniel Patrick Moynihan's questioning of the seriousness of the "health care crisis." But the Republican opposition and interest groups opposing the plan were better at shaping the message than the White House was. An early and successful spin on the president's plan was that it would lead to more bureaucracy, lower standards of care, decreased choice of provider, and increased costs. Public support for the plan began to drop in the spring of 1994, when, for the first time, more Americans opposed Clinton's plan than favored it—although, ironically, they continued to like many aspects of it (Kosterlitz, 1994). As the vote on health care reform neared, the White House stepped up its efforts, scheduling a Health Security Express bus tour and offering nightly short addresses on cable television in which the president highlighted health issues of public concern. But the public's support continued to dwindle. In its "selling of the health care reform plan," the Clinton administration tried to promote broad principles and goals, such as health security, and to avoid details on such matters as health alliances and employer mandates. This policy backfired when interest-group commercials took the opportunity to inform and persuade the public that such aspects of the plan were harmful and unwise. President Carter had also found the public difficult to persuade on rising health costs, since most people were insulated from the problem by insurance and could not get worked up over the need for change (Peterson, 1990).

Probably the best example of public misunderstanding involved the passage, then repeal, of catastrophic health insurance for elderly people in 1988. Passed by substantial margins in both the House and the Senate and strongly supported by the president, the law was not well explained by elected officials, and the public was easily led astray by opponents' scare tactics. Although the bill adversely affected primarily the well-to-do and helped the poor, many poor elderly people thought they would have to pay high premiums for services they valued little. The final blow came when the initial cost estimates of the program turned out to be much too low; the new figures predicted costs of six times the first estimates (Broder, 1994a).

Sometimes the president uses the public as a sounding board for possible solutions—solutions quickly forgotten if the cues are wrong. For example, the

Clinton administration abandoned consideration of a new value-added tax to finance its health program, because a poll conducted by the White House indicated no support for it (Peters, 1994). However, recent research on the politics of polling indicates that polling is used more for finding the catch phrases and arguments to shape issues that will win public support than for figuring out what the public wants and how to respond. Jacobs and Shapiro (2000) found that since the 1970s, the policy decisions of presidents and members of Congress have become less responsive to the substantive policy preferences of Americans.

The President and the Press

The days when a small close-knit press corps crowded around Franklin Roosevelt's desk to hear the latest presidential pronouncements are long gone. Today's White House press corps numbers in the hundreds, and it covers the president's every move, and failure to move, in seemingly excruciating detail. The first modern media president was John F. Kennedy, who used television to project the image of an energetic, talented, and handsome leader. Richard Nixon, "burned" by television in his campaign against Kennedy in 1960, learned to use it to his advantage in his effort to remake his political career in the mid-1960s. Nixon institutionalized the process of communications and put in place a series of innovations designed to control the news and put the best spin on it.

Nixon established an Office of Communications and the Office of Public Liaison, which worked to "orchestrate" the news and organize grassroots efforts supportive of the president. The Office of Communications focused in large part on local media, using them to reach the people without filtering through the larger, more cynical (and perhaps unsupportive) Washington and East Coast media. This office understood the importance of symbols to presidential activities and worked to provide short, meaningful messages that could be captured in brief "sound bites." The Nixon staff developed the notion of a "line of the day," highlighted on a given day by the president and other spokespersons. The communications staff tried to control the media's agenda and access, rewarding reporters who wrote good stories and attacking those who were critical. The communications staff met weekly with public relations staff from federal agencies to make certain the message was clear and unified.

President Reagan, using some of the staff members trained in the Nixon White House, followed the same highly coordinated, well-developed plan to control the media and reach the public. James Baker, while chief of staff, spent

35 hours a week talking to journalists. He gave an hour a day to three networks and four major newspapers (Kelly, 1993). The Reagan team was also good at "leaking" information to reporters in exchange for information from the press, such as what members of the White House press corps were working on and what they were hearing from other people in Washington.

President Clinton had a tough time getting his message across in the first two years of his presidency. Such missteps as troublesome nominees for attorney general, expensive haircuts, and aides using helicopters to travel to golf courses were emblazoned across newspapers with headlines such as the *New York Daily News's* "Bumblin' Bill" and *Time* magazine's "Incredible Shrinking President." More serious issues involving allegations of influence peddling and sexual harassment during his gubernatorial tenure followed Clinton into his second year. He seemed to suffer from what political scientist Larry Sabato (1991) called a "boom-and-bust cycle—where things are either perfect and beautiful and wonderful or they're terrible and awful," with little in between. In Sabato's view, the press tends to follow public opinion rather than help shape it, but others think media coverage helps define the presidency and form the perceptions essential to public opinion (Kurtz, 1994).

President Obama enjoyed the boom half of the cycle for his first six months in office but then began to see his popularity slip and the popularity of his proposal slip even further. His was not the Clinton problem of lack of focus or discipline. Former presidential advisers called his discipline "remarkable" (Baker, 2009, 2). This despite several times when he went off script, gave candid answers, and learned to regret them. For example, he criticized highly paid bankers who had received federal financial bailout funds and nonetheless went to expensive conferences in Las Vegas. The criticism was barely out his mouth when conference cancellations to Las Vegas and other glamour spots began. He criticized his own bowling performance by saying he should play in the Special Olympics, offending the people who sponsor and participate in such games. He had to call and apologize to former First Lady Nancy Reagan after joking about her holding séances.

President Obama had to make a surprise visit to the White House press room on a Friday afternoon to more or less eat the word "stupidly" that he'd used earlier in the week. He used it when describing the Cambridge, Massachusetts, police behavior in arresting a middle-aged, cane-reliant, black Harvard history professor in front of his own home. The arrest was for disorderly conduct—yelling at a police officer who'd come to his house suspecting that he was a burglar. Charges were quickly dropped, but police across the country were offended by the president's choice of words. He invited both the policeman and the Harvard professor (a personal friend) to the White House for a beer. As he explained in his surprise press room visit, use of the word "stupidly" had cost him dearly by pulling attention away from his health care reform agenda and moving it squarely onto race relations between blacks, police, and the nation's first black president. Consensus quickly formed among former White House press secretaries commenting on the incident: the president would have to stop expressing his candid feelings. "He'd have been better off saying something bland like 'I certainly sympathize with anyone who has to prove that he is in his own house,'" observed noted presidential scholar George Edwards III. "It takes iron discipline to remain on message" (Baker 2009, 3).

Policy Implementation

The president may spend enormous amounts of time setting the policy agenda and trying to get desired policies put into place, but the office also brings with it another important policy function: carrying out, or executing, those laws. The president is charged with overseeing the executive branch of government—some 2.7 million strong, with about 345,000 employees working in the Washington, D.C., metropolitan area.

One important way the president exercises such oversight is through appointing cabinet positions, commissions, and subcabinet posts, offices with leadership responsibility for federal programmatic functions. There are 15 cabinet posts and around 200 important subcabinet posts, all subject to Senate confirmation. The "inner cabinet" is made up of the secretaries of Defense, State, Justice, and Treasury. "Outer cabinet" members—secretaries of the Interior, Agriculture, Commerce, Labor, Education, Housing and Urban Development, Transportation, Health and Human Services, Energy, Veterans Affairs, and Homeland Security— do not generally have the access and influence of inner cabinet members. They deal with groups whose political resources are few (welfare recipients, Native Americans) and those whose well-established influence presidents could not change substantially even if they wanted to (large manufacturers, corporate farmers, organized labor). However, some outer cabinet members can exercise more power if they are particularly close to the president, such as Robert Reich, President Clinton's first-term labor secretary, or if the issue is extremely timely and salient, such as homeland security. George W. Bush also recognized four additional staff as having cabinet rank: the administrator of the Environmental

Protection Agency, the director of the Office of Management and Budget, the director of the National Drug Control Policy, and the U.S. Trade Representative.

President Obama appointed a number of "czars," including a health czar, although some thought that there were simply too many of them to give any real power. Nor is it ever clear what power a czar has, given that czars' responsibilities overlap those of cabinet secretaries, other White House advisers, and the OMB, not to mention presidential confidants such as Tom Daschle, former Senate majority leader and withdrawn nominee for both health czar and HHS secretary. He withdrew his nomination after disclosure that he had not paid taxes on limo services provided by a consulting business client. But he remained a close adviser of the president on health issues in his role as a private citizen. Historians will likely wonder: Did he work through his replacement nominees for the two jobs for which he had been nominated, or did he go directly to the president or the president's chief of staff?

Cabinet members are appointed by the president and serve at his pleasure. The popular Joseph Califano, secretary of HEW in the Carter years, discovered the tenuous nature of his position when he was rather ignominiously fired for reasons quite apart from his role as cabinet secretary (he got too cozy with potential presidential primary challenger Sen. Edward Kennedy). Or, as Abraham Lincoln said following a cabinet vote over a heated issue, "One aye, seven nays. The Ayes have it" (Light, 1984, 436). The presidentially appointed cabinet serves important functions linking the president and his plan for government with a huge body of civil servants who do the day-to-day work of implementing federal programs. Cabinet members also advise the president on issues and represent him in hearings before Congress. They chair commissions and other efforts to seek information and reach consensus. For example, in 1999 President Clinton directed the treasury secretary and the attorney general to develop a strategy on gun violence.

There is usually a fairly high turnover of presidentially appointed heads of agencies. Only 4 of the 15 cabinet secretaries in George W. Bush's first term retained those positions in his second term. Interestingly, Clinton administration appointees were longer-lasting than most. For example, Donna Shalala was HHS secretary during the entire eight years of his presidency. There were three HHS heads in the eight-year Reagan administration. Former Wisconsin governor Tommy Thompson served as HHS secretary through the first term of the George W. Bush presidency but left that position at the start of the second term.

The Bureaucracy

Presidents are important to federal agency employees. In addition to appointing the agency leadership, presidents and the OMB recommend agencies' budgets to Congress and oversee the promulgation of agency recommendations.

The bureaucracy is important to the president. It can provide useful expertise and an institutional and policy memory that can mean the difference between success and failure for a treasured policy or program. Ironically, although the president often understands the importance of "getting the bureaucracy under control," he is usually relatively uninterested in administration, and presidents of both parties tend to distrust the federal bureaucracy. Some presidents try to control federal agencies by careful selection of agency heads who share the president's ideological and policy vision. Others prefer to "work around" agencies by locating policy expertise and control in the White House rather than relying on the agencies. President Nixon tried both. He carefully selected cabinet members and other high officials to ensure that the bureaucracy would be helpful, not harmful, in his policy goals, and he also centralized control of policymaking in the White House, using agencies as little as possible.

Presidents can also reorganize the executive branch to best fit their goals and to improve overall efficiency—to some extent. For example, in 1971 President Nixon sent to Congress a reorganization plan that would have abolished the departments of Agriculture, Labor, Commerce, HUD, Interior, HEW, and Transportation and would have consolidated their functions into four new "superagencies": departments of Human Resources, Natural Resources, Community Development, and Economic Affairs. His plan went nowhere in a Congress that was lobbied by groups wanting to keep the existing agencies and in which such a shakeup would change congressional committee responsibilities—meaning that some committee chairs and members could lose authority and standing. Nixon later accomplished some of his changes with a functional reorganization corresponding roughly to the proposed superagencies, with staffers responsible for coordinating policy in those areas. Recent presidents have not attempted major reorganization—with the notable exception of the George W. Bush administration, which formed a new cabinet agency for homeland security and incorporated numerous existing offices from different departments within the new agency. Not surprisingly, the implementation of this effort was difficult and slow-moving. The reorganization proved controversial following Hurricane Katrina in 2005, which devastated New Orleans and the Gulf Coast. Some observers thought that inclusion of the Federal Emergency Management Agency (FEMA) in Homeland Security diluted the agency's ability to respond quickly and effectively.

President George W. Bush was an active user of signing statements that outlined how his administration planned to implement the law. Signed with the law, these orders sent the message to Congress that the president had his own ideas about how the law should be implemented, and as such they would be viewed by him and those who worked for him as the last word on the law before its implementation (Cochran, 2004). President Obama had criticized his predecessor's enthusiastic use of signing statements (over 1,100 during his eight-year presidency) but then used them himself to "protect" his constitutional prerogatives. For example, in 2011, President Obama issued a signing statement saying he would ignore Congress's attempt to defund the positions of four administration czars, including ones over health care and climate change (Crabtree, 2011).

The White House Staff

The White House staff typically consists of about 1,000 people. Like the congressional staff, the White House staff is an important source of expertise and political guidance—often more of the latter than the former. While most presidents fill these positions with trusted and loyal assistants and aides, sometimes the persons who are most trusted are not the best staffers. Bill Clinton's first chief of staff, longtime friend Thomas McLarty, was loyal but not best suited to the tough job of gatekeeper, and he left after 18 months. Many of the Clinton White House aides were young (in their twenties) and inexperienced in Washington norms. Not a few "old hands" were offended by what they felt was brusque or inappropriate treatment by the "youngsters." Having such young and inexperienced staffs has been a recurring problem for presidents. George W. Bush was the exception. His staffers tended to be middle-aged or older and highly experienced—several having served with his father. President Obama drew in a combination of old hands, close confidants and a few experts from outside politics, mixing some in as cabinet secretaries, others as czars, and others as staff. In a few instances he brought in old hands but put them into slots few pundits would ever have expected for them given their recent roles: former Clinton White House chief of staff and former California congressman Leon Panetta became CIA director, and in Obama's cabinet, former presidential candidate and rival Hillary Clinton became secretary of state. The president appointed an acerbic congressman from Illinois, Rahm Emanuel, as his chief of staff.

Problems can arise if aides isolate the president and tell him only what he wants to hear (Presidents Nixon and Johnson may have been treated this way), or if aides are not well informed on political relationships and mores in Washington (President Carter's aides come to mind here). President Clinton was criticized for "government by inner circle" and for relying for advice on an "adhocracy," or ad hoc groups, rather than established experts in the bureaucracy and elsewhere (Haass, 1994). Traditionally, Democratic presidents have preferred what is known as a spokes-of-the-wheel organization, whereby the president works with a few cabinet-level persons who report directly to him. Republicans tend to use a chief-of-staff model, with one person serving as gatekeeper to the presidential office. In reality, however, these organizational models oversimplify the differences in presidential interaction with staffs (Jones, 1994).

In recent years, the White House staff has grown considerably as the presidents have wanted to have more of their "own people" in central policymaking roles. For example, the Domestic Policy Council often serves as a president's window on domestic policy and the mechanism for presidential coordination of agencies. The Office of Communications in the White House is a very important vehicle for presidential links with people—especially important since Nixon. The Council of Economic Advisers is responsible for the annual economic report and provides advice to the president on economic issues. The National Security Council provides advice on defense issues. The staffs of these agencies are usually small. "The number of [White House] staff directly involved in policy choice is quite restricted," Light (1991, 55) noted. "The bulk of the staff is usually engaged in firefighting while the rest are forced to tackle one or two problems at a time."

The Office of Management and Budget

Of the agencies within the executive office of the president, the OMB is particularly pivotal to domestic policymaking. Established in 1921 as the Bureau of the Budget, its formation is viewed by some as the beginning of the institutional presidency (Moe, 1985). In 1970, it added *management* to its name and function and became the "eyes and ears" of the president (Benda & Levine, 1986). The OMB has increasingly taken on broad domestic policy coordination issues, in addition to its traditional budgetary role. Its primary function is the preparation of the president's budget; it reviews agency requests and coordinates them with presidential priorities and desires.

The OMB has long played the role of budgetary "heavy," arguing for reductions in spending or the elimination or scaling back of programs. Although most of the OMB's actions in drafting the president's budget occur behind closed doors, sometimes actions and rationales become known. Clinton's HHS secretary Donna Shalala typically requested major funding for the nation's community health centers, only to have the requests slashed drastically by the OMB. For example, in 1997 she requested $100 million in appropriations and the OMB reduced it to $8 million. When questioned about the severe cuts in a program that provides care to many of the nation's poorest residents, an OMB official replied that the agency has to operate under budget caps and said, "We have a holistic approach to public health. The system is under strain and we are being innovative. We have given increases to the Centers for Disease Control, which also serves minorities and the poor" (quoted in McGrory, 1999). In an equally telling remark, the official also noted that the Republicans in Congress could always restore the funds.

OMB officials work closely with Congress in drafting appropriations and authorization bills, monitoring spending and surpluses, working with agencies to make congressional cuts, and sometimes playing politics as they speak for the president on budgetary issues. OMB director Franklin Raines, for example, fought hard against the inclusion of health savings accounts in the 1996 Health Insurance Portability and Accountability Act (HIPAA), arguing that such accounts would "provide a tax break for the healthiest and wealthiest individuals . . . and attract them out of the general insurance market, potentially raising premiums for all other people" (*Congressional Quarterly*, 1997). Raines's successor, Jacob Lew, was even more visible and outspoken in efforts to influence Congress. He described one Republican budget plan as being "as phony as a three-dollar bill" and called another a "bankrupt approach" (OMB Director Lew, 2000). Lew threatened Congress in May 2000 with several presidential vetoes of appropriations and other important bills unless it made "significant improvements" by increasing funding or altering priorities. In conference committees, the OMB director is often an active participant in deliberations, representing the president.

When HHS secretary Tommy Thompson stepped down in 2005, he was highly critical of the OMB's role in policymaking. He asserted that the OMB acted as "super God." "They turn you down nine times out of 10 just to show you they are the boss," he told reporters in a candid interview expressing his frustrations with Washington's bureaucracy. He also complained about the White House staff, who "do not believe that anything smart or original can come from a secretary or a department" (Pugh, 2005, 4A).

The Presidency and Health Policy

Since Harry Truman, every president, Democrat or Republican, has proposed major health legislation, much of it involving national health insurance. Most presidents have wanted to expand the federal role in health; the Reagan and Bush administrations of the 1980s proposed the addition of protection against catastrophic losses under Medicare and several additional Medicare benefits, in an effort to make public coverage more efficient and better targeted. Presidents vary in their efforts to inform the public and influence Congress and in their success at doing so. President Ford offered a major plan and (largely because of economic considerations) never pursued it with Congress. President Clinton pulled out all the stops in drafting a comprehensive plan and encouraging its adoption. President Obama's plan goes further than most in access reform but moves cautiously on cost control and even more cautiously on quality reform.

One reason for the notable lack of success of presidential proposals for health care reform may be the different constituencies. For the president, concerned with a broad, national constituency, national health insurance is easily understood and explained as making broad policy changes that will improve the efficiency and effectiveness of health care for all Americans. For a member of Congress, national health care reform comes down to the effect on her local hospital, medical school, or small businesses. Each legislator sees the issue in terms of pharmacists and optometrists and nurses and drug companies and dry cleaners—many of the health care sector's components—rather than the entire issue. When the national program for the public good is thus deconstructed into its 535 component parts, problems arise, and these have thus far stymied the enactment of a comprehensive, universal health policy for the country.

Other major sticking points for presidents have had to do with the cost of a broad, comprehensive health care program—and how to pay for it. Increased taxation is something no president relishes, yet any major change must be accompanied by the resources to pay for it. Issues of unemployment also arise, though not as closely or personally at the presidential level as in congressional districts. And all modern presidents have promoted cost controls. Going back to the Nixon—and indeed even the Johnson—administration, there was a great deal of concern about rising health care costs and how to get a handle on them. So far, answers have been elusive to presidents and Congresses alike. Finally, as Steinmo and Watts (1995) noted, there are institutional constraints against passage of comprehensive health care reforms: the fragmented political power in the United

States, congressional rules allowing a minority to block legislation, fragmented power in the entrepreneurial Congress, and the increasing importance of the media.

Although many earlier modern presidents proposed major health care reforms, none before Obama did so with the fervor and dedication of President Bill Clinton. He dubbed health care reform the "defining issue" of his presidency. With the first lady as the point person, a major effort involving more than 500 experts in a dozen or more task forces was launched to write a health care reform plan in 100 days. The effort was largely conducted in secret, without the involvement of key interest groups that would be directly affected by the reforms, and it was highly decentralized, with task forces working independently and generally without concern for potential costs and likely political support (or opposition). The result—the American Health Security Act—was sweeping in scope. It called for universal health care coverage by 1998 for all Americans. It would have made changes in the way health care is structured by setting up regional insurance purchasing alliances, mandating that employers pay a substantial amount of health insurance for employees, and creating a national health board to establish national and regional spending limits. The plan would have meant major changes for employers, insurance companies, health care providers, and consumers.

In a speech before Congress in September 1993, President Clinton challenged the members to ignore scare tactics by groups that may have benefited from the waste in the existing system and produce a program that would provide universal, comprehensive health care for American citizens. But it was too late. A plethora of interest groups, with millions of dollars at their disposal, were lying in wait to attack the parts of the proposal they did not like (while remaining largely silent on those parts they approved of). Several weeks later, some 280 days after the process began, a 1,342-page bill was unveiled to Congress, the public, and the affected interests. The timing, the process, and the product were problematic. Criticism was rampant and shrill, and questions designed to shake public support were being asked in television commercials and emblazoned across full-page newspaper ads.

The timing—nine months into the presidency—was well past the "honeymoon" period, the time when Presidents Reagan and Johnson had been most successful with their sweeping new proposals. In those nine months, Clinton had been engaged in other high-visibility issues such as NAFTA and an economic stimulus program. These issues were hard-fought, even with the Democratic Congress, and involved presidential persuasion and arm-twisting that used up valuable goodwill and support. Meanwhile, the process used to draft the health plan enraged those who were not a part of it. The press railed against the secrecy and complained about the waste of money. It was a "policy wonk's" dream— months of high-level policy deliberation. But the political realities were sorely misjudged. The product, a reflection of the rarefied air of a protected policy analytical discussion, was simply too complex and too academic, containing something to offend everyone. As noted by Light a decade earlier (1984), a president can often succeed by adopting and amending proposals already before Congress. But the Clintons chose not to take this path. Rather, they forged an ambitious, comprehensive proposal for making massive changes in the current system, with limited congressional involvement.

The public, which initially seemed supportive of the proposal, began to question the need for and complexity of national health care reform. In public polls conducted in February 1994, the same percentage of people opposed the plan as supported it. After that time, the nays began to pull ahead. Even those in favor of reforms may have had a rather modest adjustment in mind. Focus groups and some polls found that many people were interested mainly in the forms of insurance, rather than the problems of the uninsured, and in whether they could obtain insurance if they left their jobs, an issue of portability rather than whether the entire system needed a major overhaul (Clymer, Pear & Toner, 1994).

The reasons for the demise of the Clinton health care reform are many. They include budgetary constraints and an antigovernment mood that doomed any comprehensive plan from the beginning (Skocpol, 1996); the White House's inability to define the issue and frame the debate, and its lack of sustained effort (Edwards, 2000); the plan's complexity, liberal approach, and cost (Quirk & Cunion, 2000); the inability of the experts to agree on the reform (White, 1995); the lack of support from the business community (Morone, 1995); a deeply divided public, which wanted reform but balked at the actual policies (Brodie & Blendon, 1995); and low levels of support from elites (Jacobs & Shapiro, 1995).

President Clinton, given an opportunity to choose early in his term between a more targeted program to cover only large, catastrophic costs and a more comprehensive, universal approach, chose the latter (Woodward, 1994). He was simply unwilling to compromise his vision of major reform. To do so, he felt, would be to violate the trust of the people and his office. As he said later, when the prospects for success of any plan were bleak, "We didn't say, 'vote for me, in a representative form of government and I will make all the necessary decisions to solve the problems of the country, except those that are difficult, controversial and make the people mad.' That was not the deal" (Wines, 1994, A9). But it was a deal, at least in health care that was not to be. President Clinton joined his predecessors in his inability to fashion a successful health care reform package.

Although comprehensive health care reform never again was a major policy theme of his administration, Clinton did not give up. Rather, he adopted an incremental approach, and if he did not succeed in the first year, he came back year after year seeking Medicare buy-in for persons aged 55 to 64, prescription drug coverage for Medicare beneficiaries, and a tax credit to assist people caring for relatives with chronic illnesses or disabilities. In his final State of the Union address, he put it this way: "The lesson of our history, and the lesson of the last seven years, is that great goals are reached step-by-step, always building on our progress, always gaining ground" (Pear, 2000b).

President George W. Bush did not attempt a national health insurance initiative, but he was successful at the most significant reform of the Medicare program since its founding in 1965. Many felt that he chose that policy initiative because it took away from Democrats a signature issue, one on which they might have run their midterm elections had he not snatched it away. It is interesting to note here that Bush's success in health and other areas flies in the face of some conventional wisdom and political research on the presidency. He had no electoral mandate yet acted decisively; in his health proposal, he shunned incremental approaches and proposed a program with huge costs; and he turned serious attention to Medicare reform in the middle of his first presidential term, not in the earliest days. But he did have one important factor in his favor: a strong, united party in the presidency and both houses of Congress. The Republican leadership was focused and determined to give the president a Medicare package—and they succeeded. Clearly party cohesion meant that many hurdles could be overcome.

President Barack Obama a dozen years later found his efforts much more in peril over lack of that kind of unity among his Democratic congressional colleagues. Having learned from the Clinton approach that it was a bad mistake to deliver to Congress an already-written policy-wonk's dream bill, President Obama left the bill-writing to Congress. He laid down some principles: full coverage for the uninsured; control of unsustainable costs of health care, bending down the steeply rising cost curve; and choice for consumers seeking a health care plan, including a public plan choice to compete with private plans for the under-65 population. Plans began to emerge in both houses of Congress by early July 2009, and they had passed two committees in the House. Despite nearly solid Republican opposition to most of the health reform ideas being circulated (Nagourney, 2009), a head of steam seemed to be building to meet the president's requested deadline of a health reform bill from both houses before the August congressional recess. Then two sentinel events opened a valve and let much of the pressure off.

First, the Senate Finance Committee under the bipartisan leadership of Max Baucus (D-MT) and Charles Grassley (R-IA) had penned a bill that would tax employee health benefits that exceeded a certain threshold of value above the value of the average family plan. The president, perhaps too quickly, said he didn't like the idea of taxing health benefits, especially those for which union members—key Democratic supporters—had given up wages in past labor contract negotiations. Committee members were unhappy with having their difficult compromises spurned (Herszenhorn, 2009). Then the Congressional Budget Office not only let out the rest of the steam from the congressional health care reform engine but firmly applied the brakes. As negotiations peaked and House action seemed imminent in late July 2009, in response to a question from the House majority leader, CBO director Douglas Elmendorf said that none of the bills in the House would save much money. Savings would likely be only about $2 billion over 10 years, all of it during the 7th through 10th years. Fiscally conservative Blue Dog Democrats immediately rebelled, seeing large government spending on a new government entitlement.

Meanwhile, the Senate ran several new tax proposals up the flagpole, trying to find a way to pay for reform (Wayne & Herszenhorn, 2009). Each quickly found its critics (Herszenhorn & Pear, 2009a). House members began to express concern that if they passed a bill containing new taxes and the Senate talked about them but didn't enact them, House members would have made their constituents mad for nothing (Herszenhorn & Pear, 2009b). Waiting until the Senate acted before passing a House bill seemed like a good idea to many. But senators were nowhere close to a solution on how to pay for reform or to bend down the cost curve.

As members left for home, and it became clear to everyone that nothing was going to pass without meeting the Blue Dogs' demand for real cost controls, health care providers began to see that health reform was going to deliver their worst fears. It was going to cost them income. Insurers had already drawn a line in the sand over the idea of offering a public plan. Unions were angry about the prospect of taxing their health benefits. Bad economic news renewed Republicans' and some Democrats' concern that an employer mandate to pay part of employees' health care costs would cost jobs and slow economic recovery (Herszenhorn & Pear, 2009b). Physicians were very worried that shaping a response to the CBO and the Blue Dogs would mean giving an independent health care cost commission real control over both physician payment and what care would be paid for; consumer groups expressed concern that efforts to appease the Blue Dogs would reduce subsidies to poor uninsured people, putting health care beyond their reach (Pear, 2009a); and the public began to express concern that reform might interfere with their own health care access and quality. To many, these refrains sounded eerily like echoes from the Clinton health reform debates.

Yet the president ended his first year victorious in passing health reform through both houses of Congress, and by late spring the following year he signed the largest health reform legislation passed since Medicare and Medicaid were enacted in 1965. He had shown success—a deftness of touch most of the time—in letting Congress take the lead, yet keeping up an active role in sensitive negotiations through his HHS secretary, his White House health adviser, and his politically savvy and tenacious chief of staff, a former congressman and a well-known head knocker. When the unions balked at the Senate's addition of a new tax on high premiums, the president personally intervened to strike a compromise, raising the threshold for the tax, exempting specific groups of union members, and delaying implementation of the new tax.

In the end, helped by large Democratic House and Senate majorities, a powerful and effective Speaker, experienced and capable committee chairs, and his strategy of neutralizing industry opposition by buying it off with early White House deals, the president was able to do what many before him had tried and failed to do: pass health reform. It was not all he'd hoped for, and in terms of controlling cost and improving quality, it may have fallen well short of his principal goals; but it was a major reform, and he had been a key player in marshaling the congressional support needed to pass it despite determined and cohesive Republican opposition in both houses.

Conclusion

In Number 70 of the *Federalist Papers*—the collection of political tracts arguing for support of the U.S. Constitution—Alexander Hamilton argued that "energy in the executive is a leading character in the definition of good government" (Publius, [1787–88] 1961, 423). While other Founding Fathers were less enthusiastic about a strong executive, they agreed that their desired system of checks and balances required roughly equivalent components—strong executive and legislative branches.

There is variance in the perception of strength in the presidency. Some presidents, including Abraham Lincoln, Franklin Roosevelt, Harry Truman, and George W. Bush, have been willing to push the limits of presidential power and, in the process, have expanded that power—at least for the short term. Other presidents have had a harder time dealing with Congress. Certainly Bill Clinton's presidential clout was weakened by the dozens of congressional and special investigator probes, one of which led to his impeachment by the House in 1998.

The president can command the public's attention and garner massive press attention, but the public is also hearing contrary messages from other interests, and the press attention is often critical and downright negative. In health, the presidential role has long been as an initiator of change in health care access and delivery. But the president is stymied at many points and has been generally unsuccessful in achieving major health legislation since the passage of Medicare in 1965. (The adoption of the Medicare Modernization Act in 2003 serves as the sole exception here.) Republican and Democratic presidents have offered surprisingly similar proposals for national health insurance, which have met similar, unsuccessful fates in Congress.

Supreme Court justice Robert H. Jackson noted in a 1952 decision that power migrates between the branches of government, and he quoted Napoleon as saying, "The tools belong to the man who can use them" (Stevenson, 2005). President George W. Bush used those tools. President Obama—a former senator—opened his health care reform effort with a distinct deference to Congress, letting the congressional committees draft the legislation, suggesting that different craftsmen can employ different tools so long as they choose ones that work.

CHAPTER THREE

Interest Groups

A Look Back

1965

Charls Walker, a top Washington lobbyist, described lobbying Congress in the days of Sam Rayburn (D-TX; Speaker for the 10 sessions between 1940 and 1961) as highly personal, direct, and easy. In a fifty-minute meeting with Speaker Rayburn, "for forty-eight minutes we would talk about Texas, family and friends. In the remaining two, we would settle what I had come to talk about. He always knew what I was there for, and would say, 'It's taken care of, Charlie,' or 'I just can't do that for you'" (Colamosca, 1979, 16). John McCormack (D-MA), who took over when Rayburn died, was similarly low-keyed and circumspect.

In 1965, the American Medical Association (AMA) was the strongest health lobby and probably the most powerful lobby of any kind in the country. A spokesperson for the AMA could say that "medicine" opposed a bill and be correct. According to a *Yale Law Journal* article of 1954, the *New York Times* had recently claimed that the AMA was the "only organization in the country that could marshal 140 votes in Congress between sundown Friday night and noon on Monday" (Morone, 1990, 256). Yet in 1965, the powerful AMA met its first major defeat with the passage of Medicare, after spending $1.2 million (an amount equivalent to about $10 million in 2010) to fight it.

The 1965 Medicare fight was unusual, a blip on the otherwise relatively blank screen of national health insurance. By 1966 things had settled down, and the physicians' group spent $49,000 on lobbying in Washington, D.C.—a small amount even in today's dollars. That same year, the American Dental Association (ADA) spent $18,000 on lobbying; the American Hospital Association (AHA), $41,000; and the American Nurses Association (ANA), $45,000.

Political action committees were few and not very noticeable in 1965. Those that did exist were mostly associated with labor unions, PACs set up to fight federal prohibitions on labor contributions to candidates for federal offices. The American Medical Association PAC (AMPAC), formed in 1961, was one of the very few nonlabor PACs.

1981

The pace of politics and interest-group competition had picked up by the early 1980s. A plethora of health-related interest groups had opened offices in the capital, along K Street, N.W. More and more of the lunches consumed at the Rotunda, the Monocle, and other longtime power-lunch eateries huddled at the foot of Capitol Hill were being bought by professional lobbyists whose clients wore white coats to work or worked closely with those who did. President Jimmy Carter's demand for spending controls on hospitals had aroused the powerful Chicago-based AHA, which stepped up its lobbying and built up its campaign contribution base. Business lobbyists, too, had health care on their menus. Costs had caught the eye of business executives as the fringe-benefit line in their annual reports began to show a higher rate of growth than wages, sales, or profits.

Chatty lunches were only a small part of the story about what was influencing health care policy. Reelection campaign costs had mushroomed as expensive television ads became the weapon of choice in the battle for votes. Campaign costs had risen tenfold in less than two decades. With so many digits in their reelection budgets, those who were elected might not even notice the generosity of moderate-sized individual contributions. Enter the PAC, bundling the campaign contributions of interest groups, corporations, labor unions, and others to represent a single set of interests (Sabato, 1985). By 1981, PACs had become a major factor in helping to fund (and speed the growth of) the campaign vortex.

Although the AMA and a few other organizations had PACs in the 1970s, PACs did not become a noticeable feature of the political landscape until the 1980s, thanks in part to the reforms of the 1970s. In an attempt to shrink the influence of a few well-heeled givers, those who wanted more citizen-financed campaigns had pressured Congress to cap contributions from individuals and interest groups and to set up a public financing mechanism for major party candidates for president. The authorization of PACs in the 1974 law led to an extraordinary increase in their number and influence.

Health care associations took notice. Clearly there were many whose interests were not being represented by the AMA, the AHA, or the insurance companies. With their own PACs, optometrists, chiropractors, dentists, nurses, nursing homes, group practice associations, family doctors, pharmacists, drug companies, occupational therapists, and others could mount lobbying efforts or make campaign contributions to ensure that when the body politic wrote national health insurance legislation, it did not neglect the part of the human body in which they had a particular interest. Well-placed contributions could make sure the donor's services—optometry or dentistry or whatever—were included in insurance coverage proposals and the donor's scope of practice was protected from would-be poachers.

Cash became a p.r.n. (physicians' notation for "take as needed") prescription for the whole health care industry. The 1978 spending totals for federal elections alone reached huge proportions for a wide range of groups: the AMA, nearly $2 million; the dental PAC, $573,000; nurses, $100,000; for-profit hospitals, $144,000; and optometrists, $112,000.

Political action committees seemed to be taking on a life of their own. Groups without them needed them; groups that had them needed bigger ones; and PACs representing broad interests experienced splintering, as subgroups formed new PACs. But there never seemed to be enough PACs. More money chasing the same number of candidates inflated the cost of campaigns, intensifying the need for larger and larger PAC contributions and more and more fund-raising efforts by the candidates. More PACs would have to raise more money.

1993

At the start of the Clinton administration, Washington seemed to be overrun with lobbyists—many with health care reform on their minds. Groups had proliferated, mutated, multiplied, spread, bred, and fed on one another, and now they represented specialized physicians' groups, specialty hospitals, insurers, businesses, labor, corporate interests, pharmaceutical firms, home care companies, prepaid health plans, walk-in clinics, children, and people who were poor, elderly, or disabled. Nursing homes in one Southern state could not afford their own lobbyist, so they retained a Washington professional who lobbied for a variety of health care groups; enterprisingly, he then contacted the nursing home association in a contiguous state and picked up another client. The story was being repeated all over town. When White House staffers began to count noses as they sized up the potential opposition to the president's reform plan, the numbers took their breath away. They identified more than 1,100 interest groups with substantial stakes in the health care battle (Broder, 1994b). No one wanted to be left out. Every interest group in the land seemed "to have something to say on health care restructuring—from dentists to the Christian Coalition," according to the *New York Times.* "It has created a daily, unrelenting round of Health Care Events" (Toner, 1994, 1). "This is the biggest-scale lobbying effort that has ever been mounted on any single piece of legislation—both in terms of dollars spent and people engaged," said Ellen Miller of the Center for Responsive Politics, a watchdog group that keeps an eye on lobbying activities and spending (Seelye, 1994, A10).

The *New York Times* described a "typical day" in the capital—March 8, 1994— in the "Year of Health Care Events":

> [Eight hundred] doctors were massed at the American Medical Association conference; 210 restaurateurs were tromping to Capitol Hill, ventilating their opposition to the idea of requiring businesses to pay for health insurance; President Clinton was making the case for health care overhaul to the American Society of Association Executives (a kind of trade group for trade groups); Ralph Nader was denouncing the AMA at a news conference; former First Ladies Rosalyn Carter and Betty Ford were arguing for mental health coverage before the Senate Labor and Human Resources Committee; and the line of interested parties stretched down a very long hall when the House Ways and Means Subcommittee on Health began considering a health care bill. And this was all before noon. (Toner, 1994, 1)

Health care lobbying had become a team sport. The AMA was just a player. No longer could its president boldly declare that "medicine is opposed to this measure as a total package" (Campion, 1984, 275). There were no "genuine peak associations" in the health domain, concluded Salisbury and his fellow researchers (1987, 1227); they found that the AMA was best described as only one among several sets of interest-group participants, though a highly significant set.

Style changed too. "It's not about going up and tugging on Rosty's sleeve (Dan Rostenkowski of Illinois, chair of the House Ways and Means Committee) and saying 'I need something,'" a former Clinton administration functionary told the *Washington Post.* "That gets you absolutely nowhere. It's knowing how to mobilize, having access to information, making the right moves at the right time" (Boodman, 1994, 6).

2009

The phone rings: "This is AARP with an urgent alert. There is a crucial vote in the US House of Representatives this week on an historic health care reform bill. AARP supports this bill which will improve Medicare and Medicaid and significantly improve health care for millions of Americans. Dial 1800xxxxxxx and you'll be connected directly to Congressman Allen Boyd. Tell Congressman Boyd to vote yes on this historic health reform bill."

The Chamber of Commerce delivers a different message. Its television ad talks about budget deficits and how the Obama health care plan will add billions to the deficit and raise billions in new taxes and involve the government much more heavily in health care.

More quietly, the American Medical Association announces that it supports health reform. So does PhRMA (Pharmaceutical Research and Manufacturers of America). AARP expects no quid pro quo: its leadership thinks this bill is in the public's and its members' interests.

The AMA and PhRMA are not so altruistic. Physicians want pay cuts restored that are due to be imposed under a schedule of fee cuts enacted in 1997 legislation. The president and congressional leadership have promised them a $246.9 billion restoration of a 21 percent pay cut in Medicare and military health care insurance (TRICARE) fees. In exchange, the physicians' group is willing to support the reform bill, although the rumor among physicians is that AMA leadership will take substantial abuse for their support of the bill at the annual convention in Chicago next year. Some state AMA chapters, such as Florida's, steadfastly oppose the health reform bill.

PhRMA has agreed to support the bill and spent more than $100 million of its own money on ads promoting passage, in exchange for limiting cuts in its drug fees and protecting it from other changes to the Medicare Modernization Act, which it was influential in crafting and passing in 2003. Many industry critics have said the legislation gave too many financially lucrative concessions to the drug industry, and the Democrats have vowed to modify those provisions. But now the White House has cut a deal with PhRMA, and both parties to the deal hope that House Speaker Nancy Pelosi (D-CA) will be able to control the deal's critics, such as Commerce Committee chair Henry Waxman (D-CA) and others as the bill moves through the House, the Senate and the conference committee. To increase their chances of success, drug industry lobbyists have been sticking close to the Speaker. "Most health industry lobbyists, who have increased their contributions in an effort to maintain their access to her, are betting that behind the closed doors of the conference, she will yield to the Senate, which has so far resisted the public option and honored a political deal limiting the drug industry's costs in an overhaul to $80 billion over 10 years" (Kirkpatrick, 2009b).

Years earlier, President Bill Clinton and his wife had begun their ill-fated health reform effort by taking on the drug companies, angering the physicians, and more often than not locking interest-group representatives out of their deliberations and planning. The result was a frontal assault on their bill by most major health industry lobbyists. Their bill never emerged from its first committee vote.

President Obama and his White House staff sought to avoid that set of problems and to instead hew closer to the strategy of an earlier, more successful Democratic president, Lyndon Johnson. His strategy was essentially "buy them off." He gave the hospitals cost-plus reimbursement (the more you spend, the more you get paid) and gave the physicians their own major Part B in the Medicare bill as well as several provisions prohibiting government from interfering with the doctor-patient relationship. He gave the insurance companies the high-volume task of processing Medicare and Medicaid claims for payment, even though the federal government could likely have done this job more cheaply.

President Obama made similar if less grand deals, and then he needed to work to make them stick. Only the health insurance industry was the object of White House scorn. In a short-lived effort to blunt that industry's opposition to inclusion of a public option, the White House accused the industry of putting their interests above those of the nation. But even that industry tried to keep its access options open by making donations to Speaker Pelosi.

Overview

Lobbying, especially lobbying on behalf of health policy, is very big business in Washington, D.C. Those lobbying Congress for healthcare-related causes during 2009 spent more than $3.3 billion on the effort (McGrane, 2009). The drug industry alone set a record by spending more than a quarter million in the single year of 2009 (Seelye, 2010b).

There were 12,220 registered lobbyists in 2011, fewer than in 2007, when the number hit a peak. This probably reflects the shrinking economy and accompanying dwindling corporate revenues. Nonetheless, the 2011 figure works out to nearly 23 lobbyists for every member of Congress (Center for Responsive Politics, 2011b).

Numbers are important, but they don't tell the whole story. Resources—campaign contributions—are the coin of the realm, and many health interests hold many of these coins. Spending by health interests topped all other sectors both in the 1998–2011 period and in 2011 alone (Center for Responsive Politics, 2011e). Although people like to complain about interest groups, they serve a pivotal function in our democratic process. They represent us—for better or worse. The body of theory that describes interest groups and their actions reflects the changes these groups have undergone. Key elements of this theory include how and why interest groups form and why they persist. Interest groups evolved rapidly from close-knit alliances into diverse, large, and powerful players in federal (and state) policymaking. Many groups occupy somewhat narrow "niches" in policy, but they also participate in coalitions that allow them to pool their efforts to effect or deflect broad policy change. Interest groups provide information and campaign support to elected officials and use several strategies to influence policy, including direct lobbying, grassroots organizing, campaign contributions through PACs, and participation in coalitions. Although interest groups spend most of their time attempting to influence Congress, they also recognize the importance of lobbying the executive branch. Interest groups also use the courts, often as a final avenue for action when other means fall short. Interest groups play an important role in both electing members of Congress favorable to their causes and working with these members to enact the policies that the groups desire (and stop the policies they oppose). In sum, the role of interest groups in defining and shaping health care policy is pivotal. Next to Congress, interest groups may well be the most important actors in health policy.

How and Why Interests Organize

Interest groups consist of individuals who have organized themselves around a shared interest and seek to influence public policy. Interest groups include organizations as diverse as the Federation of Behavioral, Psychological, and Cognitive Sciences and the Association of State and Territorial Health Officials, as broad as the American Public Health Association and as narrow as the American Society of Gastrointestinal Endoscopy. They also include corporations and institutional interests such as hospitals, medical schools, HMOs, unions, and schools of public health.

Interest Groups and Policymaking

Lindblom (1980, 85) described interest groups' role in policymaking as "indispensable." These groups clarify and articulate citizens' preferences, warn policymakers of problems with their proposals, and suggest ways to make proposals more palatable or point out why they will damage and enrage a group's membership. Simply put, groups represent the interests of their members and supporters, whether the American Social Health Association or the Association of American Medical Colleges or the nation's Catholic hospitals.

Interest groups also serve to educate their members and others on issues and to help form a feasible public agenda. They monitor activity, public and private, and can blow the whistle on a bad idea when it is proposed. Their job is to make the case for their constituents before government, plying the halls of Congress, the executive branch, the courts, and the offices of other interest groups to provide a linkage between citizens and government. For many decades in the United States, it was political parties that provided this linkage. But in recent years, surveys show that people prefer to have more clearly kindred spirits minding the store for them. The more well-heeled the group, the more likely it is to make its own way rather than turn the job over to a broader group such as a political party. Indeed, sadly for the parties, 2009 was a major turning point in the political influence business: corporations for the first time outspent the parties. Even the U.S. Chamber of Commerce and its national subsidiaries spent more on lobbying than either political party did (the Chamber spent $144.5 million, the Republican Party spent $97.9 million, and the Democratic Party spent $71.6 million) (Ambinder, 2010).

Interest groups are as American as talk shows and much older. James Madison, in Number 10 of the *Federalist Papers*, bemoaned the mischief of "factions," which he defined as "a number of citizens . . . who are united and actuated by some common impulse of passion or of interest" (Publius, [1787–88] 1961, 78). Although Madison put a negative spin on factions by suggesting that their interests might be adverse to the rights of other citizens and to the interests of the community, the right to associate is one of the first defended in the Bill of Rights. A century later, Alexis de Tocqueville, the French visitor to the United States whose uncannily accurate observations still resonate today, observed, "In no country in the world has the principle of association been more successfully used or applied to a greater multitude of objects than in America." He continued, "Wherever, at the head of some new undertaking, you see the government in France, or a man of rank in England, in the United States you will be sure to find an association" (de Tocqueville, [1835] 1956, 95, 198).

Interest-group representation has long been a fact of life in Washington, D.C.—much to the chagrin of many in government. Woodrow Wilson said in 1913 that "Washington was so full of lobbyists that 'a brick couldn't be thrown without hitting one.' " Eighty years later, President Bill Clinton, outlining his economic plan to Congress, noted, "Within minutes of the time I conclude my address to Congress . . . the special interests will be out in force . . . Many have already lined the corridors of power with high-priced lobbyists" (both quoted in Brinkley, 1993, A14). Groups are essential to the American notion of pluralism— groups competing to put items on the agenda or keep them off and to achieve their members' goals in public policies. Ideally, as Madison speculated, groups check one another and come to agree only on the common interest. Madison's ideal has not emerged, however. Groups are not equally endowed, and they fail to provide representation for all. As Schattschneider (1960, 35) put it, the pluralists' "heavenly chorus sings with a strong upper class accent." Poor people, immigrants, ethnic minorities, the uninsured, and in particular, undocumented aliens, are often not as well represented as are middle-class business interests. Nor are all middle-class interests equal. The National Rifle Association (NRA) is a very strong national lobby whose success has never been more than partly checked by antihandgun groups and police associations; in recent years, it seems to have no equal anywhere. Powerful interests such as the AMA have a greater potential to be heard than do organizations of nurse-midwives or health care consumers.

Nor do groups always act in the public interest. Frequently, their contribution to public policymaking is to exercise a veto power over policy changes and innovation. A minority, represented by a strong interest group, can stop or delay legislation or a proposed rule. The system of government is set up that way, to make it hard to change policy: lose one round, live to fight another; move from subcommittee to full committee to house floor; repeat the process in the second house; move to the more informal setting of the conference committee; and, if you still have not succeeded, seek a presidential veto, or try to influence the agency writing the regulations, or sue the agency in federal court for violating the due process clause of the Constitution. "A lot of the best lobbyists are like paid assassins," a spokesperson for the Center for Responsive Politics told the *New York Times* (Abramson, 1998). Ellen Miller, of the same center, commented that PAC money "buys silence[;] hearings are not held or amendments not introduced" (Matlack, Barnes & Cohen, 1990, 1479). Lowi (1964) termed this ability of a strong interest-group minority to ride roughshod over majority interests "interest group liberalism." President Jimmy Carter tried to sound the alarm that it was not good for the republic. Making the growth of special interest organizations the topic of his farewell address, he said, "The national interest is not always the sum of all our single or special interests" (Carter, 1981). He called the growth of these groups a "disturbing factor in American political life."

Those who run these lobby groups do not see it that way. Karen Ignagni, enduring chief executive officer of the American Association of Health Plans and one of the most important lobbyists in Washington, described her organization's efforts as simply doing its job of professional, hard-hitting work on behalf of its membership—people with an important stake in the policy process. "Most people think of trade associations making backroom deals and buttonholing legislators," she told *Washingtonian Magazine*. "That is not the way it is anymore. You run an association with all the vehicles of a political campaign with polling, grassroots organizing, and all the earned media attention you can get. The tired view of associations from the outside is that it is lowest-common-denominator advocacy. The fact is, we are not your father's Oldsmobile anymore" (Eisler, 1999).

How Interest Groups Form and Persist

Analogies help scholars make sense out of complexities. Madison wrote Number 10 of the *Federalist Papers* at a time when educated people thought of the universe as a collection of forces pressing against one another. The point at which these forces were equal, the equilibrium, seemed somehow natural or right. Applied to politics, scholars concluded, this point of equilibrium was the public interest. Political scientist David B. Truman (1951) used the term *equilibrium* in one of the first efforts to describe why interest groups form. Some disruption or disturbance upsets the equilibrium; people then band together to restore equilibrium by exerting countervailing force. Sometimes the formation of one group might lead to a disturbance that upsets another group, which might in turn cause another group to form, until a new social equilibrium is reached. Group formation might stabilize for a while, only to start up again with another disturbance. Although this explanation goes a long way toward explaining the formation of most groups, it does not explain why groups stay together once the threat or event causing the group to form has disappeared or attenuated. It also assumes that during a disturbance, anyone can easily organize those who share that person's interests into a group; far from true.

A second explanation for group formation highlights selective benefits. Olson (1968) offered what can be viewed as a "rational choice" argument: people join groups because they will directly benefit from membership through material rewards such as the ability to serve on the staff of a hospital, to bid on certain construction jobs, or even just to receive discounted travel services or an informative magazine. Selective benefits also help overcome another problem for groups seeking public policy change: the free rider. Why join the Sierra Club when anybody can enjoy the clean water and unspoiled wilderness that the club's policy advocacy has helped produce? One answer is selective benefits: to receive maps, camping tips, and other benefits of membership. Nobody does this better than AARP, the group that in its 2011 annual report claimed 40 million members, over one-fourth of the registered voters in the United States. After paying a low membership fee, anyone age 50 or older qualifies for rental car and hotel discounts, cut-rate prices on drugs, group health insurance, investment programs, and reduced-price car and mobile home insurance.

Other explanations have also been put forward. Clark and Wilson (1961) built on the selective-benefits notion, describing three types of benefits that attract group membership: material benefits (magazines, discounts, tips, etc.); purposive benefits (those associated with ideological or issue-oriented goals without tangible benefits to members); and solidarity or social benefits, which can also include benefits from achieving worthwhile policy goals. Salisbury (1969) offered a market-oriented view. He believed that interest groups are formed by entrepreneurs who invest capital to create benefits that they offer, at a price, to a market of potential customers. In effect, an "exchange" takes place between leaders who provide the incentives and members who provide their support. Exchange theory is useful because it explains not only how groups begin but also how they retain their membership and survive. According to Jack Walker (1991), 80 percent of U.S. interest groups have emerged from preexisting occupational or professional communities. He could have been looking at health groups, where the link to jobs is clear: groups representing health professionals, health providers, and the health industry dominate the field.

Today's interest groups have moved beyond membership fees as the sole source of support. AARP gets substantial resources from insurance and mutual fund companies. The AMA secures about two-thirds of its resources from real estate and business transactions (Ainsworth, 2002).

Interest groups can be launched directly or indirectly by government action. More government equals more groups. Jack Walker (1991) noted that groups are created more as a consequence of legislation than as an impetus for it. Government policies provide new benefits or jobs to people who form groups to protect (and expand) those benefits or jobs. The American Farm Bureau Federation and the U.S. Chamber of Commerce are the two best-known examples of groups started by government agencies. An example in the health sector is the National Association of Community Health Centers. Federal grant dollars helped establish neighborhood health centers across the country, and the centers then formed an association to lobby Congress for more funding. The federal funding agency facilitated the survival of the fledgling group by giving it additional grant money. An example of a lobbying group formed to protect a group's interests was the Tobacco Institute, formed to fight the regulation of cigarettes (Walker, 1991); the American Association of Blood Banks organized to fight a proposal for a national blood system (Tierney, 1987).

Natural gas interests did not have much of a lobbying presence when legislation affecting their industry came up for debate. Provisions hurting them were adopted. They responded quickly, trying to insert their interests into the legislation before it finished its journey through the process: "They just didn't have the right setup as an industry to protect themselves and promote themselves like they should," a natural gas provider CEO told analysts. "And so they pulled together a war chest of something like 80 million bucks, which may be less than what coal's got at their disposal[;] I'm not sure, but it put them in good stead" (to alter Senate proposals before final passage) (Overby, 2009, para. 6).

Ironically, complaints about the power of interest groups can help spawn more. As Democratic lobbyist Tony Podesta put it, "The irony of it is that every time the president says we lobbyists have all this influence, people who don't have a lobbyist want one. He exaggerates our power, but he increases demand for our services" (Lichtblau, 2010b).

Interest groups also seek to protect the status quo. In fact these groups often have the easiest jobs, since those wishing to change policy must mount a major informational and persuasive effort and must deal with uncertainty—a natural enemy of risk-aversive politicians (Baumgartner et al., 2009). An example of lobbying to protect the status quo was the Doctors Hospital at Renaissance in McCallen, Texas. The physician-owned hospital was singled out by President Obama for its inefficiency: too many tests, too many procedures, because physician-owners benefit from both their fees and their stock ownership. The hospital fought back with campaign contributions to both sides of the partisan aisle, but especially to the Democratic chairs controlling key committees and the Democratic Senatorial Campaign Committee, to which it gave nearly a half million dollars at a single reception on March 30, 2009. "These guys who have been raising tons of money for contributions; I am sure that some of my colleagues have been willing to hear them out," commented Rep. Pete Stark (D-CA), a critic of physician-owned hospitals (Sack & Herszenhorn, 2009). Interestingly, instead of "solving" the problems described by the president, the hospital stepped up its campaign contributions.

Economic interests play a big role in interest-group formation and continuation. Health economist Paul Feldstein (1977) noted that health associations pursue policies that allow a monopoly position for their members. This applies whether the group consists of professional members or nonprofit organizations. Feldstein argued that health interest groups will likely support policies that increase the demand for their services, enable them to be reimbursed as price-discriminating monopolists, lower the price of complementary inputs, increase the price of substitutes, or restrict additions to their supply. Simply put, economic interests support policies to help health care providers get more patients, set their own prices, reduce their costs, make their product the best deal, and freeze out the competition.

One example of how economic interests operated in the 2009–10 health reform case relates to a proposed public option, whereby the government would compete with private insurers for clients. The Service Employees International Union strongly felt that the private insurance industry needed competition and supported the public option to require the federal government to offer a health insurance plan of its own, presumably cheaper than industry plans, as a way of forcing the insurance industry to lower its prices. This was classic unwanted competition, in this case from the federal government. The private insurers hated it. They were sure it would eventually steal all their business by selling insurance cheaper than they could. The hospitals and physicians also hated it because it threatened to pay lower prices than private insurance. The measure underwent serious restrictions to make it less of a threat as it went through House and Senate, and as the final vote neared, it seemed to be surviving. But it did not. At the last minute, when Senate majority leader Harry Reid (D-NV) was desperate for a few last votes, independent Connecticut senator Joseph Lieberman demanded that it be dropped as the price of his support, and dropped it was.

Other industry lobbyists are often called upon by their clients to pursue a much more industry-specific legislative goal. One good example comes from the environmental field. Following the running aground of the oil tanker Exxon Valdez off Alaska's pristine coastline in 1989, Congress enacted a trust fund to help pay for future clean-ups and, ideally, some advance preparation for future clean-ups. The program is funded through an eight-cent tax on each barrel of oil produced in this country. But industry lobbyists did not simply roll over and let their firms be taxed without a quid pro quo. The law that created the tax also limits their and the government's liability to $75 million for each spill, a sum exceeded several-fold in the first few days of the BP Gulf Coast spill (Wald, 2010).

Nor was there anything new in this kind of industry-Congress pact. BP's land-lord for the oil rig that collapsed in 2010 sued in court to limit its liability to just over $26 million, the salvage value of the destroyed rig lying at the bottom of the Gulf. The basis for this suit was a congressional act in 1851 that limits the liability of a vessel's owners to the value of the vessel and its cargo. Congress had wanted to promote the U.S. maritime industry in competition with other countries, apparently at the expense of victims whose claims for damage may exceed the value of the sunken vessel and its cargo (Long & Gonzalez, 2010). Physicians have long sought similar limits on liability for medical malpractice, arguing that without it, many physicians will stop practicing.

Nonoccupational Interest Groups

Most interest groups represent occupations and companies, but others are brought together by ideology or a common purpose. PublicCitizen, which bills itself as "promoting health, safety and democracy," is an example. The group lobbies Congress, joins lawsuits against corporations, and also sues government agencies such as the FDA and the EPA (Environmental Protection Agency) when it feels they have failed to act to protect the public. Many such groups are small in both numbers and resources, but they often garner considerable public and media support for their public-interest lobbying. In the past 25 years, more and more of these citizens' groups, with no direct connection to a business or profession, have sprung up in Washington and in the states. One recent study of 98 randomly selected issues before Congress over four years found that citizen groups were the most frequent participant type (Baumgartner et al., 2009). These authors concluded that citizens groups don't have the resources of the more prominent groups but play an important role in policy development, especially in providing information. Poor citizens groups often align themselves with richer business groups and win at about the same rate, according to the authors.

A few well-known citizens' groups target health issues; these groups include Planned Parenthood, the Health Research Group, the National Women's Health Network, and the National Citizens' Coalition for Nursing Home Reform. Another citizens' group—Families USA—was particularly prominent in the 2009–10 health care debate. AARP is the largest—and best-known—of the citizens' groups. Unlike most citizens' groups, AARP is well funded and highly visible. In the 2009–10 reform debate, AARP endorsed the reform plan and then worked hard to promote its passage, boasting to readers of its *AARP Bulletin* that it had

E-mailed 336,757 letters to legislators;

Made 150,000 phone calls to legislators;

Mobilized 1,364,195 AARP members to participate in tele-town hall meetings;

Collected 1,130,000 signatures on petitions to Congress; and

Pulled 130,000 members into in-person town hall meetings. (Rand, 2009, 17)

The AARP also brought local staffers from roughly 15 states to Washington. Their job was to press the case for passing reform, that is, "spreading the gospel with members that they have relationships with," AARP senior vice president David Sloane told a reporter (Frates, 2010). One staffer met with a freshman congressman he knew personally who had initially voted against reform. After the meeting, he became the first of his vulnerable group of Democratic members representing conservative districts to switch his vote to yes.

Although AARP fits Jack Walker's definition of a citizens' group, its role of protecting current and expanding future benefits under Medicare seems to fit the spirit of an occupational or professional group protecting its concentrated interest in regulation (or, in this case, subsidies) and imposing costs over a broad population base.

Much smaller and narrower in their advocacy is the subset of citizens' groups that Foreman (1995) called grassroots victims' organizations, made up of persons who are directly and often suddenly and tragically affected by a health hazard or a disease. Such groups, such as Parentalalert.com, formed by parents of statutory rape victims; or S.T.O.P., an organization supporting victims suffering from long-term consequences of food-borne illness; or the National Autism Association, can achieve limited, targeted policy success. People with cancer, in particular, have from time to time successfully drawn thousands of their peers to march and rally on the Washington Mall and descend on Congress. MADD (Mothers against Drunk Driving) is not exactly a victims' organization, because it includes many with strong moral and ideological views, but it is greatly helped by victims, some of whom are willing to draw upon their tragic experiences to try to influence policy.

One of the most successful grassroots groups is the National Breast Cancer Coalition, which over a 15-year period grew from small groups of women meeting in living rooms across the country to a well-financed, highly organized group with considerable visibility and legislative effectiveness. Casamayou (2001) credits its success to a mixture of strong leadership and extraordinary passion for action—notably, more funding for breast cancer research. Post-traumatic stress disorder (PTSD) groups were by 2010 beginning to resemble the fragmented early days of breast cancer groups and showed the potential to coalesce into an important advocacy force. Although most people might assume that members of PTSD groups are mostly military veterans, many are victims of crime, especially rape. Other PTSD groups support police traumatized by their experiences. They will need strong leadership to marshal their differing yet related advocacy concerns.

Anecdotal evidence suggests that single-issue citizens' groups can eventually succeed in health policy—largely by persistence. The federal requirement that states enact a 0.08 percent blood alcohol level as the standard for drunk driving was passed in 2000, after 16 years of aggressive lobbying by MADD and many earlier defeats under pressure from the restaurant and alcoholic beverage industries. Likewise, citizens' groups succeeded in getting Medicare coverage expanded to include preventive services—again after a very long and persistent effort. Yet, the absence of a well-organized group of near-seniors to push harder for expansion of Medicare to the 55-and-older group probably contributed to deletion of that provision from the health reform bill in the Senate in 2009.

Fragmentation, Coalitions, and Changes in Affiliation

For many years the interest-group world was dominated by "peak associations," umbrella organizations representing large groups of farmers, businesses, or labor unions. In the 1990s, the landscape became much more varied, with the larger organizations still in existence but sharing space with smaller, more focused groups, often splintered off from peak associations. For example, complementing the AMA at the time of the Clinton administration's health care proposal efforts were at least 80 medical specialty groups representing surgeons, pediatricians, emergency room physicians, ophthalmologists, plastic surgeons, and others. Similar diversification occurred in the hospital industry, where the interests of small community hospitals, large nonprofit hospitals, teaching hospitals, and inner-city hospitals differed so substantially that a single organization (the AHA) could not fully represent them all. By the time of the Obama health plan effort, specialty groups and hospital splinter groups made separate demands, gave their own money, and put forward their own lobbyists. What frequently happens is that the larger umbrella organizations must take less specific, more general positions that minimize conflict, while the more specialized, smaller groups are free to adopt more specific positions targeted at their members. Rep. Pete Stark (D-CA), a longtime health advocate, described the situation this way: "I think that the specialty [physician] groups are often more effective because their issues are more focused. The AMA suffers from the same problem the American Hospital Association does. When you try and represent everyone, you basically can't represent anyone" (Carney, 1998).

Sometimes even the Catholic Church has a problem singing from the same page of the hymnal with its Catholic hospitals. In 2009, as Senate leadership struggled desperately to strike a compromise between its prochoice liberals and its anti-abortion conservatives—especially Nebraska Democratic senator Ben Nelson—critical support came from the Catholic Health Association, representing hundreds of Catholic hospitals. The compromise required states to bar public spending for abortion or use only private funds for abortions while prohibiting public funds for that use. The hospitals said the compromise could "achieve the objective of no federal funding for abortion" (Kirkpatrick, 2009c). But on the same day, the United States Conference of Catholic Bishops called the compromise "morally unacceptable." Physicians found themselves similarly split. While the AMA provided critical support for the bill in both Houses, a quarter million medical specialists broke ranks and decisively fought it (Sack, 2009).

Interest-Group Coalitions

The proliferation and fragmentation of interest groups and the rising stakes have made the formation of coalitions especially important. In these coalitions, interest groups can maximize their resources and their lobby strength. They can work to influence a wider array of policies than groups working alone. They can also help with a group's visibility and image. One interest-group lobbyist put it this way: "Coalitions show that we are in good company. They allow other groups to see us as a contributor to the community. Smart people on Capitol Hill frequently think of us as the 'go to' group" (quoted in Heaney, 2004b, 1).

Some coalitions are long-standing; subgroups have worked together over many years and have fought numerous policy battles. Such interest groups can be considered "policy communities," networks of interest groups active in a particular domain or representing similar constituencies. Sometimes these coalitions are well funded and well staffed. An example is the 100-plus-member National Health Council (NHC), founded in 1920 to improve the health of the nation and give priority to people with chronic diseases and disabilities. The NHC encompasses voluntary and professional health societies, patient advocacy groups, national organizations, and business groups with strong health interests. For the 2009–10 health reform it sent letters to members of Congress urging them to follow NHC reform principles, including coverage for all, cost control, elimination of preexisting condition exclusions and annual and lifetime insurance payout caps, and access to long-term care and end-of-life care (NHC, 2010). The legislation that ultimately passed met many of these criteria.

More typical are temporary coalitions, formed to work together on one issue or policy, then disbanded when the issue dies or becomes law. Anticipating the importance of health care reform legislation in the 2008 presidential campaign and subsequent administration, in 2007 a group of 35 U.S. companies formed a coalition to promote a market-based approach to reform and to emphasize personal responsibility for taking preventive steps to improve health. Safeway Inc. CEO Steve Burd stated: "We believe there's a real sense of urgency in solving this problem and we intend to be active participants in this debate" (Pelofsky, 2007, para. 3).

Opponents of competitive bidding for medical equipment and services, such as home health providers, formed the Coalition for Access to Medical Services, Equipment, and Technology (Carey, 2003). Twenty-five state medical societies and a group of rural physicians formed the Geographic Equity in Medicare Coalition to encourage higher payments to rural hospitals (Goldstein, 2003). Coalitions are so important that several congressional leaders have designated staff to assemble and keep in touch with coalitions, and some lobby firms specialize in a brokering service to help assemble coalitions (Birnbaum, 2004).

Sometimes coalitions bring together unusual collaborators. For example, to fight the 2003 drug reimportation bill, PhRMA joined with abortion opponents in a direct-mail campaign that focused on conservative House members. The jointly sponsored material warned that the drug reimportation measure would make the RU-486 abortion pill as "easy to get as aspirin" (Stolberg, 2003).

The consummate example of divergent interests joining was when Families USA (a liberal consumer group) persuaded PhRMA (the drugmakers' coalition) to join them in promoting a three-pronged strategy for health reform in 2009. "Although our views do not always converge, we share a common belief about a fundamental goal of healthcare reform: Every American deserves high-quality, affordable health coverage and care," said PhRMA president and CEO Billy Tauzin and Families USA executive director Ron Pollack (PhRMA, 2009).

Groups are free to join multiple coalitions, and many do. The U.S. Chamber of Commerce is a member of at least 300 coalitions on issues ranging from highway construction to expansion of the nation's visa program (Birnbaum, 2004). Heaney (2004b) identified 231 health coalitions, many of them small. His work focused on 80 coalitions made up of six or more groups. The coalitions ranged from Citizens for Better Medicare and the Coalition for Fair Medicare Payment to the Coalition for Genetic Fairness and the Friends of Indian Health. Heaney found that patient advocacy groups and groups representing medical service providers were most likely to participate in coalitions, and business groups were least likely. But coalition membership is widespread. More than 90 percent of the interest-group representatives interviewed by Heaney reported membership in one of the coalitions in the study.

Sometimes coalitions are useful for helping highly visible groups get support for their preferences from other, more "legitimate" groups. For example, in 1993 the Pharmaceutical Manufacturers' Association (PMA) formed a coalition of citizens' groups and public health advocates that opposed limits on Medicaid spending for prescription drugs. A PMA spokesperson acknowledged that the coalition was formed to give the association more credibility with Congress than if the PMA itself made the apparently self-serving arguments (Pear, 1993). Later the association added *research* to its name to add to its status, becoming PhRMA.

Niche Theory

In contrast to the pluralistic notion of interest groups' competing against one another to reach some type of accommodation, in some interest areas the groups tend to stake out policy domains that are theirs and are recognized as such and accommodated by other groups. A group does this by finding a recognizable identity, defining a highly specific issue niche for itself, and fixing its political endowments (that is, recognition and other resources) within that niche. Groups with special expertise can establish a niche, unthreatened by other interests. Clearly, such a staking out of territory has a practical appeal, since one interest group cannot influence everything. Another important reason for finding a niche is the instability of the policy world. Without the security of friends in Congress and the bureaucracy, and with forces such as citizens' groups, the president, the press, and the decentralization of Congress all exerting their influence, interest groups can attain some sense of security by staking out a policy niche and concentrating their resources there (Browne, 1991). For example, the Association of American Medical Colleges (AAMC) focuses on policies affecting the nation's 136 medical schools. This association has not often ventured into broader health care issues, but it has been perceived as the dominant force in issues related to medical education. Similarly, many patients' organizations focus only on a particular disease or condition, refusing to participate in larger battles such as the health care reform debate.

Niche politics prevail when the issues are narrow and involve few interests. Cigler and Loomis (1991, 392) thought the "bulk of group politics" took place within these policy niches, or policy communities. As long as discrete policies do not cross niche boundaries, these accommodations can continue, even as more and more groups are added. A study of lobbyists and the issues they deal with confirmed this idea. Baumgartner and Leech (2001) found a highly skewed pattern of lobbying when they examined the 1996 Lobbying Disclosure Reports. A few issues involved a very large number of lobbyists (an obvious one was health care reform), but most issues were much lower-key. The top 5 percent of issues accounted for more than 30 percent of the lobbying; in contrast, the bottom 50 percent accounted for only 3.5 percent. In other words, most issues involved few lobbyists. Not surprisingly, business was overrepresented in issues that drew few or no competing interests.

Niche politics can benefit both the interest group and the member of Congress. Both enjoy the benefits of low transaction costs. Interest groups with well-defined niches do not have to explain to legislators which groups they represent and what they stand for—thus they are able to use time with a legislator to pursue policy objectives. Members of Congress benefit for the same reason: they do not have to listen to explanations and descriptions of the group. These saved transaction costs are especially important given that the competition for legislators' time is becoming more and more severe as groups increase in number but members of Congress, of course, do not (Heaney, 2004a).

The ability to deal with one set of negotiators for an industry can also make it possible to broker a quid pro quo between bill drafters and industry representatives. PhRMA played that role with the White House in its dealings with the Obama administration over health care reform. Hoping to ward off limits on generic drug prices and also wanting to block reforms permitting importation of drugs from other countries, PhRMA executives offered $80 million worth of drug price concessions to Medicare. The money would come in the form of rebates to the federal government on the drugs it buys and 50 percent discounts to seniors who fall into the gap in Medicare Part D drug coverage called the "doughnut hole" (Connolly & Shear, 2009).

The deal was welcomed in the White House because it represented a chink in the armor of the health care industry lobby arrayed against reform. When PhRMA decided to deal, it meant other groups had to rush to the table to avoid being left out. The Democratic House leaders were much more skeptical. They greeted news of the PhRMA deal and others that followed with skepticism and threats to ignore them. But the White House made it clear that the president would do his best to encourage Congress to stick by the deals, and in the end, most of the PhRMA deal remained intact when the bills had passed both houses. Drug imports were blocked, and costs of direct-to-consumer advertising remained tax deductible (Ethridge, 2009; Wilson, 2009).

Billy Tauzin, PhRMA CEO and former Republican House Commerce Committee chair, after a White House meeting in August in which he was once again reassured that their deal would stick, said he had been told: "If you come in first, you will have a rock-solid deal . . . They wanted a big player to come in and set the bar for everybody else," Tauzin explained. He said he was told to negotiate with Senate Finance Committee chair Max Baucus and the White House would endorse whatever deal they struck, although Tauzin added that the White House had tracked the negotiations closely. Such a deal could not have been negotiated without the ability of this niche player to speak authoritatively for an entire industry. Similar deals struck with the insurance lobby—a more loosely organized set of players with varying interests, fell apart. "The insurers never made any deal," Tauzin said, meaning that not all of the insurance industry's players had signed on to an agreement reached by some of them (Kirkpatrick, 2009a).

From Iron Triangles to Issue Networks

The dominant political model of interest-group influence for many years was the iron triangle: congressional committees, interest groups, and bureaucrats—the three vertices of the triangle—did all decision making. This triumvirate was so strong that it tended to prevail over all other actors, including the president. Sometimes called subgovernments, policy subsystems, or policy monopolies, these relationships were considered impermeable and lasting. Major decisions, it was said, were made by a few experts who benefited from working closely together. The interest group benefited from close access to decision makers and implementers. The bureaucracy benefited by ensuring adequate appropriations and public support. Congressional staffers benefited by garnering the substantive and political resources of these key actors—making members of Congress look good to other members and to constituents.

President Obama suggested that a variant of this kind of relationship had been allowed to form between the oil industry, Congress, and the bureaucratic agency that was supposed to be overseeing offshore drilling; this suggests that lax bureaucratic oversight may have contributed to the BP Gulf oil spill.

Though intuitively persuasive, the notion of iron triangles proved to be simplistic and generally wrong as U.S. policymaking moved into a world of competing interests, complexity, and tough choices. When congressional power became decentralized, interest groups could not simply work with leaders or with a few committee chairs and a handful of legislators to maximize the likelihood that their positions would prevail. Today's interest-group world is much more complex and less easily defined. In what are called issue networks (Heclo, 1978) or policy subsystems (Stein & Bickers, 1995), policy is shaped by loosely connected interest groups and experts within and outside government, working together on some aspect of public policy. The definition of these entities is somewhat nebulous, because members of issue networks or policy subsystems can have varying degrees of expertise and commitment to the policy and can move in and out of the policy domain. Issue networks are sloppy and unpredictable and very difficult to describe, much less predict or explain. Another aspect of the shift to networks relates to the complexity of such issues as health care policy. Because jurisdiction over health care is widely shared among many congressional committees rather than focused in one or two committees, most interest groups now tend to work with four or five separate committees or agencies and, on some issues, with committees not generally in their purview.

Empirical studies of interest groups have increased our understanding of these entities by charting the acquaintance networks of groups identified as influential in several key policy domains, including health (Heinz et al., 1990; Salisbury et al., 1987). The researchers looked for interest groups that were influential in more than one of several different fields: health, labor, agriculture, and energy. They found none. Had the research been done 30 years earlier, they would have found that the American Federation of Labor–Congress of Industrial Organizations (AFL-CIO) was influential in multiple issue areas, such as health, income, poverty, aging, housing policies, and labor relations. Likewise, for each issue, the researchers found few examples of mediators or facilitators who worked closely with a variety of colleagues concerned with the same issues. Instead, influential people talked with people who agreed with them, based largely on their organizational or client interests. The researchers dubbed this phenomenon a network of interest groups with a "hollow core" or empty center, sans actors who could bridge various aspects of policy. Again, 30 years earlier, they might have found such mediators or coordinators in the form of the Farm Bureau in agriculture and the AMA in health care policy.

In short, the interest-group world has changed. It seems to have swung from a tightly knit, closely coordinated, impervious, and closed world to an atomistic, uncoordinated, and highly permeable one. Nevertheless, it would be misleading to say the iron triangle has completely disappeared from the scene. For some complex, nonsalient issues or those with little opposition, the iron triangle may still prevail. Veterans' policy is heavily dominated by the associations for veterans with disabilities and a few other veterans' groups, a small number of House and Senate committees, and the Department of Veterans Affairs. Few others concern themselves with policy decisions affecting veterans. When veterans' groups decided that Clinton's Veterans Affairs secretary, Togo D. West Jr., had not fought vigorously enough for the agency's budget, their attacks led West to write a memo to the president indicating that he would resign before the end of his term. Meanwhile, he promised the groups he would seek additional funding, sent a plea to the OMB, and braced himself to battle for more money in the coming budget cycle (Becker, 1999). Similarly, at the state level, groups representing people with mental retardation or developmental disabilities often work closely with legislative supporters and agency staff to achieve policy goals that are rarely questioned by other policymakers.

How Interest Groups Influence Decision Making

Lobbying today looks much like a political campaign. Issues are defined through research and polling; public support is garnered through media campaigns and heavy use of the web, often targeted to constituents of key members of Congress; and organization is paramount at the local or grassroots level where the voters reside. Simply knowing the committee chair is not enough (Andres, 2004). It all starts with information.

Information

Information provided by lobbyists may help legislators make (and defend) public policy *and* get reelected. The information may include data on the problem, on the impact of the proposed new policy, and, importantly, on the effects of the new policy on the legislator's constituents. Wright (1996) argues that the NRA's success over the years has flowed from a large membership that presents compelling information to members of Congress about the electoral consequences of their stands on gun control. Wright says of legislators that "to stay apprised of the political situations at home and in Washington, they must frequently turn to others for information and advice. Among those they turn to are organized interests" (199).

More and more interest groups are commissioning research to support their positions. As one lobbyist put it, "Commissioning studies gives us a more persuasive position to argue from" (Stone 1994, 2842). Trying to influence key provisions in the Obama health plan, or defeat it altogether, the health insurance industry commissioned a consulting firm to write a research report showing estimates of rapidly rising health care costs and significant increases in the federal deficit if the bill passed (Seelye, 2009). Oddly, that report—controversial and dubbed by reform advocates as biased and inadequate—was no longer available on the well-known consulting firm's website once health reform had passed.

Nor are ethical rules always a constraint in such efforts. One leading Harvard University researcher's slide presentation promised a drug company that his research would "support the safety and effectiveness" of its drug in young children. Attorneys general in several states sued drug companies for money spent on this type of drug, contending that it was not actually effective, while Sen. Charles Grassley (R-IA), ranking member (and former chair) of the Senate Finance Committee, who has made it a cause célèbre to reveal conflicts of interest between university researchers and drug companies, reported that the faculty member involved had received $1.6 million from the drugmaker between 2000 and 2007 but reported only $200,000 of this income to university officials (Harris, 2009c).

Months later Senator Grassley revealed that physicians at leading medical schools had been putting their names on articles written by drug industry ghost-writers (Singer, 2009d). But that was not the end of the story. By November, a *New York Times* investigation found that several members of Congress were reading speeches on the House and Senate floors that had been ghostwritten for them by the drug industry. Speeches differed only between Republicans and Democrats, with members from the same party giving the same speech (Pear, 2009b).

Interest groups have also found the Internet extremely useful in providing information to policymakers, journalists, and the public. The Internet has dramatically lowered the per-unit distribution costs and has proved a great boon for less wealthy groups, especially those with large constituencies. Groups also use the Internet for mobilizing supporters, fund-raising, and fostering grassroots activism (Bosso & Collins, 2002).

The AMA has been actively engaged in providing information on an issue near and dear to physicians' hearts: malpractice reform. The association has not shied away from strong language, arguing at various times that states are in a full-blown medical liability crisis. In fact, the GAO found mixed evidence in five states that were identified by the AMA as in crisis. Other observers have pointed out that malpractice claims and awards have declined, rather than increased, in several "crisis" states identified by the AMA (Herbert, 2004). But for those seeking change, the task is most difficult. They must be able to answer questions about how the change will make things better. Those supporting the status quo have the information advantage.

Information is most useful in the early stages of consideration of a bill, when members of Congress must get up to speed on the issue and its likely impact on their district. Later in the process things change. "We've long passed informational lobbying; now we're at the break-your-arm lobbying," said Sen. John Breaux (D-LA) late in the 1994 health care reform debate (Seelye, 1994, A10).

Gaining Access

To make use of what they see and learn, lobbyists must meet the most important proximate goal of their profession: gaining access. "The lobbyists are the hired guns, opening doors and gaining access and influence for their clients," says Mary Boyle, the vice president of the government watchdog group Common Cause (Lichtblau, 2010b). A chance to tell their story is essential to most lobbying strategies. To the interest group, access may mean telephone calls and regular meetings with members of Congress and their staff. Sabato (1985, 127) quoted one PAC official as saying, "Frequently all it takes is the opportunity to talk to a legislator 10 or 15 minutes to make your case. He may not have 10 or 1 minute to hear the other side." Wright (1990) found that the number of lobbying contacts was a better predictor of legislators' votes than the amount of campaign contributions.

Asked by a columnist what the SEIU was doing for the bill as it neared its final tests, SEIU president Andrew Stern (one of health reform's strongest supporters) said:

> You can't get through to a congressional office right now. We're on mail, phone, member meetings in the field, letters to the editor. Our top leaders have been on the phones reminding these Congress people, like [Rep. Jason] Altmire, that when they first came into our office because they were running and wanted our support, they said they were running for Congress because they wanted to

fix health care. We're reminding them that they were right then and the time is now. Or [Rep. Bill] Foster, who we ran a significant independent expenditure for, we're telling him what it is our workers thought they were working for him for.

I have never seen our members and our leaders on the phones like this. We had members who worked three to six months on these people's campaigns. They were there when they first ran for office. We've been essential to how they got to where they are. And we're privileged that we get face time with them. (Klein, 2010)

Asked if he was using the threat of supporting a primary opponent in the next election if a member did not support the reform bill, Stern answered: "The last time it was threatened—and it was more hollow then—was NAFTA. But the third rail that's being discussed today is whether if you have two candidates, a Democrat and a Republican who are both representing insurers, whether you'd run a candidate representing reform. That line has never been crossed by major groups like unions. But we're crossing it now" (ibid.).

Access may be as informal as getting together in a coffee shop—especially one across from the White House. The *New York Times* found that Obama White House staffers had met there with lobbyists hundreds of times over 18 months as a way to avoid having the lobbyists listed on the publicly released visitors' log kept at the White House. One lobbyist who had taken part in several such meetings explained that the president's staff members want to "follow the president's guidance on reducing the influence of special interests, and yet they have to do their job and have the best information available to them to make decisions" (Lichtblau, 2010a).

Simply getting legislators, staff, and the media to pay attention to an issue may be the biggest obstacle facing interest groups today (Baumgartner et al., 2009), and it is the area where well-endowed interests are the strongest.

Revolving Door

Lobbyists are paid as skilled professionals, commanding annual salaries of up to a million dollars, and those with the right backgrounds face a seller's market. A Washington headhunter said she could not believe what a hot property a former senior aide at the Health Care Financing Administration (HCFA; now the CMS) turned out to be when he sought a lobbying job: "I felt like I was representing Michael Jordan," the headhunter said. "The demand for knowledgeable people who can track what is going on on Capitol Hill and [in] the government and can figure out the pressure points that companies should be touching in Washington has greatly increased," said another placement-firm spokesperson (both quoted in Abramson, 1998). Former members of Congress or senators—who continue to have lifelong access to the floor of their former house—are in even greater demand, especially if they were respected as members.

And that demand translates to salaries, very high salaries. Many top executives at lobbying groups (trade associations, professional associations, unions, think tanks, and nonprofits such as AARP) representing health and all other interests make well over $1 million per year. The 10th annual salary survey of such groups done by the *National Journal* and its survey partner *CEO Update* showed that for the two years ending in 2009, 89 top executives made more than $1 million. Top earners included PhRMA's Billy Tauzin, who made $4.48 million; Blue Cross Blue Shield CEO Scott Serota, $3.99 million; Chip Kahn, president of the American Federation of Hospitals (for-profit hospitals), $2.33 million; Karen Ignagni, president of American Health Insurance Plans, $2.08 million; Richard Umbedenstock, American Hospital Association president, $2.06 million; and Steven Anderson, CEO of the National Association of Chain Drug Stores, $1.83 million. The highest earner was not in health, however. That was Mark Lackritz, head of the Securities Industry and Financial Markets Association, at $6.76 million, followed by John Castellani, president of the Business Roundtable, who made $5.57 million. Mr. Tauzin was third (Vaida, 2010).

Framing Issues

The form and content of the interest group's message is crucial. Baumgartner and Jones (1993) referred to this as the "policy image," or definition of an issue. There are many examples of health groups' "framing" an issue so that support of the issue is seemingly in the public interest. In a typical example, a PhRMA-funded group called Citizens for the Right to Know argued that the high price of drugs was due to drugstores' overcharging clients rather than any actions the pharmaceutical industry might have undertaken (Ainsworth, 2002).

The framing usually skirts the issue of self-interest and the ways in which groups will benefit from or be harmed by any changes. An example of rather sophisticated framing—targeting different audiences—is provided by the case of a tobacco company that wanted to prevent the Food and Drug Administration from regulating cigarette manufacturing and sales. It organized three groups. Smokers were organized around the theme that the government should stay out of their lives. Small stores were mobilized around the notion that FDA involvement would lead to more taxes and more regulation. More originally, gay rights groups were organized with the message that the FDA's preoccupation with tobacco might distract the agency from approving new drugs for HIV/AIDS (Goldstein, 1999).

Probably the most commonly cited effort at framing (and the most successful) was the adoption of the term *partial birth abortion* to describe a standard late-term abortion procedure. Prochoice advocates were never able to overcome the damage implied by the term. Another success was dubbing inheritance taxes "death taxes." Less successful have been efforts to brand pornography as a public health problem (Perrin, et al., 2008). Lobbyists' efforts to avoid restrictions on texting and cell phone use involved reframing concern over distracted driving to encompass all sources of distraction, in hopes that new laws will not specifically address web-based devices. Lobbyists argued: "Why don't we modernize the education curriculum to teach drivers to deal with all in-vehicle distractions?" Others argued that restrictions on cell phones while driving was an example of excessive governmental intervention in private lives. But reform advocates weren't buying it: "It's the same debate we had a decade ago with respect to distracted driving," said a California Senate advocate of cell phone restrictions. "The number of cell phones increased, the number of minutes increased and the number of deaths on California highways increased" (Richtel, 2010).

During the 2009–10 health care debate, the National Women's Law Center as well as the first lady framed health reform as a women's issue. "A recent study by the National Women's Law Center found that 25-year-old women have been charged up to 84 percent more than their male contemporaries for individual health plans—plans that specifically exclude maternity coverage," the group said in an ad. Their case was helped by Republican senator Jon Kyl (AZ), who asked during a hearing why he should pay for a plan that covered maternity care when he didn't need it (Halloran, 2009).

Media, Message, and Polling

Media and message were important in a recent battle of interests over a tax on sodas and related soft drinks in New York. The Alliance for a Healthier New York, a coalition advocating the tax, spent between $2.5 million and $5 million, while their opponents, characterizing themselves as New Yorkers against Unfair Taxes but funded by the American Beverage Association, spent $9 million in just the beginning months of the campaign (Hartocollis, 2010).

Perhaps the names of the coalitions alone helped defeat the tax, but the media firm hired to develop a strategy went further. "As part of a comprehensive outreach effort, we recruited over 10,000 citizens and 158 businesses to join New Yorkers Against Unfair Taxes," said a spokesman for Goddard Claussen, the media firm that had invented Harry and Louise, the mythical couple that was a major factor in defeating the Clinton health plan in the 1990s. The campaign also noted that the soda tax was regressive, hitting poor people harder than rich people, and that it was a tax on just one source of calories: "If what you want to do is tax calories, why don't you tax all calories? Let's start with those peanut butter cups, or perhaps potato chips, or McDonald's, Krispy Kreme." The tax went quickly and decisively down to defeat. Reviewing their efforts, the public relations firm spokesman commented: "I think, at the end of the day, this was a fair fight." Proponents saw it differently: "We were outgunned," "I think that their marketing was really sophisticated and effective" (Hartocollis, 2010).

The battle over 2010 health reform was more balanced in both media and lobbying spending. Spending by groups favoring and opposing health reform began early in the debate and continued even after the legislation went into effect, totaling $210 million on television advertising. Spenders included insurance companies, drugmakers, unions, hospitals and other providers, both political parties, and many others. The drug industry accounted for $120–$130 million of the total (Seelye, 2010a). PhRMA and other supporters were opposed by the health insurance industry and by the Chamber of Commerce, which also spent heavily and lobbied fiercely, both directly and through grassroots and media buys.

Advocates remembered the success of the Harry and Louise ad series that helped defeat the Clinton health plan. So in 2009, Families USA, a nonprofit advocacy group, hired the two actors who had played Harry and Louise to announce, "We're back." This time their message was in support of the Obama push for health care reform (Singer, 2009c).

Sometimes media ads are targeted primarily to policymakers and other elites, including journalists. One way to do this is through "advertorials," or sponsored messages placed in the media by organized interests to create a favorable environment for their group or their issue. Brown and Waltzer (2002) classified advertorials into three types: image advertorials, designed to create a favorable view; advocacy advertorials, which explain the group's views on controversial issues; and journalism advertorials, which target the press. Journalists are important to interest groups, not only to help frame an issue in the way desired by the group but also for "priming," or helping to characterize an issue in a positive (or negative) way. In advertorials targeted to journalists, the group may also hope to get on the journalists' lists of sources to call on for comment in stories relating to the group's interests.

Another approach is to target ads to the constituencies of key members of Congress. In the 2009–10 health care debate, the big-spending markets for health care reform advocacy ads were the hometowns of Senate majority leader Harry Reid (D-NV) and of several other members of the Senate Finance Committee (Pershing, 2009a).

Polls and focus groups are also part of this comprehensive lobbying approach. President Obama made extensive use of polls to shape his messages supporting health reform, even to the point of using specific phrases that had polled well. "I mean, I'm looking at polling, like, all the time," one top White House adviser told the *Washington Post.* "Our job isn't to tell him what to do. Our job is to help him figure out if he can strengthen his message and persuade more people to his side," the president's chief pollster explained (Shear, 2009).

The Party–Interest Group Connection

Some interests are more comfortable with one party than the other, or with one subgroup of one of the parties. Health interests traditionally give more to Republicans than Democrats. But they are not stupid. With health reform on the agenda, and Democrats in charge of the White House and Congress, the health industry for the first time in many years gave more heavily to Democrats than Republicans following the 2008 election and the run-up to health reform (Mayer, Beckel & Kiersh, 2009). But the Democrats to whom health interests gave most heavily were a particular subgroup whose views were likely to quite closely parallel those of the health industry, especially health insurance interests. "The Blue Dogs are carrying water for the industry instead of their constituents," charged the campaign manager of a liberal reform-supporting group. While conservative Democrats known as Blue Dogs rejected that characterization of their legislative motives, they did not deny that their views and those of the health interests overlapped, justifying the roughly 25 percent more contributions received by Blue Dogs than by other Democrats. "The idea behind giving to a group like the Blue Dogs is that you believe that they will agree with your positions most of the time," countered Charles W. Stenholm, a former Texas congressional representative and a founder of the Blue Dog group (Eggen, 2009).

Labor unions were on the other side of that equation. Unions gave about 25 percent more to members who voted for the health reform bills, almost all Democrats, than they gave to those who voted against the bills, almost all Republicans.

Similar patterns of support could be seen on both sides of the abortion debate: prolife groups gave to their supporters (Republicans and many Blue Dog Democrats), and prochoice groups gave to Democrats who voted against new restrictions on abortion access and financing (Beckel, 2009).

But money likes to follow power. As the 2010 midterm elections neared, so did the partisan tide of campaign-giving corporations. In 2009, Democrats received 61 percent of health PAC giving, but in the first quarter of 2010, health interests split their giving equally between the two major parties (Farnam & Leonnig, 2010). Their bets on Republicans proved accurate as the House majority switched to the GOP and the Senate Democratic margin narrowed after the 2010 election.

Direct Lobbying

The old adage "It's whom you know" has traditionally been very important in the lobbying business. Lobbyists rely heavily on legislative "friends" or advocates and spend much of their time trying to retain or increase the intensity of legislators' commitment to an established, favored position. Groups also target committee and subcommittee members, chairs, and party leaders, because they set the agenda and provide policy cues to other members (Hojnacki & Kimball, 1998). The point is to convert these supporters of a group's interests into advocates who will then persuade other members of Congress of the value of the group's position. However, lobbyists sometimes must cast their legislative nets wider than the already converted and spend at least some of their time on uncommitted members, or fence sitters. In close votes, they can make the difference between success and failure (Hall, 1996). Of course, most policy conflicts do not become close floor votes. Instead they are resolved in subcommittee or committee markup sessions or informally. In these settings, legislators friendly to the interest groups receive most of the lobbyists' attention as they mutually support one another's efforts in pressing an issue important to them.

Groups without paying members seem to prefer to hire external lobbyists, in part because lobbying may be backed by corporate or union treasuries rather than personal contributions to PACs. Spending on lobbying is less regulated than campaign or other PAC contributions. The 1995 Lobbying Registration Act required groups that spend more than $20,000 on lobbying to report their expenditures. But there is no limit on the amount a group can spend.

Although President Obama railed against lobbyists for slowing down congressional progress on health reform, the truth was that lobbying efforts by industry and other groups was as likely to favor health reform as oppose it. Spending by groups in favor of reform totaled $99.5 million in 2009, while groups that wanted to stop reform spent $85 million, according to tallies by the Center for Responsive Politics. The drug industry alone spent $26 million on lobbying and grassroots efforts supporting reform in 2009 (and more on other health issues) (Seelye, 2010a).

Special-interest provisions characterized the Obama health reform effort as it emerged from the Senate, reflecting deals that included promises of lobbying and advertising on behalf of the reform bills. PhRMA, of course, preserved its tax deduction for direct-to-consumer advertising, thought by critics to encourage the use of newer, more expensive drugs that are often no more effective than existing, cheaper drugs. Both PhRMA and media interests fought to fend off a proposal to prohibit deductions for advertising during a new drug's first three years (Wilson, 2009), and drug reimportation was again blocked in accordance with the PhRMA–White House deal (Ethridge, 2009).

A proposed 5 percent tax on cosmetic surgery dubbed the "Botax" roiled plastic surgeons. Once mobilized, the 7,000-member group sought to quickly dispel what they regarded as a misperception that likely led to the plan to make their industry the source of $5.8 billion over a decade. The group argued that cosmetic surgery patients, contrary to popular opinion, are not rich. They claimed that nearly two-thirds of such patients earn only $90,000 per year or less (Mckinley, 2009). The surgeons had an alternative money source in mind: tax tanning salons instead. And Congress obliged. "We suggested that the tanning tax would be a better alternative to the cosmetic tax and hopefully will reduce the incidence of skin cancer down the road" (Martinez, 2009).

Sealing the Deal

Lobbyists can and do participate in the legislative process at all levels: in encouraging introduction of a bill and in helping to shape the language of that bill through committee and house votes. But even if a lobbyist is unsuccessful in one or both houses, the effort continues in conference committee and finally in lobbying the White House and the executive branch during the writing of rules or other implementation-related issues.

Lobbyists are frequently present at strategy sessions with House and Senate party leaders, determining the best way to achieve mutually desired goals as the bill moves through the legislative process. While this generally benefits both legislators and interest groups, sometimes it can backfire. Heaney (2004a) reported one such instance: in 2003, the American Society of Clinical Oncology (ASCO) was allowed to negotiate directly with members of a conference committee over reform of average wholesale prices for oral cancer drugs. During the negotiations, the ASCO sent out a grassroots e-mail alert urging opposition to the direction in which the conference committee was headed (a direction not known to others outside the conference room). When a congressional staffer received the group's e-mail, he alerted Rep. Nancy Johnson (R-CT), who terminated the negotiation with the group.

Members of Congress must balance the desires of interest groups with those of their own constituents. After all, they want to keep their seats, to continue being reelected. Some political scientists have examined how members of Congress can maintain their popularity with constituents while at the same time keeping interest groups happy—often with policies that are not in the broad public interest. Lohmann (1998) argued that legislators can benefit more from catering to a well-informed minority (interest groups) than to an ill-informed majority (including their own constituents). They benefit because their constituents are generally not well versed in the policy choices of members of Congress, whereas interest groups are better equipped to monitor an incumbent's activities. Lohmann thus concluded that public policy is biased toward special interests because of an information asymmetry between the general public and those interests.

Day to day, good lobbyists work with key officials in the executive branch as well as Congress, but they focus more of their attention—and often rack up more successes—on Capitol Hill than elsewhere in Washington. Former AHA president John McMahon put it this way: "Congress has a greater understanding and more sympathy with our problems" (Iglehart, 1977, 1527). The understanding stems, in no small measure, from the important role of hospitals in the economies of local communities; the standing of hospital administrators, boards, and staffs in the legislator's district; and the likely campaign support derived from hospitals and their employees. Probably the most effective lobbyists are hometown folks directly lobbying their representatives in person. A senator from Utah, say, may not make time to meet with a lobbyist from a large conglomerate or interest group but will agree to see the manager of a company branch located in Utah or a delegation of local physicians. "We have a hospital in every district in the country, and in many communities we're the single largest employer. The grass roots and the ground game is always the most important thing in terms of influencing and interacting with legislators," the vice president of the American Hospital Association told the *Washington Post* (Eggen, 2010b).

Yet in 2009–10, relationships changed slightly. Hospitals still wielded important influence in Congress, but the Obama strategy of cutting deals up front with key interest groups made the White House actually the more important player in deal-making. The president himself, and particularly his chief of staff Rahm Emanuel, dealt with any important health industry group that was willing to deal, and those who could act decisively got commitments to make the deals stick as the legislation went through Congress. The insurance industry couldn't get unity among its interests and became the enemy of the White House. PhRMA came in first, made a firm offer of lobbying help, advertising, and broad support in exchange for protections, and the hospitals cut a deal to bear $155 billion in payment cuts over the coming decade, $45 billion less than the president had sought at the outset of negotiation (Eggen, 2010b).

Hospitals, joined by the American Medical Association, also worked hard to defeat a favored proposal of President Obama: he wanted to expand Medicare by allowing people over age 54 to buy into the Medicare program—a longtime Democratic Party ideal. But hospitals and physicians feared they would lose revenue because some members of that age group already had private insurance and would now become lower-paying Medicare patients (A. Goldstein, 2009). At such times, the $2 million that the hospital lobby had given to primarily Democratic candidates during the previous election became important in helping them gain access to key members and make their case against the proposal (Eggen, 2010b). Their key point was that rural hospitals especially would be badly hurt by the anticipated loss of revenue due to a switch of some near-elderly patients from private payment to Medicare. Rural hospitals are a particularly important constituency group for the members of the Blue Dog coalition in the House. The Medicare expansion proposal died after barely a week of discussion.

Sometimes lobbying means cutting deals that seem to have little to do with the legislation actually pending. The 1997 Balanced Budget Act cut $115 billion in Medicare provider payments over five years. Unlike other health care providers, physicians suffered few major cuts. It soon emerged that in the early 1997 debates, an AMA official had sent Speaker Newt Gingrich a letter asking that physicians be spared from disproportionate cuts. The day the letter was written, the AMA announced it would support the Partial-Birth Abortion Ban Act, a bill banning late-term abortions that was strongly supported by many Republicans. While AMA officials denied any "deal," many physicians, Democrats, and fellow lobbyists were not convinced, particularly since the AMA did not discuss its pending position with the leading specialty group of obstetricians and gynecologists, and the position seemed to run counter to the AMA's own policy that lawmakers should not dictate specific medical procedures (Carney, 1998).

Of course the deals lobbyists make can sometimes be canceled by other actors in the political drama. This was the case for PhRMA, which greatly feared that its deal cut with the president and the Senate in August 2009 would not survive the often changing policies and controversies facing the measure that fall. "The White House is not necessarily in coordination with the Senate and the House, so it's confusing and now it's a bit of a crapshoot," said pharmaceutical expert Peter Pitts at the Center for Medicine in the Public Interest (Thomaselli, 2010, 2).

Republicans, especially former presidential candidate John McCain (R-AZ), were strongly opposed to the PhRMA deal and singled it out as "particularly egregious" (Thomaselli, 2010, 4). Yet in the end, with pressure from the White House and some key supporters in both houses, the PhRMA deal did indeed stick: "Now, the health care bill is law . . . the final bill is essentially a complete tactical victory for PhRMA. In other words, what looked like a potentially crushing setback has become an amazing victory" (McCaughan, 2010).

Lobbyists also buttonhole congressional staffers. It gives them someone to work on when the legislator is too busy, but they also recognize the reality that staffers make many of the decisions on specific issues of concern to interest groups. Groups often sponsor staff seminars in exclusive resorts, where lobbyists have a chance to fully discuss issues of common interest.

Even the White House chef is not immune to lobbyists' attention. After decades of bitter, implacable, uncompromising opposition to health reform, the National Restaurant Association decided to take a more positive approach in 2009, focusing in particular on the new nutritional rules to be included in the reform legislation: "What we are trying to do is see how we can be at the table. If you are not at the table, you are on the menu," Sweeny said. Rather than go Christmas shopping, the group's lobbyist visited the White House and spoke to the Obama family chef on December 22—the evening before the crucial House health reform bill vote. Employing her "mitigation and damage control" strategy, she told Chef Sam Kass that her association "should play a leading role" in details of the nutrition bill as well as First Lady Michelle Obama's campaign against childhood obesity (Hamburger, 2010). Shortly afterward, Ms. Sweeny's group was one of 13 trade associations asked to meet with Obama health czar Nancy-Ann Deparle to lay out conditions under which they could support the reform bill. When the law passed, it exempted mom-and-pop operations; contained no tax on the industry's high-profit item, soft drinks; and gave more time for reporting compliance than initially planned. Sweeney's visit to the chef seemed to have left her industry with a good taste in its mouth.

Lobbying the Executive Branch

The president isn't the only executive-branch official who is the focus of lobbyists' attention. Interest groups may lobby for specific changes in rules and regulations or to influence the appointment of an agency head. While access is as important in executive-branch lobbying as it is in lobbying Congress, contributions to assist that access are illegal. Therefore interest groups rely heavily on knowledge of public policies, solutions, and processes. The issues are often more technical and narrower than those dealt with by Congress. But they are no less important. A large majority of interest groups consider their lobbying efforts with agencies at least as important as lobbying Congress (Kerwin, 2003). However, in sheer numbers, congressional lobbying still dominates. In one count of lobby efforts over a six-month period, interest groups, on average, lobbied on 11.1 issues per group in Congress and 1.4 issues in the executive branch (Furlong, 2005). But economic organizations representing businesses and corporations are much more likely to lobby the executive branch than are public interest groups—which makes sense given the rather technical nature of executive-branch deliberation.

Furlong (2005) provides examples of the types of issues subject to lobbying in the executive branch: Medicare reimbursement for pathogen-inactivated blood, FDA-produced guidance documents for the reprocessing of medical devices, and Medicare/Medicaid reimbursement for treatment of obesity-related health conditions. In each case, it is easy to discern a particular group's interest and how the decision might affect the profitability of its enterprise.

To get their point across, interest groups can provide written comments on proposed rules, attend and participate in public hearings, contact agency officials, serve on advisory committees, or petition for rulemaking. They can also use a variety of electronic mechanisms to communicate, including e-mail, website posting, blogs, tweets, Facebook, bulletin boards, chat rooms, and interviews with the media.

Health insurance companies moved to trying to shape the rules interpreting how the 2009–10 health reform would affect them, immediately after its passage. "The health insurance industry has shifted its focus from opposing health reform to influencing how the new law will be implemented," said Sen. John D. Rockefeller IV (D-WVA), a strong reform advocate. Two provisions, of more than 40 in the law directing agencies to write rules, call for consumers to "get value for their dollars." These bar unreasonable premium increases and require companies to meet minimum loss (payout) rates. In response to the latter, "insurers are lobbying for a broad definition of quality improvement activities that would allow them to count spending on health information technology, nurse hot lines and efforts to prevent fraud," reported the *New York Times* health expert Robert Pear (2010a).

Other interests immediately began lobbying for a long list of issues, according to the Kaiser Family Foundation's Kaiserhealthnews.org (Appleby, Carey & Galewitz, 2010):

- The National Federation of Independent Business (NFIB) wanted to maximize tax credits as well as flexibility in "grandfathering" in certain exceptions from the new law;
- AARP was watching closely to see how rules were written concerning closing the "donut hole" in Medicare drug coverage;
- The American Nurses Association wanted to be sure nurses were broadly recognized as health care providers;
- Families USA (joining with providers, insurers, and others providing health care services) wanted to see the law result in broad health insurance coverage under Medicaid or subsidized insurance;
- The National Governors Association (NGA) wanted states to have as much flexibility as possible to experiment with high-risk pools;
- America's Health Insurance Plans (AHIP) wanted a broad definition of spending for health care;
- The American Hospital Association wanted to be in on how states set up and managed health insurance exchanges that would eventually negotiate with the hospitals over payment rates; and
- The American Medical Association wanted to be sure that Medicare cuts didn't cut physician pay.

Interest groups often form coalitions to fight regulations, much as they do to fight legislation. When the Occupational Safety and Health Administration (OSHA) was drafting indoor air quality standards for a proposed ban on smoking in most work areas, the ADA, the NFIB, and the National Restaurant Association formed a coalition to fight ventilation-system requirements (Stone, 1994). In one study of approaches used by interest groups to influence rulemaking, more than 60 percent of the groups reported that they very frequently or always formed coalitions. Other mechanisms used very frequently or always were written comments (77%), informal contact with agency staff (55%), and mobilization of grassroots support (46%) (Kerwin, 2003).

Another strategy involves appointing a commission as a stop-gap measure to avoid unfavorable legislation. When an interest group sees no chance of defeating a proposed reform, a last resort is often to request a delay in final action while a commission, a task force, or a committee is established to study the issue and report back to Congress. With deft lobbying, the industry can then influence the commission to come to conclusions and recommendations that dull the reform effort. Or, if the industry is very fortunate, the commission drags on and eventually produces a weak report, and zeal for reform is lost because reformers have moved on to other topics.

A case in point is table salt. Reformers, including First Lady Michelle Obama, New York City mayor Michael R. Bloomberg, the Institute of Medicine, and (perennially) the U.S. Centers for Disease Control and Prevention (CDC), argue that salt consumption leads to 150,000 premature deaths per year, largely due to heart and circulatory system disease. They advocate restrictions on salt content of processed foods, the major source of salt in the American diet. Salt is a key ingredient because it hides bitterness and other bad tastes endemic to processed foods, according to experts. Indeed, experts have been arguing since the 1970s that salt consumption should be radically reduced. The industry's response has been "delay and divert," according to *New York Times* interviews. That is, over the years it has employed a variety of arguments and strategies to put off the day of reckoning, arguing initially—much like Big Tobacco—that its product did not cause harm. Then the industry suggested that food companies could not produce acceptable flavors without substantial quantities of salt, and finally it claimed that consumers were addicted to salt and could not be denied it. Meanwhile, the *New York Times* revealed that the salt industry had nominated a majority of the members of a U.S. Agriculture Department committee studying the issue and had provided the committee with industry-sponsored research showing that "the country could save billions of dollars more in health care and lost productivity costs by simply nudging Americans to eat a little less food, rather than less salty food" (Moss, 2010).

But even without such a full-court press, lobbyists are often happy to play in the smaller, more predictable arena of the federal agency instead of Congress. In one sense, lobbying midlevel personnel in the executive branch is easier than lobbying Congress: agency staff tend to be much more stable, and long-term relationships can be developed more easily with these staffers than with the more highly mobile congressional staff. It is also easier to get an appointment. And lobbyists carry a big stick not very well hidden under a thin veneer of deference and conviviality in their dealings with bureaucrats. That is, when they are not able to sway an agency, lobbyists often go back to Congress and get the elected officials to remind the civil servants who's really in charge. For example, Congress sided against HHS and with the United Network for Organ Sharing—a group of regional private, nonprofit organizations that harvest and allocate human organs—in passing legislation that blocked the much-delayed HHS rules intended to alter the criteria for determining who receives organs.

Agency staffers know that lobbyists possess access-to-power weapons, and they are loath to simply ignore lobbyists' requests. Staffers may choose to resist and carry the fight forward, but they are likely to make a careful job of it when they know their administrative and political bosses are going to hear the other side of the story from lobbyists, often with very little opportunity to present the agency perspective before members of Congress call the secretary and blast him with anger or hold a press conference and denounce the agency's abuse of power.

Appealing to the Courts

When all else fails, interest groups can turn to the courts. Litigation can be a powerful tool for influencing policy. Though often an expensive route for achieving change, it may be the last resort for a group unable to get satisfaction through the legislative and executive branches. As Berry (1984, 197) noted, "When an industry's profits are liable to be significantly reduced by a government policy, it becomes worth the cost of litigation for a trade association to challenge the policy in court." Berry also made the case that interest groups use the courts when they think the lack of popular support for an issue makes lobbying Congress or the executive branch fruitless. Interest groups can delay the implementation of a policy in the courts, sometimes hoping that, during the delay, changes in Congress or the administration will result in a more sympathetic body.

Interest groups can also go to court to prevent state actions that may harm their business and may spread to other states if not stopped. PhRMA has challenged state laws in Vermont, Maine, and Michigan that, according to the group, would violate the federal Medicaid statute and jeopardize the quality of health care that Medicaid patients need and deserve (PhRMA, 2004). These state laws called for manufacturers' "rebates" as a means to control rising drug costs for Medicaid—which might be viewed as threatening to drug companies' profits. PhRMA noted on its web page that "as part of its advocacy on behalf of the millions of patients that the pharmaceutical industry serves, PhRMA occasionally, and reluctantly, determines that an issue can be resolved only through the courts" (ibid.). Ironically, when this type of approach failed in several important cases against various states, PhRMA went back to Congress and got what it wanted. The MMA of 2003 took Medicaid drug purchasing away from the states and placed it in the hands of small area-specific pharmacy benefit managers— considerably more attractive negotiating partners for PhRMA than the states had proved to be.

Sometimes interest groups use litigation as a way to force administrative action, hoping that federal agencies will settle out of court rather than risk uncertain court decisions. Groups representing people with disabilities have been especially successful in these out-of-court settlements. For example, Vietnam War veterans and chemical manufacturers that produced Agent Orange, a suspected carcinogen, settled a massive class-action suit out of court in 1984.

Interest groups choose (or avoid) the judicial route based on their political standing in the electoral process, the extent to which the group can frame its interests in terms of rights, and the demographic characteristics of the group's membership. Traditionally, groups turn to the courts if (1) they are politically disadvantaged or (2) they have organizational resources such as a full-time staff, attorneys, the money to pay the legal costs, and organizational networks closely coordinated with affiliated groups or other interest groups. The AMA fits the second definition. It has its own Litigation Center, which actively brings cases against hospitals, managed care companies, and federal and state governments (Lovern, 2002). Groups that are often in conflict are more likely to use the judicial remedy than groups that engender no conflict. Interest groups are also more likely to use the courts when their areas of interest coincide with issues over which courts have clear jurisdiction (Walker, 1991).

Finally, interest groups sometimes work with executive-branch agencies to bring "friendly" suits. For example, the American Lung Association initiated a lawsuit against the Environmental Protection Agency, seeking to force the agency to review and tighten its air quality standards because of the effect of polluted air on people with asthma. The suit was friendly because the agency welcomed judicial confirmation of its ability to revisit existing standards (Wood, 1999).

Health groups spend less time pursuing their goals in federal courts than do civil liberties groups, but they do pursue this route on occasion. One reason for health groups to sue is to delay the implementation of regulations, a mechanism noted above. Starr (1982, 407) called this the "little known law of nature [that] seems to require that every move toward regulation be followed by an opposite move toward litigation." For example, the Association of American Physicians and Surgeons sued over the constitutionality of professional standards review organizations (PSROs). The AMA sued when the proposed utilization review regulations were issued, and it sued again to block the health-planning law from being implemented. And the AAMC sued over regulations imposed on medical schools.

Lawsuits have not generally been lobbyists' preferred strategy, but a recent development may change that in some situations: Corporations have begun pouring substantial sums into the election of state court judges. Recent judicial elections have toppled spending records in most states, and most judges are elected at least once, often more frequently, in almost all states. "State judicial elections have been transformed," presenting "a grave and growing challenge to the impartiality of our nation's courts," according to a nonprofit report documenting the growth of campaign spending in judicial elections (Mosk, 2010, para. 5).

Grassroots Lobbying

Interest groups recognize the importance of using their own members as constituent-lobbyists. Members of Congress value their constituents' views and weight them heavily in making their decisions. How better to influence a legislator's vote than by sending your message through her constituents? Although it seems only recently to have hit the big time, the grassroots strategy has been employed for decades. Skocpol (1992) told of the successful effort of the National Congress of Mothers in 1920 to write letters, visit members of Congress, and get publicity in local papers in support of a federal program to promote maternal health education (the Sheppard-Towner bill). To assist the women in their effort, the official National Congress of Mothers magazine included blank petitions on its last page.

Grassroots lobbying is important to legislators because it provides information about the preferences of their constituents; it is important to groups because it builds a coalition of support among their members (Hojnacki & Kimball, 1999). With the Internet, Facebook, blogs, tweets, and cell phones, reaching and organizing the grass roots have become an increasingly important part of lobbying efforts and one primarily orchestrated by lobbyists. Part of its importance is in persuading legislators that an issue "is really a constituent issue," said one lobbyist (Fritsch, 1995). There was little doubt that constituents cared when a group calling itself FreedomWorks organized a series of enthusiastic, even rowdy, protests against health reform throughout the reform debate, especially in the summer of 2009. By disrupting town meetings and other hometown congressional events, the group frightened many members of Congress and helped defeat one incumbent senator in a special election. Dick Armey, a former House majority leader and head of FreedomWorks, defended the group's actions: "The widespread protests over health-care reform could not happen unless people were 'truly scared.' This is a real grass-roots uprising that is to some extent helped by FreedomWorks, but it would be there without FreedomWorks. It's what they call in the cyber world 'viral'" (Eggen & Rucker, 2009).

In health care, grassroots campaigns are carried out both by the highly placed and well endowed and by the most narrowly focused and sparsely financed groups. The AMA has long been a master of grassroots campaigning. But the American Academy of Anesthesiologist Assistants (AAAA) also gets into the act. The AAAA devotes much of its web-page presence to how to do grassroots lobbying, along with materials to support it, such as "how to communicate effectively with your Senators and Representatives" on such topics as "Medicare's Sustainable Growth Rate" and "Rural Pass Through" (Grassroots Lobbying / AA Advocacy, n.d.).

The American Chiropractic Association (ACA) makes a similar pitch to its members and others sympathetic to its concerns. "We have plenty of very good lobbyists who come with statistics and charts. Don't do that. Tell stories about what your constituents are getting from you and your services. Facts tell, but stories sell" (Begala, 2009).

As the abortion debate heated up during the 2010 reform debate, the National Right to Life Committee (NRLC) called for an "eLobby, seeking 250,000 emails to Congress" as well as urging friends to join the effort through "personal contacts, email, blogs, social networking sites like Facebook and Twitter" (National Right to Life Press Releases, n.d.).

Although grassroots efforts are popular, there is some sentiment that they have been overused. If the effort is clearly programmed, with every postcard, e-mail, and phone call making identical pleas, the recipient may discount it. Former senator Lloyd Bentsen (D-TX) once derogatorily called an effort more "astroturf" than grassroots when, as chair of the Senate Finance Committee, he received reams of programmed responses (Toner, 1994). One user of these strategies countered, "Some members of Congress probably would like people to write letters only with quill pens and parchment by candlelight, but that's not the world we live in . . . Having worked on the Hill for many members, you certainly know when you get calls and letters that are part of an effort; it's very obvious. But the bottom line is you count them and they certainly are an expression of opinion by a voter . . . No one is being forced to do this, to pick up the telephone and dial" (Marcus, 1998). Astroturf was alive and well in the 2009–10 reform debate, but it backfired when a public relations firm wrote fake letters from real groups in support of the oil industry's agenda (Smith, 2009b).

The Electoral Link

Interest groups attempt to influence public policy choices (legislative influence) and to help determine who is elected (electoral influence). The two roles are closely linked. One key linkage is interest groups' ratings of members of Congress on a selected range of issues. Many groups determine their electoral endorsements—and campaign support—based on legislators' support of issues of concern to the group. For example, the National Federation of Independent Business polls its members to determine their top priorities before each session of Congress and sends the results to congressional offices. Just before a vote on one of these issues, the group sends a special green-edged postcard to legislators warning them that the upcoming vote will be part of the NFIB's next report card. Every legislator who votes with the NFIB's issues at least 70 percent of the time receives a small pewter trophy, inscribed with the words "Guardian of Small Business." More importantly for members of Congress, the 70 percent rating assures the NFIB's endorsement and campaign contributions.

The National Rifle Association is almost ruthless in its use of elections to target members of Congress who do not vote its way and, more recently, in demanding changes to virtually any bill, to add gun-favoring provisions. Before 2010, the NRA was narrowly focused on gun rights laws. But in 2010 the Supreme Court ruled that the Second Amendment is an individual right and subsequently ruled that the amendment's prohibitions apply to the states as well as the federal government. With that victory, the NRA found itself freed from having to fight its existential battle; it could roam freely in search of other opportunities to influence public policy in ways favoring gun ownership.

In the 2010 health reform law, the NRA demanded that Senate majority leader Harry Reid (D-NV) insert a provision prohibiting insurance companies from charging higher premiums to gun-owning homes. (Reid, whose staff said that he had long been a gun rights champion, was likely more than happy to accommodate a group quite important to his contested 2010 reelection.) The NRA also demanded a tailored exemption from a new law requiring disclosure of donors to lobbying organizations—and got it. A law reforming credit card rules was given a provision freeing people visiting national parks to pack weapons. In the same gluttony of power-wielding, the NRA caused the death of a bill that would have given Washington, D.C., a voting member of Congress instead of the non-voting representative the district has always had. The D.C. voting rights bill was deemed certain to pass until the NRA added a provision pulling the teeth of local gun laws, causing even the bill's sponsors to abandon it.

Members of Congress are keenly aware that in 2010 the NRA budget to influence elections, legislation, and rule making was $307 million; they are even more keenly aware of its membership—4 million gun owners—and the NRA's celebrated ability to mobilize them. "A lot of members are just afraid of the NRA," said one Democratic congresswoman (Nelson, 2000).

An example of the importance of elections to lobbyists relates to the OSHA proposal at the end of the Clinton administration to reduce the risk of worker injury. Business groups thought they could repeal the rules under a George W. Bush administration and so actively raised money to this end. They were right. The rules were repealed in 2001 (Baumgartner et al., 2009).

It is important to keep in mind that members of Congress are not passive recipients of lobbyists' tricks and entreaties. In fact, legislators are actively engaged in seeking funds from lobbyists and more. Apart from PAC contributions, legislators often expect contributions from lobbyists' personal funds, and members are aware that they or their friends may want to someday become lobbyists themselves.

Fueling the Election Engine

Health interests' contributions to congressional elections increased more than threefold between 1998 and 2010 (Center for Responsive Politics, 2010d). A majority of the money over that time went to Republicans, although times like the 2008–9 period saw the giving even out more.

Ranked by sectors, congressional contributions by health entities are always near the top across all industry groups. They ranked first for the 13 years 1998 through 2011 and first also for 2011 alone. Within the category of health-sector givers, members of the health professions are always generous givers, ranking third among health-sector contributors in 2010 (Center for Responsive Politics, 2011c).

Two of the largest associations representing health providers, the AMA and the ADA, were among the top 20 contributors among health associations in each of the eight congressional sessions between 1990 and 2008. Also steady contributors were the American Nurses Association, the American Academy of Ophthalmology (AAO), and the American Optometric Association (AOA), which were among the top 20 health-related contributors for seven of the eight periods. The only time they were not in the top 20 was in 2002–3, when 11 of the top spots were taken by pharmaceutical companies.

Political Action Committees (PACs)

Contributions from an interest group come from its political action committee—the campaign-funding arm of an organization or group. The first PAC was established in 1944 by a union, the Congress of Industrial Organizations (CIO), to raise money for the reelection of President Franklin D. Roosevelt (Center for Responsive Politics, 2005). Until the mid-1970s, members of Congress got about two-thirds of their campaign money from individual donors. As campaigns became increasingly expensive and public concern grew over the large quantities of unreported contributions during the 1972 presidential election, Congress passed a series of statutes in the 1970s that defined and institutionalized PACs. Following the 1974 revision of the Federal Election Campaign Act, PACs grew rapidly. Before then, 608 PACs were registered with the Federal Election Commission (FEC). Two years later, the number had nearly doubled. By the early 1990s, there were more than 4,000 PACs, a great many of them (1,795) associated with corporations. The number of PACs stabilized during the 1990s, and in 2004, at the end of the Clinton health plan debate, there were 4,184 registered PACs, a large share of them (39%) associated with corporations (Federal Election Commission, 2005). By the time of the Obama health reform debate, PAC numbers had grown, but not by much. There were 4,618 PACs at the end of 2009 (Federal Election Commission, n.d.).

Political action committees come in several varieties. Connected PACs are affiliated or coexist with some parent organization; more than 80 percent of

PACs fit this description (Wright, 1985). Unconnected PACs have no sponsoring organization and tend to be ideological in nature, often promoting a single issue. Some PACs are associated with a single business. Leadership PACs are organized by members of Congress, particularly party leaders and committee chairs. They receive money from various sources, including other PACs, and dispense it to candidates (up to $5,000 per candidate per election) in ways that help their party (and often enhance legislators' own prominence and influence nationally or within their house or party). Unconnected PACs include groups such as the liberal Moveon.org PAC, the conservative Blue Dog PAC, and the Black Republican PAC. None of the 1,570 unconnected PACs registered in 2008 had an explicitly health-related title (Federal Election Commission, n.d.).

Political action committees can be permanent or temporary, devised to support or oppose a policy on the institutional agenda. Their expenditures must be independent of candidates, without any explicit coordination or consultation with candidates. Under federal rules, PACs must report their activities to the Federal Election Commission, and contributions are limited to $5,000 to a federal candidate per election. But a member of Congress with a campaign fund and a leadership PAC can receive maximum contributions to both. State-level PACs do not report their activities and have no spending caps.

Most of the health professions have PACs, including the Academy of Dispensing Audiologists, the National Association of Spine Specialists, and the Renal Leadership Council. The AMPAC, the PAC associated with the American Medical Association, gave a bit under $2 million during the 2008 election campaign, 56 percent to Democrats, and it gave over two-thirds of its 2010 contributions (at midyear) to Democrats (Center for Responsive Politics, 2010a, 2010b). These years were very unusual. Typically AMPAC gives two-thirds to three-quarters of its contributions to Republicans. But with health reform at stake, giving switched to those in charge of Congress.

Political action committees can employ one of several strategies for distributing their dollars. They can seek to change the composition of Congress to make it more ideologically pleasing—as the director of the League of Conservation Voters candidly put it, "We want to see pro-environmental members of Congress elected" (Edsall, 1996)—or they can maximize their access to legislators. The former strategy more often leads to the funding of challengers, the latter to favoring incumbents, particularly party leaders and committee or subcommittee chairs. Given that challengers are usually cash-starved compared with well-placed incumbents, PACs have the potential to be better appreciated for their contributions to these upstarts.

Nevertheless, the lion's share of PAC money goes to incumbents. Committee membership and seniority are especially important to PAC giving in House campaigns (Romer & Snyder, 1994). In the Senate, PAC funding is more closely associated with party membership and voting record (Grier & Munger, 1993). When no incumbent is running, interest groups often target dollars to attractive first-year legislators in the hope of getting more attention from them early in their careers.

But no one can neglect the Speaker—in 2009 that was Speaker Nancy Pelosi: "Industry lobbyists, speaking on condition of anonymity for fear of alienating Ms. Pelosi, say they have stepped up their fund-raising for her all year with an eye to her pivotal role in the health care endgame, hoping to stay in her good graces and glean insights into her thinking . . . She has often accepted donations from people whom she and other Democrats vilify as opponents of reform. She has taken several checks from insurance industry lobbyists, for example, including $1,000 from Karen Ignagni and $1,500 from Mary Beth Donahue, both of the industry's trade group" (Kirkpatrick, 2009b).

The timing of PAC giving can also be important. Not all money is given during the months just before or after an election. Money provided early in a campaign can give a candidate a legitimacy and visibility that scares off other possible candidates and increases the likelihood of even more campaign dollars from other sources. The ANA was the first major health association to endorse Bill Clinton in the 1992 election. Its support may have been rewarded with 12 seats on the 47-member professional advisory review committee to Hillary Clinton's health care reform task force. The AMA was not represented on the advisory review committee (Bendavid, Goldman & Kaplan, 1993). Sometimes PACs give to both sides. Some even give after the election, as a way of "buying off a mistake" (Sabato, 1985, 92).

The modern member of Congress collects money throughout her term, and PAC money can be provided at any time, such as before an important vote in a committee or on the house floor. Many PACs deny giving money for such "present needs" for a favorable vote or action. Rather, they say they give money for support they may need in the future or to gain goodwill that might come in handy later. Some people believe there is also a fair amount of "reward" or "thank you" money for votes previously cast in support of a group's interests. Some PACs admit to "punishment" money, refusing to contribute to a candidate or giving money to her opponent.

Interestingly, there is very little evidence that PAC funding directly affects a legislator's vote on a given bill. Studies examining the linkage between PAC money and roll-call voting have found either no relationship or a very modest correlation (Smith, 1995; Cigler & Loomis, 2002). Two studies of AMPAC confirmed that there was no evidence of vote buying. Rather, the PAC chose to fund members who were ideologically similar or in positions of power, particularly in the House (Gutermuth, 1999; Wilkerson & Carrell, 1999).

Further evidence of a muddled cause-and-effect relationship between giving and getting is that PAC giving tends to change direction when party fortunes change. That is, PACs try to figure out which party is likely to be in charge after the next election and then start giving to that party so they won't be left out when power changes. Two *Washington Post* reporters noted such a shift in early 2010 when first-quarter PAC contribution reports were filed. PAC giving by big corporations had shifted from 61 percent to Democrats in 2009 to about half and half during the first three months of 2010. Why? "These corporate leaders and lobbyists have got interests and clients they need to look out for, and they are reading the tea leaves just like everyone else . . . They see what's happening . . . and they don't want to get cut short," said a GOP fund-raiser (Farnam & Leonnig, 2010).

Soft Money and Issue Advocacy

But importantly, interest groups and corporations can also give indirectly to campaigns—through either political parties or issue advocacy groups. Political parties have been the benefactors of soft money that could be used for voter mobilization and certain types of issue advocacy, and until 2002 soft-money donations were unlimited. The Bipartisan Campaign Finance Act of 2002 banned soft money; and although the U.S. Supreme Court later overturned the ban, interest groups and corporations had by then turned to issue advocacy groups operating through two financing units, 527s and 501(c)(4)s.

Beginning in the 2000 presidential elections, issue advocacy groups called 527 groups (organized under Section 527 of the Internal Revenue Code) rose to the fore in presidential and congressional campaigns. These groups differ from PACs in three important ways: (1) there is no limit on how much their sponsors can donate, (2) the money given is not a tax deductible expense, and (3) they report their receipts and outlays to the Internal Revenue Service, not the FEC. The third point is important because the FEC outlays are easily tracked, while the IRS has been slow to make information available. The 527 groups advocate for issues rather than candidates. They must not specifically endorse or recommend voting against a particular candidate, but they can come very, very close—for example, by saying that a particular candidate, named in the ad, "has a lot to answer for on protecting the environment."

The number of groups taking advantage of the 527 provision grew quickly in 1999 and 2000, peaked in fund-raising and spending in 2004, and after shrinking their giving in 2006, grew again in 2008 so that total spending by these groups exceeded a half billion dollars (Center for Responsive Politics, 2010c). Most 527 spending appears to be ideologically motivated, and as a consequence, 527 groups have not thus far played a significant role in health care policy debates.

The second kind of issue advocacy group has been more popular with health interests. Groups organized as 501(c)(4) committees, or social welfare organizations, may engage in political activities as long as these activities do not become their primary purpose. Disclosure requirements for these committees are less restrictive than those for the 527 groups, and they are not required to report the identity of their donors (Dwyre, 2002). One recent example of such a nonprofit group is the United Seniors Association (also known as USA Next), billed as an alternative to AARP. Some have argued that USA Next is the foil for groups that do not want to be directly identified with a position. Groups can provide large amounts of money to a 501(c)(4) nonprofit, which does not have to report its contributors and needs only to generally outline its expenditures. Drug companies and PhRMA were large donors to USA Next, which in 2005 sponsored a controversial series of television ads implying that AARP supported gays and was against the military. At issue was AARP's opposition to President George W. Bush's reform of Social Security (Tackett, 2005). By 2010 USA Next was seldom heard from. But other groups sprang up with similar messages and with similar funding sources.

A group calling itself "60 plus" ran ads in 2009 charging that the Obama administration was planning to reform health care "on the backs of seniors," resulting in changes in Medicare that would mean longer wait times and prescription restrictions (Connolly, 2009). The group has in the past been heavily funded by PhRMA and is closely associated with conservative and Republican groups and fund-raisers, according to SourceWatch.org (SourceWatch.org, n.d.). The group announced plans in November 2009 to spend heavily against the Obama reform, initially saying it would spend $1.5 million on ads in the districts of eight Democrats with large senior populations and would make phone calls in the districts of seven more members (Pershing, 2009b). Later, as the reform legislation stalled and the PhRMA deal was threatened with being reneged upon, the 60 Plus Association announced that it would spend $500,000 for ads against 18 centrist House Democrats who had supported the reform bill (Eggen, 2010a).

The world of campaign finance is a fluid one—determined in no small measure by the U.S. Supreme Court. One of the most meaningful decisions was in January 2010, when the court ruled 5-4 that government may not ban campaign spending by corporations (Liptak, 2010a). In *Citizens United v. Federal Election Commission* (558 U.S. 50 [2010]), the Court ruled that free speech in support of or against candidates is every citizen's right under the First Amendment, and the Court has long held that for First Amendment purposes, corporations are people. Hence the campaigning restrictions could not stand despite earlier rulings by the Court to the contrary. Many think the result will be much more candidate-specific advertising by corporations. President Obama called the new Court decision "a major victory for big oil, Wall Street banks, health insurance companies and the other powerful interests that marshal their power every day in Washington to drown out the voices of everyday Americans" (Liptak, 2010a).

These uses of nonprofit groups or the spending of money embedded in corporate budgets have been dubbed "stealth campaigns" (Hojnacki & Kimball, 1998), and they can be quite effective. In fact, differences between the politics of elections and the politics of policymakers are becoming much smaller. Interest groups wage campaignlike efforts to "win," and members of Congress are constantly running for election and collecting money to run. The days of behind-the-scenes lobbying among "gentlemen" are truly over and long forgotten in today's technology-savvy, no-holds-barred campaigns.

The Success of Interest Groups

Modern lobbying is more a campaign than a social event. Interest groups target members, hone the message, and decide on the best approach based on the target group and the message. Grassroots lobbying is usually done before committee action to help "soften up" the system by demonstrating public support. Direct lobbying is still focused on the committee and entails the lobbying of allies to encourage them to become advocates, or horses. Typically, interest groups combine grassroots and direct lobbying efforts aimed at supportive members of Congress and those who have not committed to a position. If the issue has no strong district ties, groups concentrate on direct contact (Hojnacki & Kimball, 1999). In some sense, direct contacts can help close the deal on specific issues that cannot be dealt with by the grass roots. As one lobbyist put it, "The grassroots got this issue [vitamin labeling] on the radar screen, but it's the Washington lobbyists who are crucial to making a law" (quoted in Weisskopf, 1995). The statement certainly is self-serving, but it also rings true.

There is some evidence that the money tends to be more persuasive in committee activities than on the house floor, because in committees visibility is lower, more decisions are made, and there are fewer members to persuade (Hall & Wayman, 1990; Keiser and Jones, 1986). Committee members can relatively easily and without much attention table a provision or make an amendment, without seeming to "sell out." They also have many choices to make about their level of formal and informal participation on an issue, ranging from merely attending a hearing or markup session to offering amendments and advocating on a group's behalf. If groups can tie their desired policies to strong public support, their chances of success are enhanced.

Some of the nation's strongest interest groups are weakened in their bargaining ability by their own members. For groups representing a large, diverse membership, developing and maintaining a policy focus that satisfies all members can be tough. The U.S. Chamber of Commerce offers a classic case. It suffered serious splits in 1993–94 over its opposition to health reform, and the process was repeated in 2010, when the harsh criticism of the Obama plan leveled by Chamber president Thomas Donohue led to departure of two of its biggest members, Apple and Pacific Gas and Electric (Vaida, 2010).

Hundreds of different health-related interest groups participate in health policymaking today, collectively affecting a range of programs and policy issues. There are many new consumer groups and an increasing number of groups representing corporate medicine, such as prepaid health plans, hospital chains, walkin clinics, and home care companies. Relman (1980) referred to this body as the "new medical-industrial complex." There have also been huge increases in the number of businesses and other non-health-related corporate entities involved in health policymaking and in groups representing providers and corporate interests, which tend to have substantially more resources.

It is nearly impossible to overstate the barriers to reform of the health care system raised by interest groups in today's competitive policy world. They have kept many issues from reaching the agenda and have seriously delayed and modified policy action on many others. Political scientists have long recognized the power of interest groups to keep issues from being discussed and recognized as problems. For example, the excess of hospital beds was widely acknowledged and the cost implications well understood. But federal funds continued to be available to build more hospitals, largely because of the ability of provider lobbies to keep the issue off the agenda. Big business successfully kept employer mandates at bay for decades before relenting in 2010, and teaching hospitals have protected graduate medical education dollars for years, despite the need for cuts in federal health spending and the desire to give states more flexibility in making policy decisions formerly concentrated in Washington. Despite the success of the Obama health reform, provider groups were once again largely successful in fending off serious cost controls, tough quality controls on physicians and hospitals, international and (in the case of generic biologicals, even domestic) competition for the drug industry, special taxes on plastic surgery, or a public option to compete with private health insurance.

Conclusion

Interest groups are powerful actors in health policymaking, arguably second only to Congress. Yet not all interest groups are equally powerful, and even the powerful are not dominant on all issues and at all times. These groups are most likely to affect bills when the issues are nonsalient, narrow, specialized, and without public support and when the groups employ a multipart strategy that includes contributions, direct and grassroots lobbying, and coalition building. Similarly, strategies that target a few specific changes can focus attention in a way that broader consumer groups cannot.

Changes in Congress, the presidency, the bureaucracy, the media, and the public occur over time, and these changes affect interest groups. The public is notoriously fickle, strongly supporting one policy or evidencing concern for one problem, only to move on to other policies and problems a short time later (Downs, 1972). However, one advantage interest groups hold is that they are patient. If they don't succeed in one Congress—even one decade—they remain to participate in different Congresses and decades. Perhaps no better example of this patience is health care reform, where many of the same groups and even the same lobbyists made the same arguments in 2009 and 2010 that they had made in 1993–94.

Interest groups tend to take advantage of technological advances and changes in campaign finance statutes to update their approaches and present their positions. Most, if not all, interest groups use the Internet and e-mail to maintain their constituencies and get their message out to policymakers and the public. When changes are made in one aspect of campaign finance—be it soft money or Section 527 committees—the groups adjust their funding streams accordingly. They also adjust their funding strategies, if not their positions, when political changes occur in Congress or the White House.

The success of interest groups, in health and other areas, is in the details—the often complex, many times largely ignored aspects of the law or regulation that can affect millions of dollars in reimbursement or the ability of health professionals to ply their trade independently. The expertise and intensity of interest groups' involvement in the complex details are often persuasive. It is at these margins of public policy that groups can most effectively use their lobbying strategies and PAC dollars, often without the benefit of public or media scrutiny.

Some worry that interest-group spoils go predominantly to the wealthiest of groups—those not only able to contribute generously to campaigns but also able to afford the most targeted, most professional media campaigns, electronic services, and informational assistance, including polling and focus groups. While all groups can use the Internet—and small groups may have an advantage here—the Internet is a passive form of lobbying and is probably most effective when part of a larger lobbying campaign.

In this atmosphere, then, health-related interest groups seek to inform and influence national policymakers to act (or refrain from acting) in ways that benefit their membership. The field is crowded and the stakes are high. One public relations staffer described health lobbying this way: "In all the issues we've worked on, we've never, ever found an issue that so many different constituencies were so instantly interested in. On health care, the interest level is immediately there and it is very deep. You don't have to explain to people why they should care" (Rubin 1993, 1084).

As more and more health care groups come to realize that they too must be players to protect their interests, the number and variety of these groups will continue to grow. Balance may yet be achieved as the cacophony fades into background noise. Poor people will likely have to count on health care interests with a stake in serving them to press the concerns of lower-income groups about access, quality, and financing. Whatever measures are taken to reduce the influence of PACs and campaign spending on health care policymaking, interest groups will still find a welcome on Capitol Hill, at the White House, in the health care agencies of the executive branch, and often in the courts. Those who become health lobbyists are likely to enjoy a successful and well-supported career. Plying their trade, they will work in an institution that is as integral a part of the system of health care policymaking as Congress itself and those who actually provide health care.

CHAPTER FOUR

Bureaucracy

A Look Back

1965

In the 1965 negotiations over Medicare, one of the most important players, Wilbur Cohen, was a bureaucrat. As a longtime staff member in the Federal Security Agency, the Social Security Administration, and the Department of Health, Education, and Welfare, Cohen had had a hand in virtually every national health insurance proposal since the 1930s. He was well known on Capitol Hill for his knowledge of both Social Security and health insurance. Sen. Paul Douglas (D-IL) once said, "A Social Security expert is a man with Wilbur Cohen's telephone number" (Harris, 1966). Cohen helped draft the administration's bill on Medicare, consulted with members of Congress on proposed bills, and was asked to summarize various proposals to the key committees. When Ways and Means Committee chair Wilbur Mills decided to combine several proposals into a "three-layer cake" (the layers were later known as Medicare Parts A and B and Medicaid), he asked Cohen to draw up legislative language to pull the pieces together, along with an analysis of the costs, within 12 hours.

Cohen was more than a substantive expert. He was involved in meetings in the White House and on Capitol Hill to assess the standing of proposals and develop strategies to achieve legislative success. He was one of a small group of strategists who developed a plan in 1956 that prompted congressional action by persuading a well-placed legislator to sponsor a bill and elicited wide public concern about the health of elderly people through a media campaign sponsored by the labor unions (Marmor, 1970, 30). Standing outside the Senate chamber during debates on the measure in 1965, Cohen heard rumors that labor unions were supporting an amendment the administration opposed. He called the labor representative, found out the rumor was false, and was able to hold the votes of liberal senators that might otherwise have been lost (Harris, 1966).

Cohen served as a broker between the president and congressional committees and among interest groups (Marmor, 1970). He reported regularly to the president and transmitted the president's views back to legislators. The president assigned Cohen the responsibility for working with interest groups, most notably the American Medical Association and the American Hospital Association, in implementing the newly adopted Medicare program.

Although Cohen had more access and visibility than a "typical" bureaucrat, he epitomized the importance of bureaucratic expertise and guidance to both the president and Congress. In 1965, the presidential staff was small and typically dominated by political, rather than policy, experts. Lyndon Johnson, like presidents before him, relied on the staffs in the executive agencies to put presidential preferences into legislative language and to produce statistics and rationale to support it. Congress, too, relied on the federal departments in the mid-1960s. Clapp (1963, 129) called the executive branch "a leading source of information for the legislator." Executive-branch officials worked closely with congressional committees, providing them with briefings, speeches, useful documents, and strategy suggestions. Though more responsive to members of the president's party, agency personnel were generally available to assist any lawmaker in drafting legislation and often provided research to help back up their position, even if it did not reflect the thinking of the department.

In the 1960s, Congress typically gave considerable discretion to the agencies in implementing the law. Wilbur Cohen negotiated actively with interest groups on many aspects of the implementation of Medicare. In the Public Welfare Amendments of 1962, Congress specified that the federal government would match 75 percent of the cost of services "prescribed" or "specified" by the secretary of Health, Education, and Welfare, words that gave HEW enormous discretion in deciding the nature of the program—and its cost (Derthick, 1975).

In 1965, federal health spending exceeded $3 billion, with most going to the "other" category (not falling in the four program areas of Medicare, Medicaid, Veterans, and Defense health), including research and training. HEW was the major health agency, accounting for 4 percent of all federal outlays (excluding Social Security). It was divided into eight agencies: the Administration on Aging, the Food and Drug Administration, the Office of Education, the Social Security Administration, the Public Health Service (PHS), Vocational Rehabilitation Services, St. Elizabeth's Hospital, and the Welfare Administration.

1981

President Ronald Reagan was highly skeptical of the loyalty and ability of the 366,000 federal public employees working in Washington. Even though Jimmy Carter had served in office only four years, following an eight-year Republican occupation of the White House, there was a general view that the federal departments were filled with Democrats hostile to Reagan's desire to reduce the size and power of government. President Reagan's skepticism led him to adopt a very careful hiring policy, putting in place cabinet and subcabinet appointees and other top officials who were often highly ideological and very loyal to him. Extreme cases involved an Environmental Protection Agency director and an Interior Department secretary who were forced to resign early in their assignments over questionable decisions and clear preferences toward business. The Reagan administration reached down further into the operations of the agencies, filling a higher proportion of noncareer senior executive positions, than any other modern presidential administration.

In addition to "stacking the deck" with like-thinking employees, the White House also encouraged these appointees to use their administrative powers to advance White House objectives (Salamon & Abramson, 1984). They were encouraged to reinterpret the conduct of agency business to the greatest extent possible, reduce regulatory actions, and reduce the adverse effects of regulations on business. There were layoffs in many agencies, called reductions in force, or RIFs. Some 12,000 federal employees lost their jobs through RIFs in fiscal years 1981 and 1982.

In 1981, the relationship between the executive agency staff and Congress was very different from that during the Johnson presidency. With the dramatic increase in congressional staff, there was less call on agency staff to assist in drafting laws and less need for agency help in plotting political strategies. Some agency expertise was still needed, however, particularly in statistics, evaluations, simulations, and informed estimations of the effects of current and proposed programs. A congressional staff person, usually one who was new to the job and often to the issue, could rely on a seasoned agency expert to help prepare speeches, testimony, committee reports, and sections of the bill. To gain expertise, a congressional committee would often "borrow" federal agency employees for temporary assignments. Such an arrangement benefited all parties. For Congress, it was an opportunity to get topflight expertise; for the staffer on loan, it was an opportunity to affect policy directly; for the agency, it was a way to build goodwill and strong bonds with congressional members and staff.

In 1980, a new Department of Education was formed, and HEW became the Department of Health and Human Services. HHS had four operating agencies: the Public Health Service, the Social Security Administration, the Office of Human Development Services, and the Health Care Financing Administration (HCFA). By 1981, HHS accounted for approximately 13 percent of total federal outlays, with overall spending of nearly $90 billion. Federal health spending was more than $66 billion, and health care services and Medicare made up more than 90 percent of the total.

1993

The federal bureaucracy facing Bill Clinton was similar in size to that in the times of Lyndon Johnson and Ronald Reagan. The number of public employees had grown between 1965 and 1993, but largely in the state and local sectors, which had increased by more than 40 percent. The health bureaucracy played a key role in Hillary Clinton's health care reform task force. But the key decisions about the makeup of the Clinton health package were made in the White House. Donna Shalala, HHS secretary, took a back seat to both the first lady and White House adviser Ira Magaziner. Magaziner directed and coordinated the efforts of the 500-member task force assembled in the early months of the Clinton presidency. Federal agency personnel were actively involved in the task force deliberations but were outnumbered by congressional staffers and outside advisers. Some 137 HHS staff members participated in the health care reform work groups—about one-third of all the government employees (including congressional staff and representatives of other federal agencies) in the groups and more than one-fourth of the total work-group membership.

Vice President Al Gore headed an effort to make government more efficient, called the National Performance Review. The effort produced hundreds of recommendations designed to save $108 billion over five years. In the first year, the review claimed to have reduced the federal workforce by 71,000 positions and saved $47 billion. Early in his presidency, Bill Clinton announced that he intended to provide more flexibility to states in launching innovations in Medicaid and Aid to Families with Dependent Children (AFDC). The HCFA soon set about implementing the policy, which broadened the scope of the research and demonstration waivers and allowed states to ignore some Medicaid and AFDC rules to try out new approaches and policies in 1993 and 1994.

In 1993, HHS accounted for some 18 percent of all federal spending—more than $280 billion. Health care services and Medicare made up 95 percent of the total federal spending on health. The four operating agencies in HHS were now the Public Health Service, the Social Security Administration, the Health Care Financing Administration, and the Administration for Children and Families (replacing the Office of Human Development Services).

2009

During years of Republican control of both houses of Congress and the White House in the early to mid-2000s, skepticism of the role of government prevailed; agencies were cut in size and reorganized to place more political control over scientists and field staff, and decisions favoring unburdening the business of regulation were enforced.

For example, the Food and Drug Administration relaxed its regulatory vigor related to food processing businesses. Peanut butter lovers, school kids, hospital and nursing home patients, vending machine customers, and millions of others were shocked to learn in 2009 that their favorite snack food was being recalled after more than 500 people were sickened in 43 states, while at least eight others died in three more states. The peanut butter was contaminated with salmonella when processed and shipped from the Blakley, Georgia, plant where it was packaged (Harris, 2009a). Worse, the company knew that it had contamination problems but illegally sought repeated tests of its product until it got a favorable outcome, then shipped it to thousands of buyers nationwide. Previous plant inspections by the Georgia Department of Agriculture had found filth, flaking rust, rodents, roaches, a leaky roof, an oven not hot enough to kill germs, and a plant not designed for food processing. Whistle blowers had told the FDA that the plant was in major violation of food safety laws and regulations, but years dragged by without agency follow-up—until events compelled reaction. Staff shortages, split regulatory responsibilities with the U.S. Agriculture Department and state agencies, a congressional and White House disposition against agency interference in market operations, and bureaucratic inertia probably all contributed.

The newly elected President Obama, whose administration had inherited the problem, pledged to fix it. Calling the FDA's failure to inspect 95 percent of the nation's food processing plants "a hazard to the public health," he vowed to fix the problem with more staff and a Food Safety Working Group of departmental secretaries to advise him of needed statutory changes, coordinate enforcement efforts, and assure that laws were obeyed (Harris, 2009b). Six months later a second salmonella outbreak—this one in Iowa eggs—sickened 1,500 people in several states. Whose fault was that? Again, the same factors had been in play.

Congress took two decades to write a new law, the Bush administration was in no hurry to implement the changes, and the changeover in bureaucratic leadership with the coming of President Obama had held things up to the point where the new rules did not go into effect until after the outbreak.

Understanding the Public Bureaucracy

The president, members of Congress, and the courts, the traditional triumvirate of power in the United States, tend to overshadow another group of policymakers, one that is clearly more important in the day-to-day operation and working of government: the public employees who work for federal, state, and local governments. According to the U.S. Bureau of the Census, as of 2008, the latest reporting period, there were more than 22 million public employees, 14 million of them working at the local level. Although the term *bureaucracy* encompasses both public and private sector organizations that are large, hierarchically organized, and highly specialized, in common parlance *bureaucracy* has come to mean publicly funded agencies and offices. Public sector employees are called, usually derisively, bureaucrats.

Bureaucracy conjures up images of inefficiency, waste, and red tape. Yet the evidence is not so clear-cut. For example, *red tape*, clearly understood in the abstract, is difficult to pin down. Appleby (1945, 64) described red tape as "that part of my business that you don't know anything about." A study by Herbert Kaufman (1977) concluded that although citizens object to the weight of red tape, everyone likes some portion of that weight. What is red tape to one person is, to another, an important consideration that could not be omitted. Many local officials consider regulations associated with the rights of people with disabilities to be excessive, expensive, and unnecessary, but to individuals who are disabled these requirements are essential. In their study of red tape, Bozeman and DeHart-Davis (1999) narrowed its definition to include rules, regulations, and procedures that remain in force and entail a compliance burden but do not advance the legitimate purposes the rules were intended to serve. Burdensome— yet effective—rules such as those protecting people who are disabled would not qualify as red tape under this definition.

Public administrators have much lower standing in the United States than in European and many Asian countries. In part this is a function of history. There is no mention of administration or bureaucracy or federal agencies in the U.S. Constitution, and the modern administrative state developed only recently, somewhere between the two Roosevelt administrations (Morone, 1990). In many European countries, the bureaucracy developed before the system of government and plays a strong institutional role in developing and implementing policy. The rather weak position of U.S. public bureaucracy is also explained by Americans' reverence for individualism and democracy—notions that run counter to bureaucracy and its quest for efficiency and effectiveness, not accountability.

Political Appointees versus Careerists

The top-level policymaking jobs in federal and state governments are generally filled with appointees of the chief executive: president or governor. At the federal level, the president fills more than 2,000 positions in federal departments—from department secretary and deputy chief of staff to assistant administrator. He also names members of the Federal Communications Commission and other independent commissions. Some 1,125 high-level executive-branch appointees (ambassadors, U.S. attorneys, U.S. marshals, and others) require Senate confirmation (Pfiffner, 2001).

In some states, governors make many appointments; in others, appointments are limited. Public appointees tend to be short-timers in both federal and state government; the mean tenure for a Washington political appointee is about two years. When the president leaves, so do these people, to be replaced by appointees of the new administration. Heclo (1977) dubbed political appointees "birds of passage," who understand they will not be around long and must act quickly if they expect to accomplish anything. Most public employees are civil servants, personnel who are hired and rewarded on a merit system and whose tenure does not rely on any one political party or officeholder.

Not infrequently, conflicts arise between political appointees who are pursuing a presidential goal, such as holding down costs or tightening regulation, and careerists who want to continue or expand programs they consider worthy. Following the disastrous BP oil spill in the Gulf of Mexico in the spring of 2010, President Obama ordered a moratorium on new deep-water oil leases and promised much closer scrutiny of applications. His appointee, Interior Secretary Ken Salazar, strongly supported the president and set about trying to change both the culture of the Minerals Management Service (MMS), which issues deep-water drilling permits, and its "friendly" review process for applications. Yet the MMS culture strongly supported a "partnership" view of its relationship with the oil industry, a view encouraged over many years by both Congress and several presidents, especially George W. Bush.

Thus, despite President Obama's ban on new drilling, followed by a revised ban issued by Secretary Salazar, the agency continued to issue permits and waivers during the month following the initial April 23, 2010, ban. The *New York Times* reported that its review of agency records showed issuance of 19 new environmental waivers and 17 new drilling permits for work of the type that led to the explosion in the Gulf (Urbina, 2010). A month later another news service reported that offshore drilling plans were still being approved "with minimal or no environmental analysis" (Bengali, 2010). This occurred despite resignation of the agency's career civil service director in late May. Salazar decided that the problem was the conflict between the agency's dual roles of promoter of drilling, on one hand, and safety and environmental regulator, on the other, and so he issued an order changing the agency's name and moving its regulatory authority to another agency.

Sometimes members of Congress try to separate careerists from the political aspects of a department by contacting them directly. According to Robinson (1991), some congressional committees sent packages of materials to the HCFA (now CMS) with instructions that political appointees were not to see the material. The committee wanted technical assistance but did not want to release the information to political appointees of the opposite party.

Bureaucratic Power

When we think of power, defined simply as the ability to act or produce an effect, we generally do not think of the bureaucracy. But we would be wrong to overlook it. As Norton Long (1949, 257) noted more than a half century ago, "The lifeblood of administration is power." Public employees are armed with the ability to influence legislation, interpret it, implement it, and evaluate it. They work closely with most of the central actors in the policymaking process and create linkages among them. They have their own motivations and act accordingly.

Bureaucratic power has long rested on expertise. No matter how many staff members Congress and the president may add, that staff will likely not be expert in every programmatic aspect of an issue. Agencies staffed with personnel whose job it is to deal with the details of a program, and who likely have been doing so for many years, will still have the advantage. Bureaucratic expertise is "indispensable for the effective operation of any modern political system" (Rourke, 1984, 15).

A typical occurrence in 2009 illustrates how powerful the health bureaucracy can be because staffers understand the subtle nuances of both medical care practice and Medicare payment rules. The HHS Office of the Inspector General (OIG) issued a report challenging physician billing practices under Medicare's "incident to" rule. That rule allows physicians to bill for services rendered by a nonphysician so long as the physician is in the room and the nonphysician is qualified and licensed to perform the service. The study found that many physicians were billing for more than 24 hours per day by adding their assistants' time as their own. This was perfectly legal so long as the nonphysicians were being supervised and not performing procedures for which they were unqualified. But the OIG study showed that nonphysicians had performed 21 percent of the physician-billed services, including many for which they were both untrained and uncertified—a clear violation of the rule. In response to the study, HHS changed its manual to reduce the ability of physicians to bill for services performed by nonphysicians. Although the study, using 2007 data, examined only a tiny sample of billing practices, Medicare had been billed for more than $1 million for the services in dispute, suggesting that many billions of dollars are likely to be at stake as the practice is revised by the new manual (Silva, 2009).

Federal bureaucrats also have the advantage of staying power. Executive-branch political appointees come and go, and congressional and state legislative staffers are highly transient, but careerists, by definition, stay. They stay and learn and remember. They comprise the institutional memory of what was proposed and adopted in earlier years—a valuable commodity in an area such as health, where many "new" proposals have actually been introduced several times over.

Bureaucratic power also rests on what Francis Rourke (1984) called political mobilization and Norton Long (1949) called political astuteness—the ability of an agency to garner support from the recipients or beneficiaries of the agency's programs. As Rourke (1984, 48) put it, "In the United States, it is fair to say, strength in a constituency is no less an asset for an administrator than it is for a politician, and some agencies have succeeded in building outside support as formidable as that of any political organization." One example of a politically astute health agency is the National Institute of Mental Health, which has enjoyed support from mental health practitioners across the country and has successfully separated itself from the other national institutes, becoming independent in 1966 and later forming the basis for the Substance Abuse and Mental Health Services Administration, an agency within HHS.

We need to keep in mind that power does not reside solely in the top leaders of an organization; rather, as Long (1949, 258) said, "It flows in from the sides of an organization . . . it also flows up the organization to the center from the constituent parts." Power is not just a friendly lunch between the department secretary and the chair of the House Energy and Commerce Committee. It is also the friendship between congressional committee staff and a staffer at the CMS's Office of Legislation and Policy and the support from interest groups and program recipients who want to make certain that Medicare and Medicaid are well staffed and well funded—a goal shared with the agency personnel.

In past years it was common in political science to talk about agencies being "captured" by special interests, an event most likely to occur for agencies that provide benefits to a narrow group of interests—a client agency—such as the Department of Veterans Affairs. The idea was that, since the agency's survival depended in large part on the support of its constituents, it could not be impartial but would accommodate the needs of its constituents, regulating to protect their interests. In recent years, empirical studies testing the capture theory have debunked the idea for most regulatory agencies. In fact, the studies have shown how, over time, agencies continue to regulate an industry vigorously rather than becoming increasingly sympathetic to it (Meier, 1985; Quirk, 1981). Other research has highlighted a more pluralistic interest-group model in which many groups form advocacy coalitions but find their influence curbed by external pressures from other actors and groups and by an agency's internal structure, professionalism, and leadership (Gormley, 1982; Meier, 1985).

Agencies often try hard to obtain positive and strong public support. They do it with good service, good media relations, advertisements, education campaigns in public schools, and public involvement in commissions, boards, or contests. They especially seek the strong support of "attentives," those people and groups who directly benefit from or otherwise support an agency's mission. The National Institutes of Health (NIH), for example, is supported by the research community of the health professions' schools and laboratories, high-tech industries, and broad-based organizations supporting specific diseases (such as the American Cancer Society). In the case of the NIH and other agencies, many of these groups benefit directly or indirectly from research dollars available from the agency. Some agencies have a specific, highly targeted clientele, such as veterans. Organizations of veterans have been extremely vocal and effective in maintaining programs and increasing funding for the Department of Veterans Affairs.

Some observers believe bureaucrats are becoming more powerful. Morone (1993) noted that bureaucrats are playing a greater role in formulating health care and are implementing laws with less deference to Congress. Others disagree. Rourke (1991) argued that the role of expertise has diminished as public confidence in experts has declined. Think tanks and nonprofit groups, often advocating certain points of view, have proliferated in Washington and the states and provide white papers, policy analyses, and applied research that compete with bureaucratic advice. There are simply too many experts—and they disagree too often. Whether it is conflicting "expert" testimony on the psychological profile of the defendant in a murder trial, the disagreement of scientists over the extent of the problem caused by destruction of the ozone layer, or the disagreements of statisticians over the root causes of food-borne illnesses or the impact of obesity on morbidity and mortality, the point is the same: whom is the public to believe? Possibly both sides of the argument on the importance of bureaucrats are right. On detailed, complex issues, much is delegated to the bureaucracy. On less salient, less complex issues, Congress may be less willing to delegate authority to the bureaucracy.

The Political Environment

The political environment of government agencies can vary enormously. James Wilson (1989) categorized agencies into four types based on whether they provide narrow or diffuse benefits and whether the costs they impose are narrow or diffuse (see fig. 4.1). For agencies providing narrow benefits and imposing narrow costs (benefits to a few, costs shared by a few), their political environment can be categorized as interest-group politics, best described as having interest groups on both sides of an issue. A good example of this interest-group agency is the Occupational Safety and Health Administration: labor and business often clash over the agency's actions, and the agency finds it hard to please both sides

	Narrow benefits	**Diffuse benefits**
Narrow costs	*Interest-group* · *OSHA*	*Entrepreneurial* · *EPA* · *FDA*
Diffuse costs	*Client* · *NIH* · *VA*	*Majoritarian* · *CDC*

Figure 4.1. Regulatory politics: The Wilson model. *Source:* Wilson, 1989.

in its activities and its choices. At the other extreme, some agencies that distribute broad benefits and impose broad costs have little interest-group involvement, and these may be called majoritarian agencies.

The Centers for Disease Control and Prevention is one such agency. Reduced interest-group participation might seem enviable at first glance, but it could prove problematic in times of budget cutbacks, when the agency can find it hard to muster outside support. The CDC's mission is "to collaborate to create the expertise, information, and tools that people and communities need to protect their health—through health promotion, prevention of disease, injury and disability, and preparedness for new health threats" (CDC, 2011a). Few of the activities implied in that mission statement will make money for any major industry. Creating and providing vaccinations is a losing proposition for drug companies because the research costs and potential liability exceed likely profits, so they are unlikely to lobby for more money for CDC. Health promotion may cause a small amount of spending on advertising media, if the announcements are not run as free public service announcements. So the television industry isn't likely to spend time and money lobbying for CDC. While there are many users of CDC health survey data, they tend to be universities, whose faculty isn't likely to lobby on CDC's behalf at budget time.

An agency granting broad benefits while imposing narrow costs is not in an enviable position, since the interest groups paying those costs might coalesce to oppose agency goals. Members of the broad group of beneficiaries seem, individually, to have little at stake in the benefits, but those suffering the costs are big losers. The FDA is a perfect example of this type of agency, called an entrepreneurial agency. Its mission is to protect the broad public interest. But doing so means battling with food and drug manufacturers who are financially harmed by agency actions. With millions of dollars at stake, the effort and costs of marshaling powerful coalitions to fight the agency are a good investment for the pharmaceutical industry. Indeed, the FDA has long suffered from the criticism that it pays too much attention to the industry and not enough to consumers. A case in point was the FDA's 2008 approval of a patch to help injured knees. Scientific staff of the agency had repeatedly rejected the patch as unsafe because its high failure rate necessitated new surgery to remove it. But when lobbied by four New Jersey congressmen and its own former commissioner, the agency rolled over and granted approval. In congressional testimony in September 2009, the agency's head called the lobbying "extreme," "unusual," and "persistent" and acknowledged for the first time in history that an FDA decision had been influenced by political pressure. The approval was scheduled for re-review following the congressional hearing (Harris & Halbfinger, 2009).

In the final category of agency politics are those agencies whose benefits accrue to a few and whose costs are widespread. Health personnel agencies such as the Bureau of Health Professions are examples of these client agencies. Their programs directly benefit medical and nursing schools, with costs widely spread across most of the population. Such an agency is a good candidate for "capture" by interest groups, because the goals of the agency and the goals of the groups are likely to be closely aligned. Opponents are hard to find and are unlikely to invest the effort to form an interest group to oppose the agency's actions, since the costs are so small to each payer.

Some scholars have pointed out that in recent years, the federal agency role in intergovernmental relations has increased and Congress's role has decreased. Probably nowhere is that illustrated more than in health, where federal agencies are actively engaged with the states to implement positions that are not always in line with congressional wishes. The EPA staff is engaged with states in negotiating performance indicators; the HHS staff determines whether states have met performance standards and decides which states deserve bonuses and which ones sanctions. The CMS has been criticized for not stopping states from "gaming" Medicaid through what is known as Medicaid maximization strategies and for allowing states to use waivers to spend Medicaid and State Children's Health Insurance Program (S-CHIP) dollars on adults who should not be eligible under the law. The CMS has encouraged states to enact waivers and is highly engaged in their negotiation. The Clinton and George W. Bush administrations strongly encouraged the use of waivers—to the point where when legislative change did come along, it merely acknowledged what had already become policy: states can make the adjustments they desire by working with federal bureaucrats. Thus, according to Gais and Fossett (2005, 510), "Waivers . . . allow presidents to pursue controversial policy goals without seeking approval from a slow and divisive legislative process." These authors also note that waivers allow a president to help political friends (and punish enemies) and neutralize congressional scrutiny by encouraging state delegations to support their states' waiver requests.

Bureaucratic Behavior

Rationality is an important goal of public administration. Rationality has many meanings, but Waldo's concept (1955) of rational action is appropriate to public administration: action correctly calculated to realize given desired goals with minimal loss to the realization of other desired goals. Not all decisions are rational, of course, because few decision makers have the full information, time, and resources necessary to know with certainty the consequences of each alternative. Public decision makers are under time and resource constraints. Full knowledge about the alternatives and their consequences is nearly impossible. Instead, public decision makers "satisfice," or make the best decision given the constraints. Simon (1945) described a "satisficing" decision maker as one who does not examine all possible alternatives, ignores most of the complex interrelationships of the real world, and makes decisions by applying relatively simple general rules. Simon also described this decision maker as applying "bounded rationality" to decisions. Knott and Miller (1987) argued that rationality is impossible because of the dysfunctions in bureaucratic structure. Characteristics of bureaucracy—specialization, trained expertise, hierarchy, and rules—combine to produce a variety of bureaucratic dysfunctions, including trained incapacity, goal displacement, and rigidity cycles.

Simon (1960) talked about two types of decisions: programmed and non-programmed. Programmed decisions are those that recur frequently and can be handled by standard operating procedure (SOP), the rules of operation followed by all employees in the same situation. SOP can be viewed as a way to limit bureaucratic power and to force staff to conform to organizational goals (Rourke, 1984). It is also the only practical way to run a large organization. The regional offices of federal agencies make many decisions every day about what is acceptable and unacceptable behavior on the part of grantees and recipients. SOPs help ensure uniformity among these offices and their counterparts in Washington. The emphasis on SOP is not arbitrary or necessarily convenient. As Guy Peters (1981, 76) put it, federal agencies "are responsible for public money and act in the name of the people and must therefore be accountable to the public. Accountability, in turn, may force the bureaucrat to protect himself against possible complaints, and the protection comes through adherence to rules and procedures."

Nonprogrammed decisions are those that Simon (1976, 6) described as "novel, unstructured, and consequential." They cannot be handled with SOP but must be dealt with using the staff's discretion. Decisions related to the drafting of regulations, allocation of resources, and implementation of new programs are examples of nonprogrammed decisions.

In nonprogrammed decisions, bureaucrats must balance many concerns—those of their own professions, their political bosses, their funders (Congress), and the public. Bureaucrats are also cognizant of their own agency's reputation and mission. In many cases there are conflicts among several of these "masters" and the agency's own mission that are important to that agency's survival. In health, the NIH is an example of an agency with a strong sense of mission—biomedical research—that has remained constant over decades. In contrast, the PHS has seen its mission change from caring for merchant sailors, to environmental and preventive medical activities, to responsibility for care delivery to targeted populations, preventive care, and health personnel. Although agencies must be somewhat flexible to survive, such major organizational personality changes can strip an agency of its identity and leave it floundering. The NIH, by contrast, holds so strongly to its mission that it has repeatedly resisted efforts by powerful health committee and subcommittee chairs to add new agencies with a statistical and social science focus. When one was slipped in—the National Institute on Aging—its director (despite his own training as a psychiatrist) quickly realized that his agency must focus on the biological aspects of aging rather than social science concerns, if it was to thrive in the NIH environment.

Public Bureaucracy and the Policy Process

In the early years of public administration, the roles of politicians and public employees were seen as distinct and clearly defined. Elected officials were responsible for making political decisions or policy; appointed officials handled administrative matters and the implementation of political actions. In contrast, today's public bureaucrat is involved in all aspects of policymaking: setting the agenda, formulating solutions, and implementing the policy, including translating sometimes vague congressional directions into concrete, workable programs.

Setting the Agenda

Bureaucrats, according to Kingdon (1995), are specialists who provide information and statistics that define problems in a way that can move the issues to the forefront of public attention. They can make the dimensions and severity of a problem known to Congress, the White House, and the press. Sometimes what they want to say may not be what others want to hear. Distracted driving is a case in point. Common sense tells us that distracted drivers conducting cell phone conversations and texting are dangerous, but designing a study proved problematic since researchers couldn't ethically send drivers out with phones to see if they crashed. National Highway Transportation Safety Administration (NHTSA) staff figured out a way to test the impact of distracted driving with a

$50 million driving simulator. With that they could test what happens when a distracted driver encounters an unexpected event like being cut off by another car or someone or something that darts in front of her. The bureaucrats developed the machine and designed the study (Wald, 2000).

But when they proposed it to their bosses in 2003, they were cut off at the knees despite having compiled an enormous briefing document based upon 150 articles reporting crash consequences of cell phone use, hands-free or otherwise. A *New York Times* investigation—following revelations by Clarence Ditlow of the nonprofit advocacy group Center for Auto Safety—discovered that agency leaders met and discussed the proposed study, its preliminary findings based on the literature review, and a proposed letter to state governors warning them that exempting hands-free usage from laws restricting cell phone use by drivers might not be a good idea. But fear of adverse congressional reaction prevented the letter from being sent, the study from being conducted, and the wrongheaded view that cell phones don't cause accidents from being corrected. "My advisers upstairs said we should not poke a finger in the eye of the appropriations committee," Dr. Jeffrey Runge, NHTSA head at the time of the review meeting, told the *New York Times* in 2009 after reports of the suppressed research had begun to leak out (Richtel, 2009).

A month after the *New York Times* article, the Secretary of Transportation—recently appointed to the job by newly elected President Obama, announced a change in agency policy. He called for a forum on "distracted driving," intimating that cell phone use was as deadly as drunk driving. "This is a sea change if it leads to action," said Clarence Ditlow, Center for Auto Safety director. Several members of Congress began moves to withhold state transportation money if states did not ban hands-free phone use as well as other conversations and texting while driving (Richtel, 2009).

Formulating Health Care Policy

The health reform act of 2010, popularly known as the PPACA, for Patient Protection and Affordable Care Act, contains five pilot projects, 30 demonstrations, and 402 mentions of those pilots and demonstrations (Kuraitis, 2010). Most were suggested by the CMS bureaucrats or those working with or for MedPAC.

The CMS was also given broad new authority to experiment with payment innovations, relaxing many limitations in their previously granted demonstration project authority. They can now do short demonstrations rather than minimum-five-year projects, an option that will permit them to try an idea, perfect it, try it again, and then take it to Congress for legislative authority to implement it systemwide.

The PPACA makes an even larger grant of authority to a newly formed bureaucratic agency, a 15-member independent advisory board charged to recommend cuts in Medicare spending if spending growth exceeds the target of GDP plus 1 percent. The board makes its recommendations and Congress must vote them up or down. If down, Congress must replace them with its own cuts in equal amounts.

The congressional battle for the board's creation was hard-fought, because Congress does not like giving up its power. To constrain the new board, Congress prohibited it from making many kinds of recommendations, such as rationing or changes in eligibility, copays, or benefits through the year 2018, when presumably these restrictions disappear. Even with these constraints on the board's options, and certainly without them after 2018, this is a broad grant of authority closely equivalent to the Base Closure and Realignment Commission set up to do the politically toxic work of deciding which military bases will be kept, which ones will be refurbished and perhaps granted new missions, and which ones will be closed. Congress must vote the entire slate up or down, and if down, make its own list—a list no member wants to be accused of cooperating with if it involves closing bases in her district or state.

Another example of bureaucratic influence on policymaking is nursing home payment reform. Nursing homes are paid for today by CMS using a case-mix adjusted payment system that was the brainchild of one bureaucrat, Betty Cornelius. She began pushing the idea in the mid-1970s, then urged her agency (then HCFA, now CMS) to fund demonstration projects developing the idea, encouraged researchers to work on the problem of classifying nursing home patients and subsequently home care patients, and eventually saw her ideas become the law of the land when Congress mandated the RUGs (resource utilization groups) system of classifying patients for purposes of CMS payment in 1987 nursing home reform legislation (Clauser & Fries, 1992). The agency continues to reform the payment method, and in 2010 it implemented RUGs IV, to improve some classification issues (Provider Conference Call, 2010). This major industry-wide reform came directly from the bureaucracy and continues to be refined and managed by it, dictating performance and payment for every nursing home that accepts Medicare or Medicaid patients, with little or no congressional involvement in policy modifications.

When Congress considers measures to provide insurance for the uninsured, it needs to know how many Americans are uninsured, where they reside, and why they are uninsured. HHS can provide that information. Most if not all of the burgeoning concern with the rise in health care costs emanates from the CMS Office of the Actuary, which regularly generates reports projecting health expenditures and their underlying components. The agency is even more successful in helping develop a policy agenda for the administration than for Congress. Robinson (1991) noted that 89 percent of executive-generated Medicare legislation in 1987 could be traced to HCFA (now the CMS). Borins (1999) found that 71 percent of state and local "cutting-edge" innovations were initiated by bureaucrats. Only 18 percent were initiated by politicians.

While the counts are not yet in for bureaucratic ideas in the PPACA, because such tracing of ideas takes months and years, there is little doubt that the CMS, the MedPAC, the Agency for Healthcare Research and Quality (AHRQ), the Health Resources and Services Administration (HRSA), and other agencies will have contributed most of the ideas. Of course they are able to do this because bureaucrats are specialists, keenly interested in their relatively small aspect of policy, well connected to both academic researchers and frontline practitioners. When they hear a good idea, they are able to help get funding to permit the innovator to develop and test it, refine it, and then help promote it up the line to the White House and Congress. Some of the reforms proposed by the president and others in the Obama administration included the following, and most of them have the stamp of the nitty-gritty technical approach to a problem that is the special talent of the bureaucracy (Health Care Reforms, n.d.).

- Research on the overutilization of services and on comparative effectiveness
- Independent advisory panels
- Tax reform
- Insurance company antitrust reforms
- Preventive strategies
- Reform of coverage mandates
- Reform of doctors' incentives
- Medical malpractice liability costs and tort reform
- Rationing of care
- Payment system reform

- Health care technology reforms
- Addressing the shortage of doctors and nurses
- Addressing Medicare fraud
- Importation of prescription drugs
- Pilot programs
- Privatizing Medicare with a voucher system

The last item probably came from Congress, not the CMS, while importation of prescription drugs has passed at least one House of Congress in the past and may have emanated there.

Implementing Health Policy

Implementation may be defined as the activities directed toward putting a program into effect (Jones, 1984), or what happens after laws are passed that authorize a program policy, a benefit, or some other tangible output (Ripley & Franklin, 1986). Guy Peters (1981, 77) argued that, to a great extent, "the 'real' policy of government is that policy which is implemented, rather than that policy which is adopted by the legislature." Yet implementation is an area not widely understood—even by policymakers. Nathan (1993, 122) called it the "shadow land," the neglected dimension of U.S. governance. A report of the National Commission on the State and Local Public Service (1993) described implementation as the short suit of U.S. government. So much time is devoted to what should be done that little energy remains for the questions of how to do it. The commission thought that the public's frustrations about government stemmed from unsuccessful implementation—the failure of government to turn promises into performance.

Implementation begins when Congress, through a series of instructions—sometimes specific, sometimes less specific—delegates to federal agencies the policy it wants carried out. The federal agency then follows those instructions. Although this course seems straightforward, many things can happen to impede successful implementation:

—Agencies responsible for implementation may lack the enthusiasm, the staff, the expertise, or the resources to carry out their responsibilities.
—The congressional instructions may be so vague that the federal agency must make many important assumptions, such as designating which state programs are "acceptable" or what is "reasonable cost."

—Multiple congressional goals or conflicting instructions may make it difficult for agencies to carry out their assignments.

—Interagency rivalries may cause problems, with agency staffs fighting one another over interpretation of the law and resource issues.

—The recipients of a program (for example, state or local governments) may be uncooperative or may demand different interpretations.

—The number of people involved may slow the process: if several federal agencies and several state and local agencies must serve as "clearance points," the eventual outcome will be adversely affected.

—Time can be a problem; for complicated measures, such as those relating to clean air and clean water, the process of collecting information, writing draft regulations, and encouraging public comment can add years to the process of rulemaking.

—State and local agencies, communities, or recipients of the program can slow implementation if they disagree with any aspect of it.

—Congress can change its mind, or at least enough of Congress to make implementation difficult.

Republicans had bragged that if they won big in the 2010 November elections, they would try to repeal major sections of the president's health reform act. But even if they did not take over one or both houses, they would make sure that "not one dime" was available in agency appropriations to implement sections of the law that they did not like (Pear, 2010e). They were able to make good on their promises in a House resolution in April 2011, because they held a strong majority, but they were never able to pass a budget through the Senate, still controlled by the Democrats.

When agencies write rules, their process for revising them if they need to is more manageable and more nuanced than it would be if Congress had to change a law. And agencies do make mistakes that necessitate revisions to their rules. Sometimes they overreach in their rule writing, while at other times they do the opposite, leaving too much unwanted behavior unrestrained. HHS issued new rules relating to inadvertent disclosure of patient data to unauthorized sources. The standards for reporting disclosures to patients were set rather high, seeking to avoid burdening providers and patients with notifications of "trivial" events. Consumer groups and members of Congress reacted with outrage because the rules left it up to the provider to decide whether or not a particular disclosure would harm the patient. Urged by the White House, HHS secretary Kathleen Sebelius pulled them back (Pear, 2010d).

In another example, HHS had to back down after it issued demanding standards for what constituted "meaningful use" of electronic health records to qualify for federal subsidies provided in the 2009 economic stimulus act. Hospitals and physicians cried foul when the standards required them to meet 23 (hospitals) or 25 (physicians) criteria to qualify for any subsidy. In response, HHS softened the rules for physicians to require meeting any 15 of the 25 requirements and 5 of 10 goals. Hospitals would have to meet 14 and 5 (Pear, 2010c).

Sometimes it is Congress that overreaches. Even though an agency has been given broad discretion and authority by a congressional majority vote, individual members may feel strongly that the rules written should favor one conclusion rather than another. Typically that member influence is wielded discretely in phone calls or visits to the agency secretary or administrator, or it comes in official comments along with thousands of others, making it difficult to conclude that the member had special influence, even though it is well known that congressional comments carry substantial weight (Balla, 1998). The knee patch example given above (see the section titled "The Political Environment"), in which members of Congress pressured the FDA into overruling its scientists, is uncommon only in the fact that it so clearly produced an inappropriate outcome. Pressure that tilts a close call one way or the other or serves to move things more quickly or more slowly may be the more usual effect.

Congress does not treat all agencies equally. The amount of discretion afforded an agency depends on several factors, including the agency's resources (such as political support, expertise, and leadership) and its tolerance of other actors, especially interest groups. Meier (1985) described agency decisions as falling within or outside a zone of acceptance. If the agency decision falls within the zone of acceptance to Congress, the president, and the courts, the agency will be given more autonomy. Agencies dealing with salient, noncomplex issues are more likely to have smaller zones of acceptance, and Congress is more likely to intervene. Sometimes Congress has little choice but to allow discretion to agencies, especially on complicated, politically volatile issues, but it can still provide specific guidance.

In some cases, the enabling legislation describes in detail what information should be collected. OSHA not only is obliged to rely on what is already known about health and safety aspects of substances and activities; it must also create and use new knowledge when what is available is insufficient. Different statutes require different criteria for risk assessment and require different information to be collected—even for the same agency. Sometimes the criterion is "no known or anticipated adverse effects"; sometimes it is to ensure that "unreasonable risk" is eliminated, but using the "least burdensome requirements" (Kerwin, 2003, 59).

Congress can set deadlines for agencies' actions (although they often do not meet them). It can also impose "hammers," which call for provisions in the statutes that will take place only if the agency fails to issue its own regulation. These provisions are not the desired policy of Congress but rather ways to pressure the agency to act quickly (Kerwin, 2003).

Issuing Regulations

The single most important bureaucratic task in implementation is issuing rules and regulations for carrying out the law. Broadly speaking, regulation is government restriction of individual choice so as to keep conduct from crossing acceptable boundaries. Examples include prohibitions against selling unsafe drugs, operating an unsafe workplace, and polluting the nation's air and water. In health insurance, state and now federal laws prohibit, for example, imposing annual or lifetime limits on coverage. Regulations are made explicit in rules designed to implement, interpret, or prescribe law or policy. A more colorful definition, from former U.S. Supreme Court justice Oliver Wendell Homes, is that "a rule is the skin of a living policy . . . Its issuance marks the transformation of a policy from the private wish to public expectation" (Kerwin 2003, 2).

Federal rulemaking occurs every year, causing the Code of Federal Regulations to swell by hundreds of pages yearly. Title 42, Public Health, contains all the rules relating to health and health care concerns of the federal government. That title—just one of the Code's 50 titles—contained five volumes, five chapters, and 1,999 parts in the version revised December 8, 2011 (Code of Regulations, 2011). Of its thousands of regulations, a small fraction, perhaps 15 percent, are considered "major" rules as defined by various statutes and executive orders, including one that calls for estimation of the costs and benefits of any rules that will cost businesses or state and local governments more than $100 million. The Office of Management and Budget annually issues a report containing all these calculations. For 2011, it reported that agencies issued 66 major rules. That batch of rules was expected to produce between $18.8 billion and $86.1 billion in benefits each year, and $6.5 billion to $12.5 billion in cost. HHS issued 18 of those rules, estimated to generate $18 to $40.5 billion in benefits and cost $3.7 to $5.2 billion (Office of Management and Budget, 2011e).

Given the importance of rulemaking, it is not surprising that agencies must follow procedures set forth in federal law—in this case, the federal Administrative Procedures Act. This act requires notice when a department plans to issue a rule. The notice must be published in the Federal Register, the official notification document of the federal government. Interested parties are then allowed an opportunity to participate in the proceedings by presenting written or oral information. Hearings are often held on salient rules of great interest to many people. Draft and final regulations are then published. Some agencies are required by law to hold hearings and base final rules on the evidence in the record. Others must convene advisory groups to aid in the drafting of regulations. A 1996 federal law requires that if a regulation under development has substantial implications for a significant number of small businesses, the agency—especially if it is the EPA or OSHA—must convene a panel to develop information and secure recommendations from affected interests. The panel reports to the agency, which in turn is expected to incorporate the information into the regulation or supporting analyses (Kerwin, 2003).

Interest Groups and Regulations

When an issue enters the regulation-writing stage, it does not cast aside politics. Rather, interest groups understand the bureaucracy to be one more venue for achieving policy goals. A simple way to affect the process is to comment on the proposed rule. Agencies must read and respond to these comments in their final regulations. Typical of the level of detail in such comments were those of PHI, a nursing home industry worker advocacy group. It responded to a CMS invitation to provide comments on the nursing home reform provisions in the PPACA. Nine specific comments were offered (with the clear intent to offer more as the process developed), which included calls for

- specific measures of workforce satisfaction, turnover, and other details as part of quality assurance efforts;
- reports of nursing home staff turnover and other worker-related measures on the Nursing Home Compare website to be built by CMS;
- focusing the civil money penalties authorized in the law on workforce issues and "person-directed" care;
- prioritizing workforce concerns in national demonstration projects authorized by the law;
- using established curricula for dementia abuse avoidance training;

- coordinating the required state and federal background checks on staff;
- focusing the National Training Institute for nursing home inspectors on "patient-centered care" and culture change in the nursing home;
- using the new National Nursing Aide registry to also substantiate training in patient-centered care; and
- directing training grants to peer mentoring, coaching supervision, and other staff-related approaches.

"Enacting health reform was a big step but it was only the first step," the group's director said. "Long-term care stakeholders and workforce advocates must work closely with the agencies implementing reform to fully realize the law's potential to strengthen the quality of direct-care jobs and improve the quality of long-term services and support" (Shineman, 2010).

Although many regulatory decisions are complex, detailed, and of interest to only a few affected groups, some do have broad public interest. Perhaps the most outrageous example comes not from the United States but from Egypt's response to the 2009 swine flu epidemic (formally known as H1N1). Here are exhibited in bold relief the pitfalls of unanticipated consequences of a regulation. Thinking that it could control the 2009 swine flu epidemic (which in fact was not spread by pigs), Egypt banned pigs and killed all those the government could find. But—as regulators were told, and they dismissed as unimportant—in Egypt, pigs are the local garbage collectors. Pigs eat the city's garbage. So when they were all dead, tons of garbage began to stack up in the streets, alleys, and pathways. And what do tons of garbage bring? Thousands of rats. "Killing all the pigs was the stupidest thing they ever did. This is just one more example of poorly informed decision makers," a ministry of state for environmental affairs told the *New York Times* (Slackiman, 2009).

Congress and the President and Regulations

Another misconception of those who think the regulatory process is always smooth and compliant with Congress is the assumption that agencies will do whatever Congress asks and do it quickly and well. This is not always the case. There is often considerable delay between legislative enactment and the issuance of final regulations—particularly when Congress is of one party and the president of the other. Food safety concerns sometimes took a back seat to avoiding intrusive regulatory action during the George W. Bush administration. But when Democrats took over Congress, the party's president took over the White House, and people began dying of egg contamination, Congress and the new president wanted to know why the agency had taken so long to get regulatory enforcement in place—enforcement not particularly favored by the previous administration, under which the rule-writing had taken place. So an outraged Congress pointed the finger of accusation at the agency.

Key committees held hearings in August 2010 demanding to know why 1,500 people had gotten sick from salmonella bacteria in eggs two years after the major producer of the contaminated eggs had recorded the first of 73 contamination problems. An FDA inspection of the producer's barns after the outbreak was traced to that firm found "flies, maggots and rodents, and . . . overflowing manure pits" (Harris & Neuman, 2010). The inspection occurred under rules written before the outbreak, but which had not gone into effect until July 2010, after the outbreak happened. The hearings suggested that the agency was at fault. Never mind that the same egg producer had started the last salmonella outbreak in the nation in 1987, but Congress took two decades to strengthen the law. State regulators pleaded with the FDA to shut the producer down, but the federal agency felt it lacked authority to do much without congressional action (Neuman, 2010).

The pace of regulatory initiation sometimes picks up as a president gets ready to leave office. President Clinton's administration issued scores of regulations in its final week, including well over 50 from the EPA (McCoy, 2000). Two important sets of health rules were among those issued in the final weeks of 2000: rules ordering ergonomics programs at worksites and rules setting time limits for health insurers to make treatment decisions.

A new president is sometimes reluctant to strike down regulations that have worked their way through laborious and legally defined processes. Indeed, the Supreme Court overturned an effort by President Reagan to eliminate a rule ordering air bags or passive-restraint seat belts in cars. The EPA under President George W. Bush sought to soften regulations promulgated during the Clinton years that required companies to install additional pollution controls when expanding or modernizing older power plants. The new regulations allowed utilities to make improvements without adding pollution controls. Several states sued the EPA, challenging the changes (Heilprin, 2004). Rule changes between administrations became easier with passage of a 1996 law, the Congressional Review Act, giving Congress the power to kill final rules put in place within the preceding six months (Skrzycki, 2000b). Democrats in Congress, joined by a few

Republicans, tried to use the Congressional Review Act to challenge a regulation on mercury in 2005 but were unsuccessful. To send a regulation back to the EPA, majorities of both houses and the president have to agree on the change.

Sometimes presidents use the regulatory route to set policy without going to Congress. The EPA under President George W. Bush issued regulations setting up a cap-and-trade approach for sulfur dioxide and nitrogen oxide emissions and looser standards for emissions of mercury. The changes were not minor. For example, coal-fired power plants emitting mercury were given 11 additional years to make significant cuts under the regulation (Drew & Oppel, 2004). One problem with heavy reliance on regulatory policy is that the regulations are often challenged in court.

The Courts and Regulations

The courts do not get involved in writing regulations, but they do respond when a group or a person challenges the legality of a regulation. The Administrative Procedures Act provides for judicial review of any agency action by a person or corporation that is either wronged by the agency or has a grievance. Under this act, citizens can use the courts to prod agencies into action. When federal agencies fail to issue regulations expeditiously or within congressional deadlines, they may get sued and the plaintiffs may prevail. Some federal agencies see their regulations taken to court with some regularity. For example, the EPA's and OSHA's regulatory products are routinely challenged in court. A health-related regulation issued by the Equal Employment Opportunity Commission was blocked in 2005. The rule would have allowed employers to reduce or eliminate health benefits for retirees when they reached age 65 and became eligible for Medicare. Some 10 million retirees could have been affected by the regulation. The district court ruled that the provision was contrary to congressional intent and the Age Discrimination in Employment Act (Pear, 2005).

Regulations issued by the Bush administration also fell to a court ruling after Bush's presidency had ended. The FDA was ordered by a federal judge to ease availability of the Plan B morning-after birth control pill. Women age 17 and older must be allowed to obtain the pill over the counter without a prescription. The judge ruled that the agency in its 2006 regulations had bowed to political pressure from the Bush administration when it set the age limit at 18. The judge gave the agency 30 days to comply (Singer, 2009b).

Where the Rubber Hits the Road

Simply issuing regulations does not get an agency home free. Bureaucrats must encourage, cajole, and otherwise urge the entities to which the money will flow for the provision of service to act in an expeditious way faithful to the law and regulations. Sometimes, getting a high level of compliance is not easy. Because much of the money goes to state and local governments, they are the primary focus of much of this activity. Control by the federal bureaucracy over state and local officials is quite limited. Washington agencies can urge and educate their state and local counterparts, provide them with financial incentives, or threaten them with the loss of federal grant money, but they cannot force perfect compliance or timeliness. The relationship can best be described as bargaining: by offering a grant, the federal government achieves only the opportunity to bargain with the states: "Instead of a federal master dangling a carrot in front of a state donkey, the more apt image reveals a rich merchant haggling on equal terms with a sly, bargain-hunting consumer" (Ingram, 1977, 499). What the "consumer" can shop around for is a better political deal from another part of the federal government—often Congress or the president. (In fact, the opportunity for such relief greatly impedes states' implementation of desired federal activities [Hill & Weissert, 1995].)

Health reform brought about considerable foot-dragging by the states. Several states balked at the expansions in Medicaid included in the health reform law, even though the federal government would pay for most of them for many years. They also balked at the mandate on individuals to buy insurance, and several state attorneys general sued the federal government to bar the mandate from taking effect. Several state insurance commissioners pleaded for more time for their states' insurance companies to comply with the new rule requiring that firms spend 80 percent of their premiums on patient care rather than on administrative expenses, salaries, and profits. Florida's insurance commissioner, one of the complainers, said he got little sympathy from Washington, D.C.: "'amorphous displeasure' with the new requirement is not enough. States must provide concrete examples of adverse effects on the market, if they want relief," he said he was told (Pear, 2010f).

Regulatory Agencies

In addition to "line" agencies within HHS—such as the Social Security Administration, the CDC, and the CMS, whose primary responsibility is program management—there are agencies whose entire role is to regulate economic or social activities. The three main regulatory agencies with authority over health issues are the Food and Drug Administration, the Federal Trade Commission (FTC), and the Occupational Safety and Health Administration. A fourth regulatory agency, the Environmental Protection Agency, deals with environmental issues.

The Food and Drug Administration

The FDA is probably the best-known of the federal health agencies, certainly of the federal regulatory agencies. It regulates food, pharmaceutical drugs, medical devices, and dietary supplements. In the 1980s and 1990s, the FDA was frequently in the news for targeting smoking among young people, the ill effects of passive smoking, and efforts by cigarette makers to hide the adverse effects of their products. In recent years its attention has been on drug safety and, most recently, on bioterrorism. It has around 12,000 employees and a $4 billion budget (Food and Drug Administration, 2011). By one estimate, its jurisdiction covers more than 20 cents of every consumer dollar spent in the United States (Stolberg, 2002). Nearly half of the FDA's employees work in drug evaluation and research.

The FDA's interest in drug safety flows from its establishment in 1906, when one of its top concerns was patent medicines. The 1937 Food, Drug and Cosmetic Act required manufacturers to prove the safety of a drug before the FDA would allow it on the market. In 1958, an amendment to that law, known as the Delaney Amendment for its sponsor Rep. James Delaney (D-NY), required the FDA to bar the use of any food additive that caused cancers in either humans or laboratory animals. In 1992, federal law allowed the FDA to assess user fees on drug companies to reduce the time to review and approve new drugs. In 1997, Congress mandated faster reviews of clinical trials, review of drugs within 60 days of submission of an application, and reporting of the recommendations of advisory panels within 90 days of receiving applications.

The FDA is no stranger to controversy. Given its nature as an agency whose decisions are broad and interests are narrow, this makes sense. Its mission is to ensure the safety of the nation's food and drugs, but in doing so it must regulate some of the most powerful companies and interests. The battles are many over genetically modified foods, regulation of cigarettes, dietary supplement labeling, and prescription drug safety.

Since the 1990s, battles have been waged between companies wanting to produce genetically modified foods and consumer groups that oppose those foods. The latter group has generally lost, but often in a noisy fashion. In 1992 (at the strong urging of President George H. W. Bush), the FDA ruled that genetically modified food products would be treated no differently than foods produced through traditional methods. The decision was especially controversial because it was against the advice of nearly two-thirds of the FDA's own scientific panel, and later congressional reports criticized FDA oversight of genetically modified food products as too lax.

Under a Democratic administration little changed. In 1993, FDA rules required the industry to keep the agency informed of new products but did not require firms to label products as genetically modified. In 1994 the FDA banned farmers from labeling milk as free from a genetically modified growth hormone that is used to increase milk production. In 2000 the agency required companies to notify it within 120 days if a genetically modified food was going to market. Although a survey of consumers in 2000 found that an overwhelming majority were in favor of mandatory labeling of genetically modified foods, there is still no policy (Byrne, 2011).

The debate continued into the Obama administration. In 2010, the seafood industry introduced genetically modified salmon, bred with a growth hormone gene designed to make the fish reach full size in 16–18 months rather than two years. Tests presented to the FDA by the industry claimed that the new fish were indistinguishable from the old ones in taste, texture, color, and nutritional content. Consumer advocates cried foul, charging that sample sizes for the tests were so small that they could not possibly have tested for the allergic reactions many Americans have to one or another seafood. Critics saw the battle as a watershed, anticipating that if the salmon were approved for marketing unlabeled, other species would follow. Next would be cows genetically modified to resist mad cow disease, "enviropigs" (they produce less polluting manure), or other changed beasts. Experts debated whether FDA had the legislative authority to alter past practice, which favored no label and no restrictions on sales (Pollack, 2010).

The FDA has regulated the advertising of prescription drugs since 1962. In 1982 it declared a moratorium on direct-to-consumer advertising. Three years later, it lifted the moratorium but stipulated that ads directed at consumers must meet the standards required for information targeted to professionals. In 1997 the FDA allowed prescription drugs to be advertised on television and radio along with a list of major health risks associated with each drug. In 2004 the agency recommended that the ads describe the side effects in formats that are easy to read and understand (Michigan Consumer Health Care Coalition, 2005). By 2009 the industry had overstepped its new grant of authority. Bayer HealthCare

Pharmaceuticals promoted its birth control pill, Yaz, on popular prime-time shows like *Grey's Anatomy*. This was an unlikely venue for prescription drug ads, which typically dominate the commercial breaks on evening news shows watched by an elderly population. Bayer's ads left the impression that Yaz could help young women with menstrual problems, acne, and mood shifts. The FDA ordered the company to revise its ads, which subsequently told viewers, "The FDA wants us to correct a few points in those ads" (Singer, 2009a).

Off and on during its existence, the FDA has been accused of being captured by the pharmaceutical industry. In recent years the criticisms have arisen again. Indeed, the number of FDA warning letters to drug companies about inappropriate advertising fell from a peak of 157 in 1998 to 23 in 2004. And in the next five years, the FDA intervened in several product liability cases, arguing that the drug companies should not be held accountable for patients' being unaware of adverse side effects not mentioned on drug labels (Adams, 2005b). The FDA has actively fought reimportation of drugs from Canada and Europe—to protect the nation from possibly unsafe drugs or to protect the drug industry from lower-priced competition.

The FDA has often had an adversarial relationship with Congress, which has watched over its decisions, and its budget, very carefully. One reason for the skeptical treatment might be that, unlike the budgets for other health agencies, the FDA budget is approved by the agriculture appropriations committees—thus competing for funding with crop insurance, commodity price supports, and other agricultural issues.

The FTC, OSHA, and the EPA

The Federal Trade Commission was established in 1914 to prohibit unfair competition and prevent unfair and deceptive trade practices. In health, the agency battles anticompetitive restraints in the health care market and challenges false and misleading health care claims. Its June 2010 report on its antitrust actions in health care and health care products runs to 125 pages of recent cases in which it filed a complaint, sought an injunction, exacted a compliance order, defended its actions against a producer or provider in court, or filed an amicus curiae brief with the court in support of one side or the other (Meier, Albert & Brau, 2010). Cases ranged widely against drugmakers, hospitals, drugstore chains, physicians, chiropractors, home therapy providers, and others. Typical cases charged that if a chain hospital or drugstore took over a competitor, there would be too large an increase in the firm's share of the local market.

The Occupational Safety and Health Administration was established in 1970 with passage of the Occupational Safety and Health Act. Its director also holds the title of assistant secretary of labor. OSHA's rulemaking power is broader than that of most other regulatory agencies. For example, OSHA can adopt temporary emergency rules outside the Administrative Procedures Act procedures, and in its first two years it was allowed to promulgate consensus industry standards as rules (Meier, 1985). OSHA may undertake rulemaking processes on its own initiative or in response to an individual petition.

OSHA is a federal agency that Democrats love and Republicans hate. Democrats think OSHA protects working men and women, and Republicans think it targets businesses and treats them unfairly. In its early years, OSHA concentrated mainly on safety issues, until a House committee directed the agency to shift its emphasis from safety to health standards enforcement (Thompson, 1983). The relationship of OSHA with Congress and businesses has been rocky. In OSHA's first six years, about 100 bills were introduced each year that would have restricted the agency, many involving exemptions of farms and other small businesses from OSHA rules.

OSHA fared very poorly in the Reagan and George H. W. Bush administrations, which targeted the agency for cuts and reduction in its monitoring activity. However, under the Clinton administration, the agency stepped up its enforcement of workplace safety laws and strongly supported a major revision of the Occupational Safety and Health Act, the first since its initial passage in 1970. With a Republican administration and a Republican House in 2001, OSHA once again became the focus of efforts to reduce its scope and reach, but the efforts were unsuccessful in the Senate. OSHA instead moved toward more voluntary compliance and partnership programs with small businesses, corporations, and industries, including the construction industry.

In 2010 one of OSHA's key concerns was with the exposure of workers in the workplace to infectious disease. Mine safety found a place on the agenda as well, following mine accidents in West Virginia and Utah. International attention to the issue arose after the Chilean mine collapse in which 23 miners were trapped below ground for months. While OSHA jurisdiction is limited to the United States, the drama of the trapped miners tended to focus attention on mine safety, already a concern here.

Regulation of environmental hazards and pollution comes from the Environmental Protection Agency, which regulates air pollution, water pollution, hazardous wastes, and pesticides. The EPA, like the FDA, is a highly visible, important agency that affects businesses, environmental proponents, energy interests, states and localities, and the general public. Under Democratic administrations, the agency often runs afoul of business and energy interests. Under Republican administrations, the critics are largely states and localities and environmentalists. The Obama administration's EPA sported a long list of issues of concern to the agency, which was headed by a very activist administrator. The list included drinking water, water pollution, wetlands, watersheds, air pollutants, home air and radiation, climate policy, carbon footprints, toxins, solid waste, superfund sites, brownfields, oil spills, toxic substances in the home, recycling and reuse, residential water conservation, green buildings, smart growth, green communities, energy efficiency, fluorescent light bulbs, green power, indoor air pollution, health risk assessment, ecosystems, noise pollution, and more.

The Many Masters of the Bureaucracy

In recent years, political scientists have argued among themselves about the source of bureaucratic accountability and control. Some (Calvert, Moran & Weingast, 1987; Fiorina, 1981; Weingast & Moran, 1983) have argued that Congress is the real master of the bureaucracy. Its long-standing ability to authorize programs, appropriate agency funding, approve executive appointments, and monitor activities has been amplified in recent years by its tendency to micromanage the implementation of programs through detailed legislation. Thus, say these scholars, Congress is clearly chief puppeteer, holding most of the strings. A counterargument is that the president is the primary overseer of the bureaucracy, through the appointment process and budgetary and regulatory direction (Moe, 1985; Rockman, 1984; West & Cooper, 1989–90). Others have argued that the existence of so many masters undercuts the power of any one and that the bureaucracy is relatively autonomous because Congress and the president are simply too busy or too bored to adequately oversee its activities (Wilson, 1989).

Hammond and Knott (1996) concluded that there are conditions for which each argument seems to fit. One institutional actor cannot determine the policy outcome, they argued; rather, the results are the product of interactions among the president, the House, the Senate, and the congressional committees.

The Bureaucracy and Congress

Congress is important to federal agencies because it authorizes the legislation that sets up the programs, outlines the duties of the federal bureaus, and appropriates funds to carry out the programs and staff the agencies. With these laws, Congress must decide how much discretion to give agencies—whether to "hardwire" or "softwire" the process (Epstein & O'Halloran, 1994). When Congress hardwires the program, it provides detailed directions to the agency; when it softwires, it gives the agency considerable discretion in carrying out Congress's will. Either way, the idea is to curb bureaucratic "drift," the gradual shift of the bureaucracy's activities away from the original congressional intent.

Congress can provide oversight in two ways. In setting up the agency, key and enabling coalitions can make certain structural choices and arrangements to ensure that current and predicted future needs are met. These choices, in turn, affect the ability and willingness of future legislators to influence the administration to further their own ends (Horn, 1995). This is called an ex ante approach. Congress can also conduct ex post activities that change the authorization or appropriations in ways that best suit the congressional interests of the moment. The problem with this second approach is that the transaction costs are very high. Congress might find it more efficient to set up an agency agenda "to perform like on automatic pilot," making precisely those decisions it desires (Calvert, Moran & Weingast, 1987, 500). Congress does not have to closely monitor or scrutinize agency proceedings.

Congress does not speak with one voice, and often in the clash of ideas, the bureaucracy is caught in the crossfire when the 535 elected officials who make up Congress choose to act in their own self-interest—apart from the institutional function of oversight. These individual choices of legislators to engage in agency oversight are less studied and understood. Hall and Miler (1999) argued that these individual actions are taken, often in the form of signals to the agency, to aid supportive interest groups. Sometimes these signals are subtle, such as letters to agency heads, and sometimes they are played out in hearings and in the press. Personalities can come into play as well. Alabama Republican Richard Shelby in 2010 put a hold on all of President Obama's nominations because he was frustrated with the failure to award a military contract that would have produced jobs in his state. His holds meant that each of 70 nominations would require 60 votes, necessitating some Republican support, which was unlikely to come. "It boggles the mind to hold up qualified nominees for positions that are needed because he didn't get two earmarks," the president's press secretary said (Phillips & Zeleny, 2010).

For example, the FDA has a long history of attracting congressional wrath, sometimes for being too lenient and sometimes for being too strident (Johnson,

1992). In 2004, Rep. Maurice Hinchey (D-NY) introduced legislation stripping $500,000 from the FDA chief counsel's office budget as punishment for the agency's assertion in numerous court proceedings that its labeling determinations preempted state law. He accused the FDA of using the courts in a "pattern of collusion between the FDA and the drug companies and medical device companies in a way that had never happened before" (quoted in Lasker, 2005). The bill did not go beyond the introduction stage, but the message was sent. In 2005, Sen. Tom Coburn (R-OK) put a hold on the nomination of Lester Crawford as commissioner of the FDA in an effort to make him obey a 2000 law that Coburn had sponsored. The law required the FDA to change condom labels to give more information on the "effectiveness or lack of the effectiveness in preventing" sexually transmitted diseases (Johnson, 2005).

Although the bureaucracy is responsive to the concerns of Congress and others, Congress is often unresponsive to the bureaucracy and unwilling to acknowledge agencies' needs and capabilities. Leaving office at the end of the Bush administration, CMS administrator Kerry Weems lamented the lack of money and staffing given the agency to do its inexorably expanding job. He noted that the agency had fewer employees than it had had a decade before and too little money to pay its bills to providers in a timely fashion (Inglehart, 2009).

Despite its willingness to oversee and even ridicule administrative implementation efforts, Congress does little "up front" to make certain that implementation goes smoothly. As one FDA official noted, "Comforting the bureaucracy isn't very important on the Hill" (quoted in Johnson 1992, 105). Derthick (1990), in a case study of two programs in the Social Security Administration, highlighted the congressional lack of concern over administrative problems. Congress has little interest in the capabilities of the implementing agency or department or in problems that might arise between agencies or between a federal agency and its state and local counterparts. "It does not occur to presidential and congressional participants that the law should be tailored to the limits of organizational capacity. Nor do they seriously inquire what the limits of that capacity might be" (184). Congress changed its mind several times in the months preceding implementation of the Supplemental Security Income (SSI) program. On December 31, 1973, the day before the law was to take effect, the president signed a bill that increased benefits and changed the program for a last time before the checks were mailed.

Sometimes Congress seems to act as though it wants its agencies to fail. Kerwin (2003) gave one example. The Department of Transportation, which was assigned the task of establishing mandatory alcohol testing for public transportation workers, was denied additional funds or personnel for that purpose. When the department sought to get another agency to loan some of its staff for the effort, the House Appropriations Committee intervened, pressuring the second agency to rescind its offer of help. Why? Congress wanted to show Transportation that it was serious when it said it would provide no more money to the agency. Apparently, what was right for the country was not necessarily right for these senators' states—making implementation more difficult.

The Bureaucracy and the Presidency

One of the assignments given to the president in the Constitution is to make certain the laws are faithfully executed, notably by the bureaucracy. The president can do this in several ways. The first, and perhaps most important, is through the appointment of agency leadership. Second, the president has some leverage over agencies through the development of his budget—although Congress is free to ignore the president's budget and often does. The president has leverage in an agency's priorities, and its goals are expected to reflect those of the president. An agency will generally want to receive a maintenance, if not increasing, budgetary allocation, and so, with some exceptions at the individual level, the agency leadership brings its considerable weight to bear in testimony and meetings with Congress to pursue a program favored by the president. Finally, the president has leverage over agencies through the role of White House staff, particularly the Office of Management and Budget. The OMB oversees the issuance of regulations and agency policies that affect the budget.

Selection of agency heads can be difficult if the policy positions they have taken in the years before appointment invite controversy, or if their remarks can be construed to be controversial, whether they intended them that way or not. CMS administrator candidate Donald Berwick, a nationally regarded expert on health care quality reform, was accused by Republicans of advocating health care rationing. In fact, what he said was: "The decision is not whether or not we will ration care—the decision is whether we will ration with our eyes open" (Pear, 2010b). He went on to explain that insurance companies make arbitrary decisions every day about what care to deny. He'd prefer to see those decisions made out in the open according to effectiveness and efficiency criteria. This explanation was not enough for Senate Republicans, who steadfastly opposed him. He served in an interim capacity for 17 months but ultimately left Washington when he was unable to achieve Senate confirmation.

The relationship between the president and the federal bureaucracy is often adversarial, at least on the part of the president. Harry Truman was reported to have complained, "I thought I was President but when it comes to these bureaucrats, I can't do a damn thing" (Nathan, 1983, 3). Richard Nixon in his second term tried to control the bureaucracy by putting Nixon loyalists in key policy-making roles in federal agencies. Ronald Reagan adopted a jigsaw-puzzle management approach, whereby information was given to career bureaucrats only in pieces so they would not be able to see the larger picture (Pfiffner, 1987). There has also been a trend toward installing political appointees further and further down the policy chain as a way of ensuring compliance (Rourke, 1991). But there is little evidence of deliberate bureaucratic sabotage. Rather, career bureaucrats tend to want to please newly elected presidents, even those with whom they may not agree. As James Wilson (1989, 275) put it, "What is surprising is not that bureaucrats sometimes can defy the President but that they support his programs as much as they do."

Of course, presidents can take a proactive role in setting up offices and using bureaucrats to advance campaign promises or dearly held policy goals. For example, George W. Bush set up new faith-based offices in 5 federal agencies nine days after his inauguration. Subsequent executive orders added offices in 10 more agencies, each with a director and staff and with a mission to increase the capacity of faith-based organizations to compete for grants at all levels of government. Administrative rules were issued to overturn restrictions on religious institutions receiving federal dollars, on the use of government money to build and renovate places of worship, and on using religious beliefs as a criterion for recruiting and retaining staff (Gais & Fossett, 2005).

Once a measure becomes law, the president's interest often wanes. Only on rare occasions—for example, when a regulation is controversial, highly valued by an important interest-group ally, or potentially counter to other goals, such as cost cutting—will the president get involved in writing regulations or other implementation processes. There are some exceptions, however. Jimmy Carter, in 1978, concerned about inflation, ordered a weakening of the regulations protecting workers from cotton dust (Thompson, 1983, 22). Similarly, the Reagan and Bush administrations of the 1980s were concerned about the impact of environmental and health regulations on businesses. President Clinton took on implementation of S-CHIP as a major focus—meeting with governors, setting up high-level interagency task forces, using the media to highlight the importance of the issue, and offering technical assistance to states in signing up children for S-CHIP and Medicaid.

Although the bureaucracy is clearly in the domain of the president, savvy bureaucrats cultivate congressional leaders of both parties. "Every program I had was bipartisan," said former HHS secretary Donna Shalala. "I was passionate about supporting the President's policies but I was bipartisan in administering the department" (CMS, 2005). She also said she always made it a point to get to White House meetings early so she could make and keep friendly relations with the staff there, knowing that they could make or break her policy initiatives.

Yet political bosses do interfere with the FDA. To the shock of liberal supporters, in 2011 HHS secretary Kathleen Sebelius—to whom the FDA administrator reports—overruled the FDA's recommendation to permit the "morning after" pill to be sold on open drugstore shelves to girls of any age without a prescription. The secretary averred that the industry had not proved that young teens would be able to take the drug safely. Critics charged that no other over-the-counter drug had been put to such a test. The secretary's action to overrule the FDA—which makes its decisions after careful consideration and consensus by an expert advisory scientific panel—set a precedent. No other president had acted to overrule the FDA on one of its recommendations (Edney and Armstrong, 2011).

The Bureaucracy and the Courts

The judiciary plays an important role in bureaucratic policymaking, a relationship that Judge David Bazelon called "an involuntary partnership" (Rosenbloom, 1981, 31). The courts oversee bureaucratic actions to make certain they are not violating due process, legislative intent, individual liberties, or equal protection of the law. Many regulatory agencies spend years developing legal theories, collecting data, and preparing analyses that will stand up in court.

In the past few decades, courts have stepped up their oversight of administrative regulatory decisions, often questioning both the process and the substance of administrative activities, abandoning their traditional deference to bureaucratic expertise. One example is a 1999 U.S. Court of Appeals ruling that prevented the U.S. Agency for International Development from forcing U.S. organizations receiving its grants to pledge their opposition to prostitution. The court ruled that the order exceeded the agency's statutory authority and violated the organizations' constitutional free-speech protections. Grant recipients feared the pledge would prevent sex workers around the globe from working with them to prevent the spread of AIDS and other sexually transmitted diseases (Human Rights Watch, 2011).

Here the court was quite clear in its reasoning that the agency had misread the law. Yet the courts' role in interpreting and directing the agencies toward how best to conform to the law is criticized by some as muddled. Agencies prefer a steady and predictable line of decisions from the courts so that they know both how to avoid trouble and how to prepare their defense when they think they might be moving too close to the line. They rely on the doctrine of *stare decisis,* which roughly translates into "let the decision stand" and refers to the expectation that the courts will feel themselves bound by prior rulings and the theories they reflect.

For the states, one of the most troublesome court rulings concerns the interpretation of the federal Employee Retirement Income Security Act. The courts have ruled that the 1974 law preempts state laws that relate to employee benefit plans, including their health coverage. However, recent court cases have narrowed the sweep of the ERISA preemption, making it clear that ERISA does not preempt all types of state health care legislation. A Supreme Court case in 2004 was a setback in some ways. The Court overturned a Texas law that allowed enrollees of HMOs and other insurers to sue in state court, claiming that ERISA preempts the state law (Butler, 2004).

But the states are just as likely to turn to the courts seeking a mandate directed at a bureaucratic agency that they feel is not acting aggressively enough. In 2007 the Supreme Court overruled lower courts and blatantly rebuked the Bush administration's EPA's interpretations of the Clean Air Act. The agency had concluded that its statutory authority did not extend to regulation of greenhouse gases: tailpipe emissions, thought to account for about one-fourth of all heat-trapping gases (Greenhouse, 2007). The states (Massachusetts, California, and others, as well as environmental protection groups) felt the law clearly gave EPA the needed authority. The argument came down to whether or not carbon dioxide should be considered a "pollutant" within the broad meaning of the Clean Air Act. The court majority saw it as not a close call. "The statutory text forecloses E.P.A.'s reading," Justice John Paul Stevens asserted in the majority opinion, noting that such gases are acknowledged even by the EPA to cause global warming. They "fit well within the Clean Air Act's capacious definition of air pollutant," his majority opinion added (ibid., 1).

An interesting sidelight of the ruling was the minority opinion, however. The 5-4 ruling rejected the minority opinion that the court had no business evaluating the validity of the EPA's statutory interpretation. The minority argued that states and others in the suit should be seeking their remedy from Congress and the executive branch, not the courts.

While the states and environmentalists hailed the decision, nonetheless, by 2009, the EPA had not acted to change its rulings, hoping instead that Congress would obviate the need for agency rule-making as Congress and the nation took up a debate over whether or not to adopt a cap-and-trade approach to regulating greenhouse gases. Under such a strategy, industries are awarded a number of pollution permits loosely related to their current contribution to air pollution. Clean plants can sell theirs to dirty plants, forcing dirty plants to choose between the price of the permits and the cost of installing cleanup equipment and adding cleanup procedures to their plant operations.

Agencies are not simply victims of the courts; they also use the courts to uphold their pronouncements or punish those who violate federal regulations. The EPA, for example, has brought civil suits against companies that fail to comply with the Clean Air Act. Some state agencies use the courts to get increased funding from their legislatures (Rosenberg, 1991). If agency directors' pleas for more money for a program fall on deaf ears in the legislative appropriations process, they may encourage a court order mandating spending to ameliorate the situation with the needed funds.

The Health Bureaucracy

The primary health agency in the federal government is the Department of Health and Human Services. At least 15 other federal agencies also have health care–related outlays. HHS controls over one-quarter of all federal outlays, up from just over 3 percent of the U.S. budget in 1961 thanks largely to the growth of Medicare and Medicaid expenditures. In 2011, HHS's budget was more than $911 billion (excluding Social Security), of which at least 85 percent was spent on health. The HHS budget was projected to pass $1 trillion in 2014. HHS administers the two largest categories shown in figure 4.2 (Medicare and Medicaid) and most of the "other mandatory programs" category, which includes everything from the federal employees' health program (which HHS does not administer) to maternal and child health, information technology, programs directed to rural areas and public hospitals, and immunizations and epidemiology.

The oldest federal health agency is the Public Health Service, whose lineage dates back to the 1798 Marine Hospital Service. It became the PHS in 1912. The

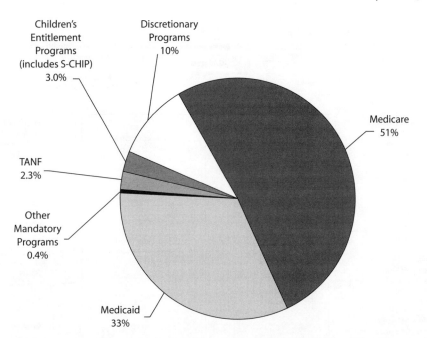

Figure 4.2. HHS 2011 expenditures by category. *Source:* Advancing the Health, Safety and Well-Being of Our People: FY 2011 President's Budget for HHS, p. 1, www.hhs.gov/asfr/ob/docbudget/2011budgetinbrief.pdf.

agency was originally concerned with the provision of medical care to merchant seamen and later took over the responsibility for quarantining people who had infectious and communicable diseases. The PHS is no longer a department within HHS but a unit under the assistant secretary for health (see the HHS organizational chart, fig. 4.3). Other early federal health agencies were the National Hygienic Laboratory, established in 1887 (which became the National Institutes of Health in 1930); the Food and Drug Administration, established by law in 1907; and the Children's Bureau, established in 1912. These early agencies were primarily concerned with public health. The interest in children's issues— evidenced by establishment of the Children's Bureau and passage of the Sheppard-Towner Act of 1922, providing funding to states for personal health services to pregnant women and to children—was a turning point in the federal government's duties and responsibilities, a turn away from public health and toward personal health services.

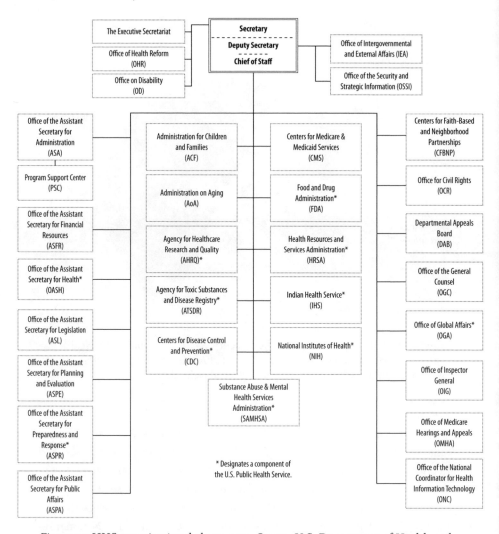

Figure 4.3. HHS organizational chart, 2011. *Source:* U.S. Department of Health and Human Services, www.hhs.gov/about/orgchart.

Until the 1950s the United States had no overall, comprehensive health agency but rather departments operating independently, reporting to Congress and the White House. The Department of Health, Education, and Welfare was created in 1953. President Truman had attempted to create this consolidated agency for several years but had been thwarted by interest groups, including the American Medical Association. The AMA agreed not to oppose HEW when President

Eisenhower promised that the government would "stay out of medical affairs" and that the AMA could choose the department's special assistant for medical affairs (Harris, 1966, 65).

The Health Care Financing Administration was created in 1977 to combine Medicare and Medicaid under one administrative agency. In 1980, HEW became the Department of Health and Human Services, when the Department of Education was created. In 2001 HCFA was renamed the Centers for Medicare and Medicaid Services.

Today's HHS has a workforce of 72,923 full-time equivalents and is made up of 11 major line agencies, each with a set of programs authorized in legislation. Overall, the programs total more than 300 (HHS, 2011). They range from the large and highly visible—including the Centers for Medicare and Medicaid Services, the Food and Drug Administration, and the National Institutes of Health—to those less well-known to the public and to Congress, such as the Agency for Healthcare Research and Quality, the Substance Abuse and Mental Health Services Administration, and the Health Resources and Services Administration. The largest of these agencies is the CMS (until 2001 the HCFA); it oversees the Medicare and Medicaid programs, which provide benefits for more than 85 million people, and, with the HRSA, administers the State Children's Health Insurance Program.

Although the CMS is the largest of the agencies within HHS, it is also the one most disliked by Congress and the president. In part this is because of the arcane rules that surround Medicare and Medicaid. "The legislation . . . for HCFA, is essentially flawed," said Donna Shalala, former head of HHS. "It's contradictory, it's rigid, and they [Congress and the president] blamed HCFA for what was a bad piece of legislation" (CMS, 2005).

Among the federal health agencies, the CMS is by far the biggest spender, by itself accounting for outlays of more than $808 billion in fiscal year 2011 for Medicare, Medicaid, S-CHIP grants to states, fraud and abuse control, and administrative expenses. The distant second in health agency spending is the NIH, the principal biomedical research agency of the government, with appropriations of more than $32 billion in fiscal year 2011. The NIH is made up of a director's office and 27 institutes and centers, ranging from the National Cancer Institute, authorized in 1937, to the National Center on Minority Health and Health Disparities and the National Institute of Biomedical Imaging and Bioengineering, both established in 1981.

The National Cancer Institute is the oldest institute, predating the formation of the NIH itself by seven years. Its organization is more autonomous than that of the other institutes, with the director reporting directly to the president, through the OMB, bypassing the NIH director and the HHS secretary (Epstein, 1979). The unusual organizational system was put in place by 1971 federal legislation launching a national effort to cure cancer. As Samuel Epstein noted in *The Politics of Cancer*, the effort was sold to Congress in a campaign that claimed the cure for cancer was imminent and only a massively funded national effort was needed to conquer the disease by America's 200th birthday. The National Cancer Institute's autonomy was so important that it needed to be "removed from the 'bureaucracy' of NIH" and be free to find the cure for cancer (Epstein 1979, 326). This organization suited President Nixon, who was suspicious of federal agencies and preferred a direct relationship with the rejuvenated and well-funded agency. The National Cancer Institute remains the only institute directly accountable to the president. The cure for cancer still evades us.

One of the most recent changes in the federal health agencies was the recasting and restructuring of the National Center for Health Services Research, first in 1989 into the Agency for Health Care Policy and Research, with a new mission, then in 1999 into the Agency for Healthcare Research and Quality, again with a new mission. The Agency for Health Care Policy and Research was formed to showcase and more generously fund health services research on the outcomes of diagnostic and therapeutic interventions. One of its most controversial concerns was the development of clinical practice guidelines, a task that soon ran into political problems when the agency issued a set of guidelines for the public in December 1994 saying, in effect, that most of the back surgery performed in the United States was unnecessary. In 1996, the agency ended its clinical guidelines program.

The new agency title, Agency for Healthcare Research and Quality, includes the word *quality* to highlight its new responsibility to coordinate all federal quality-improvement efforts and health services research, and it drops *policy*, which the agency thought created the misconception that it determined federal health care policies and regulations. The agency's restated mission is "to improve the quality, safety, efficiency, and effectiveness of health care for all Americans" (AHRQ, 2006).

Reflective of the American health care system's preoccupation with medical interventions—despite the fact that most morbidity and mortality is due to lifestyle choices and socioeconomic precursors—one of the smaller budgets of a health agency is the CDC's; it had a mere $6.3 billion in 2011. The agency started in 1946 with 400 employees and concentrated primarily on malaria, mostly using DDT. It now bills itself as "the nation's premier health promotion, prevention, and preparedness agency and a global leader in public health" (CDC, 2011b). Its nationwide and worldwide mission charges it to

- monitor health,
- detect and investigate health problems,
- conduct research to enhance prevention,
- develop and advocate sound public health policies,
- implement prevention strategies,
- promote healthy behaviors,
- foster safe and healthful environments, and
- provide leadership and training.

Working with national and international partners, the CDC collects health and behavior data at the county and state levels as well as conducting surveys of households representative of the nation's population to monitor changing health status. Housed principally in Atlanta, with offices in Washington, D.C., and elsewhere, it has more than a dozen centers within its organizational structure, ranging from centers on global health, infectious disease, HIV/AIDS, viral hepatitis, sexually transmitted disease and tuberculosis prevention to centers for chronic disease, environmental hazards, and prevention of birth defects, among others. Despite its very limited budget, it was a key player in identifying the viral nature and key behaviors that led to HIV/AIDS infections in the earliest days of the pandemic, when the National Cancer Institute was the lead agency for the problem because it was widely thought to be a form of cancer.

Conclusion

In the United States, unlike in many other countries, a life of public service in the executive branch has never been highly regarded. Rather, bureaucrats are often the butt of jokes, cartoons, and snide remarks from friends, family, and customers. Nevertheless, bureaucrats are key actors in forming, implementing, and evaluating policy, in health as in almost every other area of public concern. Bureaucrats provide the expertise and institutional history that are essential to Congress and the presidency, which may have ideas but little sense of how they might actually work in the real world.

The linkage that bureaucrats provide between truth and power is essential. Nevertheless, the health bureaucracy, like its legislative and presidential counterparts in other areas, is suffering under a public skepticism about government and government programs. Its role as scapegoat, especially useful to members of Congress, state legislators, and presidential candidates, has hurt the health bureaucracy in the public's perception. Many people worry that the unattractiveness of the public sector will repel the best and brightest young people and lead to a weakening of government expertise. With so many baby boomers nearing retirement, these concerns may be realized very soon. Nor is the situation helped by frequent hiring freezes and periodic reductions in force that plague the agencies from election cycle to election cycle.

In health, bureaucrats have helped draft major legislation such as Medicare and Medicaid; HHS was the lead agency for passage of President Obama's Patient Protection and Affordable Care Act; bureaucrats designed and offered solutions such as diagnosis-related groups (DRGs) and resource utilization groups; and they have been responsible for implementing every national health program since 1887. They regulate the operation of the health care industry, safeguard the health of the nation's workplaces, and protect consumers from unsafe foods and drugs. At the state level, they oversee the insurance industry, license health care professionals, and monitor provider services and facilities. Bureaucrats work closely with Congress, the president, and interest groups but are also policy actors in their own right, with their own preferences and goals, their own expertise and political support. Federal bureaucrats are also key intergovernmental actors, working closely with state and local officials and nonprofit groups to achieve policy goals and allocate funding. Some scholars contend that this component of bureaucratic power has strengthened in recent years with increased use of waivers, rules, demonstration projects, and selected interpretations of congressional direction. Gais and Fossett (2005) worry that what they call "executive federalism" can use these tools to pursue presidential goals and build coalitions with political friends at the state level in a way that exploits state differences and political ties to the detriment of broader intergovernmental effectiveness.

Yet the wide availability of expertise, the technological advances that allow members of Congress to obtain data quickly and in an accessible form, the proliferation of specialized health lobbies armed with detailed information and technical analyses, the difficulties in attracting smart new employees, and budgetary constraints—all may adversely affect a stronger bureaucratic role in policymaking.

Political partisans have long recognized the importance of bureaucracy but have often attempted to work around or ignore what they cannot control. Scandals that give rise to questions about the independence of federal agencies from political interests and interest groups are troubling markers of what may be an undermining of the public's and Congress's faith in public servants working in Washington and around the country.

Such cases clearly reflect the downside of a politically responsive bureaucracy. American bureaucrats typically want to please their political masters; they fear consequences to their budgets, staffing, and statutory authority if they show themselves to be too independent. At the lower ranks, just below the top-level political appointees, career bureaucrats are imbued with civil service tenure that in the best of circumstances should steel them against trading their integrity for political favor. Yet even if these rank and file workers risk supervisory wrath and do their jobs as called for, they can be overridden by the departmental secretary or undersecretary or minions of assistant and deputy assistant secretaries who are political appointees put in their jobs because they are in favor and in ideological agreement with the president and his supporters.

Unfortunately, most Americans do not make the distinction between careerist and political appointee among bureaucrats. When an agency's political leaders embarrass it in the news media by failing to show an appropriate level of independence in the face of political pressure, they blemish the reputation of the career bureaucrats who day to day typically do their jobs with the integrity expected of them. The correcting mechanisms are elections, unless someone is willing to bear the burden, the glacial pace, and the uncertainty of a lawsuit to compel bureaucratic action. The disgruntled must work to vote out the president and get a Congress more willing to insist that agency leadership follow the law rather than bend with political winds.

CHAPTER FIVE

States and Health Care Reform

A Look Back

1965

In the early 1960s, state governance was largely embarrassing. Governors were generally elected every two years or were allowed only one four-year term, and they had little power when they did assume office. Thanks to citizens' concerns about vesting too much power in a few persons, states had successfully spread decision making over a spate of agencies, commissions, and boards that were not directly accountable to anyone. When Daniel Evans, on taking office as governor of Washington State in 1965, called a cabinet meeting, 60 people came (Sanford, 1967). Legislatures were even more poorly prepared to deal with state problems. Legislative pay was a pittance, there were no or very few staff members, and the legislature was in session for only a few days every other year. Many states were run by special interests. In some states, railroad interests dominated; in others it was power companies or racetracks, oil or insurance companies.

Cities were often ignored by legislatures composed largely of members representing rural parts of the state. In 1960, more than 6 million people lived in Los Angeles County and fewer than 15,000 lived in a rural county in northern California's mountains, yet each was represented by one state senator. In Vermont, a town with a population of 38 had the same representation as the city of Burlington, with 35,531. Translated into legislative control, 11 percent of the people in California could control the state senate; 12 percent of the people in Vermont could control the state house of representatives (Grant & Omdahl, 1993). The reason for this maldistribution was twofold. First, many states had not changed their legislative district lines, or redistricted, for decades. In 1963, 27 states had not redistricted their legislatures in 25 years, and 8 states had not redistricted in more than 50 years (Sanford, 1967). The Vermont house had not redistricted since 1793. Second, many states copied the federal legislative model, with an upper house based on geographic units; the obvious geographic units were counties, and states often assigned one senator for each county.

State officials often ignored the problems inherent in states' legislative structures. As Sanford (1967, 35, 36–37) put it, "The states . . . have failed to advance with their citizens into the modern world . . . When twentieth-century growth began to overtake us, the machinery of state government was outmoded, revenue resources were outstripped, and the state executive was denied the tools of leadership long supplied the President of the United States."

Despite their lackluster leadership, states were key players in health in the early 1960s, serving as the primary providers of mental health and (with local government) public health services. By 1965, change was in the air. States were scrambling to reapportion their legislative bodies to respond to the U.S. Supreme Court decisions in *Baker v. Carr* (1962) and *Reynolds v. Simms* (1964), which applied the principle of one person, one vote, to both houses of every state legislature. In 1967, more than half the states had constitutional revisions on their ballots to reorganize the legislature, make changes in the executive branch, improve the judicial branch, and change the relationship between the state and local governments.

Between 1965 and 1975, states underwent a remarkable transformation. Their legislative, judicial, and executive offices became vibrant and responsive. Their state employees were energized, and state capitols became places where exciting programs were launched and carried out, thus attracting many of the brightest and best young people to Albany, Lansing, and Tallahassee. Changes were made in state constitutions to unshackle local government and to balance the state's tax system so it would weather economic difficulties and maintain equity among the citizenry. States began to tackle the tough issues they had often avoided in previous years—from the environment to economic development, from education reform to controlling health care costs.

1981

By the start of the 1980s, state legislatures had greatly improved their staffing and more adequately represented all citizens of the state. The legislatures had more women and minorities and, compared with the 1960s, greater partisan competition, with Republicans picking up seats in the South and Democrats in the North. There was a tremendous jump in the number of women serving in state legislatures between 1969 and 1980, from a total of about 300 to nearly 800 (Patterson, 1983). Membership in legislatures for ethnic and racial minority groups also increased during this time, although their proportion of all legislators was small—about 4 percent. State after state strengthened the powers granted to governors, giving them stronger budgetary authority, longer terms of office, and the ability to serve multiple terms, to appoint more cabinet members, and to have a strong line-item veto (Beyle, 1989). Overall, states had made a remarkable, though not widely heralded, recovery in their ability to deal with tough problems. Indeed, in the mid-1980s, the Advisory Commission on Intergovernmental Relations (ACIR) described states as moving from fallen arches to arch supports of the system. The ACIR noted that states were "more representative, more responsive, more activist and more professional in their operations than they ever have been" (ACIR, 1985, 364).

Furthermore, states were becoming the sources of innovative policies, particularly in health. In the 1970s and 1980s, states became concerned about the rapidly increasing costs of health care to their budgets and instituted reforms such as rate-setting systems, negotiated contracting, and diagnosis-related groups. They also adopted risk pools for health insurance, right-to-die acts, and mandatory seat belt laws.

1993

The makeup of state legislatures in 1993 was much more representative of the population in gender and occupation than in earlier decades. More than 20 percent of the 7,424 state legislators were women—five times as many as in the 1960s (Thaemert, 1994). In five states—Arizona, Colorado, New Hampshire, Vermont, and Washington—women held more than one-third of the legislative seats. In others, women were still somewhat rare. In Alabama, Kentucky, Louisiana, Oklahoma, and Pennsylvania, women made up less than 10 percent of the total (that was the percentage of U.S. Congress members in 1993 that were women). But overall, compared with the U.S. House of Representatives and with previous years in the states, female representation in state legislatures in 1994 was greatly enhanced. State legislatures had fewer attorneys, business owners, and farmers than in the 1960s and more legislators whose legislative service was a full-time job. Some 15 percent of all state legislators were full-time—up from 3 percent in 1976.

In 1992, a sitting governor was elected to the presidency—the first time since Governor Franklin Roosevelt was elected in 1932. Bill Clinton, governor of Arkansas, not only understood state governance but also was actively involved as a spokesperson for states through the National Governors Association, which he had headed and for which he served as leader in the development of several policy positions—including those on welfare reform and health care.

States had become increasingly active players in the health care field. Ideas discussed in Washington, D.C., in 1993–94 were already in place in several innovative states; other states were considering ideas such as a single-payer system, generally viewed as too radical for national consideration. The role of states in health care reform was more than a parochial concern; it was a central issue in congressional hearings, news conferences, and Sunday morning television talk shows. Washington clearly could not monitor and implement the program on its own. It needed states.

2009

Although health reform was in the air during the years of run-up to the presidential election, the states had long since grown tired of waiting. They'd heard that kind of reform tempest before, only to be disappointed when nothing happened except that their uninsured population continued to grow. By July 2009, three states had decided to do it themselves, and 14 more were moving in that direction.

Maine, Massachusetts, and Vermont had enacted and were implementing laws that would provide insurance to nearly everyone in their states. Maine had acted so early—2003—that by 2009 it had substantially implemented its plan, covering 23,000 individuals and 725 small businesses, all of whom were voluntarily enrolled. The plan's target date for full implementation had been set at 2009. In 2006, Vermont passed comprehensive reform legislation intended to achieve nearly universal enfranchisement through sliding premium subsidies that would be available to persons with incomes up to 300 percent of the poverty level.

But it was the Massachusetts plan, enacted in 2006, that drew policy attention in 2009, as it became a model copied by national reformers. The Massachusetts plan included both an individual mandate and state-level insurance exchanges, features that were eventually included in the PPACA. By September 2008, the state had enrolled well over 430,000 uninsured individuals.

Other states, including Connecticut, Iowa, Kansas, Minnesota, New Jersey, and New York, expanded insurance to uninsured adults or uninsured children. Their actions and those of Massachusetts, Maine, and Vermont were pathbreaking and bold and highlight the innovativeness possible in a federation such as the United

States. States don't have to wait for permission from the national government to act, and in recent years they haven't.

But 2009 was all about national health reform and the PPACA, signed into law in March 2010. The politics of national health reform—and the state role in it—were fascinating. The associations representing state officials—particularly governors and state legislators—were not active players in the debates, in large part due to the inability to reach bipartisan agreement. But the Republican Governors Association and the Democratic Governors Association had no such constraints; they played an important role informing their federal counterparts on what would work and what would not and serving to help focus public opinion around agreed-upon positions. Also, individual governors lobbied their own senators and house members on what was best for their states (and how their actions would later play out in those states) (Dinan, 2011; Conlan & Posner, 2011).

Governors, state legislators, and other state officials (particularly state insurance commissioners and attorneys general) knew that along with the political clout, they had another card to play. The states would be pivotal in implementing any health reform and in doing so would no doubt determine its success or failure.

Overview

Bold problem-solving in health care is a venerated tradition in the states. States have long had a broad role in health. One analyst called the scope of state activities in the health area "truly awesome and capable of reaching into almost every facet of health care delivery" (Clarke 1981, 61). States are responsible for the funding and coordination of public health functions, the financing and delivery of personal health services (including Medicaid, mental health, public hospitals, and health departments), environmental protection, regulation of providers of medical care and the technology they employ, regulation of the sale of health insurance, rate-setting, licensing, and cost control. States provide health insurance for their own employees and retirees and play a pivotal role in educating and credentialing health care professionals.

State institutions are similar to national entities in their structure and purpose. However, several differences are important in understanding why state and federal policies can be so divergent, including, at the state level, direct democracy, the requirement for a balanced budget, and the very muted role of the press in state capitols. States differ from one another in very significant ways, including their willingness to enact innovative legislation and their implementation of Medicaid programs (Olson, 2010).

Federalism and Intergovernmental Relations

To understand states and health policy, one must understand federalism and the intergovernmental relations that define states' roles and responsibilities in health and other areas.

In its earliest years, the United States was governed by the Articles of Confederation, which set up a weak national government and strong states. The national body (unicameral, with equal representation from the states) had no power to tax, enter into commercial treaties, retaliate against discriminatory foreign trade policies, or enforce the provisions of existing treaties. Congress relied on states to act, and it needed state cooperation to discharge any functions. There was no national government; instead, the United States "consisted solely in the congregation of envoys from the separate states for the accommodation of certain specified matters under terms prescribed by the federal treaty" (Diamond, 1985, 30). The states issued their own money and had their own trade policies with other states. When there were interstate disagreements, Congress was virtually powerless to deal with them.

While acknowledging that the confederation did not work, the delegates to the Constitutional Convention of 1789 were not yet ready to establish a fully national government. They compromised in the wording of the Constitution, which divides responsibilities between the two levels of government. Certain functions, such as interstate commerce and national defense, were assigned to the national government; others, such as the selection of presidential electors who would choose the president, were left to states. The strongest language in favor of states came in the Tenth Amendment: "powers not delegated to the United States by the Constitution, nor prohibited by it to the states, are reserved to the states respectively, or to the people." Yet the Constitution authorizes the national Congress to "provide for the general welfare" and to "make all Laws which shall be necessary and proper" for executing this and other powers given to the legislature. The commerce clause is also crucial: anything defined as interstate commerce, or crossing state lines, is in the federal domain. Finally, the supremacy clause clearly states that if federal and state laws are incompatible, the federal law prevails.

Federalism was the key means by which the Founding Fathers sought to ensure that power would not be concentrated in one set of government officials.

Instead they wanted to establish a balance of powers, so that one level of government would have a "check" against the undue power of another. They set up a system of government in which both governments were sovereign and powerful. As James Madison described it, "The federal and State governments are in fact but different agents and trustees of the people, constituted with different powers and designed for different purposes" (Publius, [1787–88] 1961, 294).

The broad parameters allocating powers between the national and state governments soon led to the important role of the courts in defining those powers. The first major decision on this, *McCullough v. Maryland* (1819), was made when Maryland leaders questioned the power of the federal government to establish a national bank in Baltimore, a power not specifically listed in the Constitution. This celebrated decision established the notion of "implied powers": the national government was not limited to those powers clearly outlined in the Constitution; Congress could also become involved in areas that were "implied" in such vague phrases as "providing for the general welfare" or "necessary and proper." By so broadly construing the intent of the Constitution, the Supreme Court allowed the responsibilities of the federal government to encompass a broad array of activities and programs. Until the 1990s, the Court generally came down strongly on the side of the federal government.

An important point to keep in mind about federalism is that it is a system of rules for the division of public policy responsibilities among a number of autonomous government entities (Anton, 1989). In the United States, these entities are the national and state governments. The autonomous nature of the relationship is crucial: states are not administrative units of Washington, D.C.; rather, they have their own responsibilities and duties, many of them overlapping those of Washington. The relationship was once described as cooperative federalism, with federal and state governments interacting to achieve common goals. The metaphor commonly used is of a marble cake, with the government units representing the halves of the cake and programmatic activities, such as education, welfare, and health, "marbling" through them.

The states were the dominant actors in federalism in the country's first century. With the Civil War came a nationalizing effect, expanded later during Franklin Roosevelt's New Deal and still further by Lyndon Johnson's Great Society. States had become key actors in implementing an activist federal domestic agenda, largely thanks to federal grants that provided incentives for state action in social programs, transportation, urban development, special education, community development, and job training.

Ronald Reagan, in his vision of "New Federalism," preferred a different view of the relationship between federal and state governments. His call for a sorting out of responsibilities, whereby the national government would handle only those functions purely national and the states would handle most other areas, was similar to dual federalism, a system with another cake metaphor: a layer cake, one layer representing the responsibilities of one government, the other layer those of the other government, with little cross-layer mingling. The models differ in the extensiveness of the federal role, but they share the view, established in the Constitution, of state sovereignty.

Federalism has another important policy strength: improving the possibility of policy innovation. States can try out new ideas and techniques or philosophies that, if successful, can later be adopted by other states or on a national scale. Indeed, states are regularly referred to as the "laboratories of democracy." Compared with the federal government, states' smaller size and proximity to the people make them proving grounds for innovations in policy and governance. Moreover, the likelihood of finding a significant innovation is greater with 50 different states devising different policy programs than if we relied solely on the action of one federal government.

The important role of states is established in the U.S. Constitution and ratified by history. As in most dynamic relationships, changes occur over time. In the 1960s and 1970s, Washington was very strong and states rather weak in capacity and resources. In the 1980s and 1990s, the federal government was fiscally constrained with a $3 trillion budget debt, while the states were reasonably fiscally secure and administratively capable of taking on problems, including health care. In the early years of the twenty-first century, states were constrained by falling revenues and increasing demands, while Congress, free from pay-as-you-go budget restraints, reduced taxes, increased defense and homeland security spending, and ignored calls for Medicaid reform and fiscal relief. In the second decade of the century, the states continued to be constrained and Washington was beginning to think about living within its means.

Congress and the president cannot "commandeer" states to do anything. However, they can provide incentives through federal grants, or punish states that do not act in a desired way by withdrawing federal dollars, or simply preempt state actions. Preemption must be based on some constitutional purpose such as interstate commerce or protecting the public welfare. And preemption is increasingly being used, even by conservative Congresses and presidents.

Federal Grants

During the nation's first century, government at any level did very little. The people did not particularly want government services, and governments had few taxes through which to raise the resources to provide services. The federal government's role was largely restricted to "war and danger" and some limited pork-barrel funding. States were more active, particularly in economic development activities: they built roads and bridges, dredged canals, set forth civil and property rights and family and criminal laws, and provided education (Walker, 2000). For the federal government, a turning point was the imposition of the income tax in 1913; finally, it had resources. And with the coming of the New Deal, Franklin Roosevelt's effort at overcoming the Depression, it also had a cause. The federal government wanted to help citizens find jobs and bring home a salary, setting them on the road to financial recovery. Yet it could not do this solely from Washington. It was easier for Washington to give grants to states and localities so they could provide the services. Thus, in the 1930s the age of the federal grant began. Between 1933 and 1938, 16 federal grant programs were enacted.

Yet not until the 1960s and 1970s did federal grants reach their heyday. Again, the federal government wanted action: to alleviate poverty, to equalize educational opportunities, to clean the nation's air and water, and to ensure adequate health care for underserved populations. But, alas, this too could not be done from Washington. So the 1960s saw Congress enact hundreds of new federal grants: 150 in 1965 alone. Between 1965 and 1970, the dollars provided in federal grants doubled; the total doubled again between 1970 and 1975 and nearly doubled again over the next five years (table 5.1). The growth after 1990 was substantial: an increase of $142 billion between 2000 and 2005 alone. In 2010, federal grants jumped by $180 billion over the 2005 figure, largely from the stimulus program designed to help states suffering from sharp drops in revenues (and increased demands for services) because of the distressed economy. In 2010, grants peaked at 17.6 percent of federal outlays, then dropped to 15.7 percent in FY 2012 when the stimulus funding ended.

Medicaid—the federal-state program for poor children, the disabled, and the elderly—is by far the largest federal grant program, making up 45 percent of federal grants to states and localities. Besides Medicaid, federal grants go to programs ranging from highway beautification to Head Start, from water purification to prevention of terrorism. Federal health programs include block grants for substance abuse, mental health, and maternal and child health; funding for

Table 5.1.   Federal grants, 1965–2012

Year	Amount of grants ($ billions)	Percentage of state & local expenditures	Percentage of federal outlays	Constant dollars, 2005 (billions)	Grants to individuals (% of total)
1965	10.9	15.5	9.2	65.9	34.1
1970	24.1	20.1	12.3	123.7	36.2
1975	49.8	24.0	15.0	186.9	33.6
1980	91.4	27.4	15.5	227.1	35.7
1985	105.9	22.0	11.2	186.9	47.3
1990	135.3	18.9	10.8	198.1	57.1
1995	225.0	22.8	14.8	283.6	64.2
2000	285.9	22.2	16.0	326.8	63.9
2005	428.0	24.5	17.3	428.0	64.0
2010	608.4	n.a.	17.6	527.1	63.2
2012*	584.3	n.a.	15.7	488.4	66.0

Source: OMB, 2011a, table 18-2: Trends in Grants to State and Local Governments.
Notes: n.a., not available.
*Projected.

AIDS programs through the Ryan White Comprehensive AIDS Resources Emergency Act; and funding for antibioterrorism activities. Health grants accounted for nearly half of all federal grants in fiscal year 2012—up from about 6 percent in 1965. (See fig. 5.1.)

Federal grants were a boon to states and localities, since they provided the resources to pay for services that could not be, or would not have been, offered without the additional money. They also helped professionalize state and local workforces in many areas, including health. States increased the salaries of their employees and challenged them with innovative and much needed programs, funded in part by federal dollars. Federal grants also equalized services in a way that states could not accomplish on their own. Medicaid, AFDC, and other federal grants are designed especially to assist poor states or states with poor citizens, which have few natural resources to tax.

Most federal grants are categorical: money provided to states and localities must be used for rather specific functions, from funding clinics for patients with black lung disease to providing curriculum assistance to the health professions. Sometimes the grants are competitive; states and localities submit proposals, and only a small number receive funds. More often, the grants are distributed to all states or localities based on a formula that includes such "need"

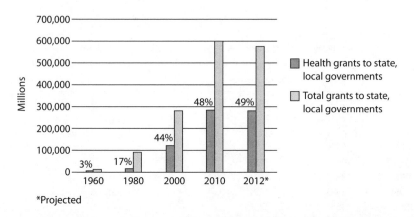

Figure 5.1. Growth in health grants as share of total federal grants to state and local governments. *Source:* OMB, 2011a, table 18-2: Trends in Grants to State and Local Governments. *Projected.

measures as counts of poor persons, rural highways, waterfront land, or dilapidated housing.

In 1966, a new type of grant, the block grant, came into existence. Block grants allowed states and localities more discretion over how the dollars could be used. Typically, Congress would specify the policy area in which the funds could be spent, but the state or locality could decide, within the broad category, which programs best fit their own needs. The first block grant was in health, legislated in the Partnership for Health Act in 1966. Other health-related block grants are for maternal and child health; alcohol and drug abuse and mental health; and preventive health care.

The most recent block grant was the State Children's Health Insurance Program, enacted in 1997. States and localities typically like block grants, but Congress is generally less enthusiastic; it is much harder for members of Congress to take credit for programs funded under this grant device, and oversight is difficult. Block grants usually suffer from these political flaws in their struggle for funding. The substance abuse, mental health, and maternal and child health block grants have not increased substantially since their inception and remain relatively small in dollars. For example, the preventive health block grant funding peaked in 1999, with funding in FY 2010 totaling only $102 million for the 50 states. A Clinton-era block grant, Temporary Assistance for Needy Families (TANF), is a case in point. Congress was unable to come up with a multiyear reauthorization and relied on temporary extensions for more than three years—in the process leaving states and the program recipients with considerable uncertainty. S-CHIP was also mired in politics for its reauthorization in 2007, with stopgap measures funding the program until its final approval—in an expanded form—in 2009.

In 2009–11 the federal government provided a massive stimulus program of short-term funding to states for education, social services, and infrastructure and an increase in Medicaid federal matching funds. The Recovery Act of 2009 funding was designed to "bolster state budgets through the worst of the recession and avoid greater cuts to state services and tax increases (OMB, 2011a, 280). The state fiscal stabilization fund in the Recovery Act provided $53.5 billion in relief, most of it targeted to state and local education programs. The Recovery Act provided $84.5 billion in additional funding through a temporary increase in the federal government's share of Medicaid. A 2010 law extended the enhanced Medicaid funding through mid-2011, providing an additional $14 billion in relief to states (OMB, 2011a, table 18-2).

In 2011, as in earlier years, some attention was given to the possibility of making Medicaid a block grant—giving states a set amount of money and letting them administer the program within those parameters. While often supported by Republicans, including Republican governors, who argue that the flexibility in block grants is key, these proposals seldom advance beyond rhetoric.

In 2010–11 some states, led by Florida, turned down, gave back, or refused to apply for millions of federal grants. In Florida's case, the total was at least $54 million. Florida legislators tied their willingness to leave federal dollars on the table to their ideology in general and the federal suit challenging the constitutionality of PPACA in particular. "The legislature didn't feel it was appropriate to take money from a bill that was unconstitutional," said Republican state representative Mike Horner (Shrieves, 2011). Other states were beneficiaries when the moneys were allocated to them.

Regulatory Federalism

Federal budget deficits, an aging population, projected slow economic growth, and shortfalls in Medicare and Social Security all loom as the nation proceeds through the second decade of the 21st century. Potentially higher taxes and substantial reductions in federal spending raise questions of how the federal government will exercise its role in federalism. The nation has had some experience with similar circumstances and actions that may well foretell the future. When

national lawmakers can't accomplish what they want with spending induce-
ments, they have a tendency to try to do so with regulatory punishments.

In the 1980s, when federal budgetary restraints began to take hold, new
federal grant spending became a liability and federal regulation—whereby states
and localities could be coerced into acting in certain ways—became more appealing. Regulations and requirements have long been a part of federal grants,
going back to the Hatch Act of 1939, which prohibited partisan political activity
by federal employees and by state and local employees funded with federal grant
dollars. The past few decades have seen a new type of regulation, in which Washington enlists state and local governments in national efforts on behalf of particular disadvantaged groups or to advance certain policies, such as environmental
protection. Four types of intergovernmental regulation are popular: crossover
sanctions, partial preemption, direct orders or mandates, and preemption.

Crossover sanctions are regulatory mechanisms that impose a financial penalty in one area based on defects in another. Particularly popular is imposing
penalties in the highway trust fund if states do not make desired federal changes.
Early crossover sanctions dealt with transportation matters (such as lowering
the speed limit and changing the minimum drinking age). Then a second generation of sanctions tied the loss of a state's highway trust-fund moneys to non-
transportation issues such as the control of junkyards and municipal air. One
of the most compelling crossover sanctions called for states to strengthen their
standard for drunk driving or lose 2 percent of their federal highway trust-fund
money. States face well over a dozen different financial penalties under which
they can lose from 5 to 100 percent of their highway trust funds for failure to
comply with federal requirements.

Occasionally the sanction is connected with a non-highway-funding source.
For example, the 1992 Synar Amendment punishes states that do not meet negotiated targets for reducing tobacco sales to minors through a 40 percent reduction in their substance-abuse block grants. A variation on the crossover sanctions
was introduced in 2005, when the Senate version of the highway bill called on
states to adopt stiff penalties for repeat offenders, those with very high blood-
alcohol levels, and those whose licenses had been suspended for drunken driving
but who drove anyway. States that failed to enact legislation setting forth specific
penalties for these three groups would see up to $600 million diverted from high-
way construction to programs aimed at highway safety (Wald, 2005).

With partial preemption, the national government establishes rules and regulations calling for minimum national standards for a program. States can admin-

ister the program if they follow the standards; in states that fail, or do not wish to do so, federal agencies will administer the program. This type of intergovernmental mandate is often used in the environmental area, in laws pertaining to such issues as safe drinking water, surface mining, and clean air. It also applies to state occupational health and safety: half of the states have chosen to administer that program; half have chosen not to do so. The Health Insurance Portability and Accountability Act of 1996 contained partial preemption provisions. The law included new access, portability, and renewability standards for group and individual market insurers. If states did not pass laws that enforced those provisions, the federal Department of Health and Human Services stepped in (Ladenheim, 1997). The PPACA contained a partial preemption regarding the establishment and administration of insurance exchanges. If states act by a given date, they will establish and run these exchanges; if states do not meet that deadline, the federal government will handle exchanges in those states.

In direct orders or mandates, the federal government orders lower governments to take certain types of action. More than 50 percent of all federal statutes preempting state and local authority enacted over the nation's 200-year history were adopted during recent decades. Particularly troublesome for states is the tendency for Washington to mandate without federal financial assistance to pay for the newly required service. Many of these mandates are in the area of environmental protection. Although states pay some of these environmental costs, they mainly shift the burden to local governments. The effect on smaller jurisdictions can be devastating. An Environmental Protection Agency mandate requiring localities to monitor a particular substance in sewage discharge cost a small North Carolina town of 3,000 residents more than $30,000 a year through an increase in their property tax. The 1990 Americans with Disabilities Act is another unfunded mandate that costs states and localities billions of dollars. The Drug-Free Workplace Act of 1988 also imposed substantial costs by requiring all federal grantees and contractors (including, of course, states and localities) to ensure that their workplaces were drug-free and that they offered antidrug programs for employees (Gais & Fossett, 2005). But the largest federal mandate is Medicaid: Congress has substantially broadened the scope and reach of the program over the past decade. Although the federal government shares the cost of Medicaid with the states, changes made in Washington force states to fund their share of the program expansion. While nominally, the states are acting voluntarily, since they are not obligated to participate in the Medicaid program, realistically, they are far too committed to the services it pays for to back out now; this means they must accept changes forced upon them by the federal government.

Congress at times feels guilty about its heavy-handed conduct and vows to do better. One of the first measures to pass the Republican-controlled Congress in 1995 was a bill to limit unfunded mandates. The 1995 law provided that any proposed bill is out of order if it will cost state and local governments more than $50 million. But alas, the provision can be overruled with a majority vote. And mandates in place in 1995 were not affected by the law. Though clearly a step forward, in the opinion of many state and local officials, the law does not guarantee that unfunded federal mandates will end; in fact, as many as two-thirds of the major mandates that Congress imposes on states are exempt from the law. Also, one assessment of the early implementation of the measure found that passage of significant new mandates and preemptions continued. State and local governments' biggest success may have been in changing how the mandates were to be implemented rather than whether they should be enacted (Posner, 1997).

While states complain about mandates, there is some evidence that they respond to them more than to incentives such as grant funding. Sometimes lesser approaches also work. The federal government can "signal" to states to act, through messages and instructions. CMS officials were often very engaged with their state counterparts to instruct them on legal ways of maximizing Medicaid access and even promising lenient treatment in the federal quality-control process for states' mistakes in determining Food Stamp eligibility. Gais and Fossett (2005) reported that not all states responded to these efforts, but many did, and enrollments rose quickly.

Finally, the federal government can simply take over a state function or preempt the states. Over the eight years of the G. W. Bush administration, there were 57 preemption votes in Congress, in areas including air pollution, contaminated food, and the regulation of the Internet. One of the preemptions concerned specific types of medical liability involving prescription drugs and medical devices. The Justice Department contended that consumers cannot recover damages for injuries from vaccines and medical devices approved by the FDA. While the administration initially said that FDA approval set the minimum standard and that states could provide "additional protection to consumers," in 2004 the Justice Department argued that FDA approval "set a ceiling as well as a floor"—preempting a state law or state court finding that a drug or device is unsafe (Pear, 2004). However, a 2009 U.S. Supreme Court ruling (*Wyeth v. Levine*) rejected the argument of federal preemption, concluding that "it is not impossible for Wyeth (the maker of the drug in question) to comply with its state and federal law obligations" (J. Goldstein, 2009).

In May 2009, President Obama issued a memorandum to federal agencies asking them to proceed with caution before preempting states and requiring agencies to revisit previous regulations of the past ten years. Early in President Obama's term, the administration decided to base new nationwide motor vehicle tailpipe standards for carbon on the state with the strictest standard—California—rather than preempting that state and others that wanted to exceed federal standards (Conlan & Posner, 2011).

Although Republican ideology is typically more supportive of stronger states and a reduced federal government presence, ideology and politics often interfere with federalist beliefs. For example, while President George W. Bush came to the White House directly from the governor's mansion in Texas and, in his campaign, had argued for smaller government, he was strongly supportive of federal legislation to limit jury awards for pain and suffering in medical malpractice court cases. "It's a national problem that requires a national solution," he told a group of health care professionals (Stolberg 2002, A16). Support for this position is especially noteworthy given that more than half of the 25 states with no damage caps have constitutional provisions that bar legislation limiting recoveries by plaintiffs in civil cases (Jost, 2003). Supporters of federal malpractice laws say there are no problems with such preemption in an area where states have traditionally prevailed. They cite the federal government's primacy in interstate commerce as constitutional justification (Adams, 2003a)—an assertion that might be challenged should federal law be enacted. Ironically, the Congressional Budget Office estimates that federal malpractice law reform would save only about 2 percent of total health care spending, largely because most of the proposed reforms have already been enacted by so many states (CBO, 2009a).

Disregard for federalism issues cuts across party lines. In 2005, Democrats sponsored legislation in the Senate to "force" states to report the names of companies with 50 or more employees who received government-funded health care (namely Medicaid). The measure—designed to pressure Wal-Mart to improve employee health coverage—may be politically pleasing to federal legislators, but it flies in the face of federalism. In fact, Maryland enacted a bill that would have required Wal-Mart to spend more on employee health benefits. Similar bills were introduced in several other states (Joyce, 2005).

Most observers of federalism would describe the U.S. model as nationally dominant—that is, that the national government has assumed preemptive power. However, increasing state activism and institutional capacity has given support to the role of states as laboratories of democracy—in health and other policy areas. But the final arbiter of decisions related to which governmental level does what is the U.S. Supreme Court. Since the country's beginning, the Court's decisions have served to shape the contours of federalism and the allocation of power.

The U.S. Supreme Court

By 5-4 majorities, the U.S. Supreme Court, in 1992, began to reconsider the distribution of power between federal and state governments. In *New York v. United States* (1992), the Court resurrected the Tenth Amendment's residual-powers clause to invalidate a provision of a federal law requiring states to "take title" to their low-level radioactive wastes. In a 1995 case, *United States v. Lopez*, the Court failed to buy the notion that a federal law banning the sale of firearms close to school grounds was justified under the interstate commerce clause. It was the first time in six decades that the Court found Congress exceeding its power under the interstate commerce provision. In *Seminole Tribe v. Florida* (1996), the Court defended the sovereign immunity of states by striking down a federal law that authorized private suits against states in federal court (the Eleventh Amendment states that the judicial power of the United States shall not be construed to extend to any suit in law or equity, commenced or prosecuted against one of the United States by citizens of another state). A 1999 ruling in *Alden v. Maine* extended state immunity from private suits to state courts.

Some observers viewed these developments with alarm, as indicating that the Court was committed to expanding state sovereignty at the expense of the federal government's policymaking and enforcement authority. However, others believe the decisions, while important, were more of an adjustment than a "sea change" (Brisbin, 1998). Indeed, the Court did not always rule "in favor" of states. Several examples:

—In *Bush v. Gore* (2000), the Court found in a 5-4 vote that states may not, by later arbitrary and disparate treatment, value one person's vote over that of another, a decision that overruled the Florida Supreme Court and stopped a recount under way that might have resulted in a different president sitting in the Oval Office in 2001 (Savage, 2001).

—In *Tennessee v. Lane* (2004), the Supreme Court upheld Congress's power to subject states to monetary liability under certain provisions of the Americans with Disabilities Act.

—In *Gonzales v. Raich* (2005), the Court ruled that marijuana consumption and cultivation was a matter of interstate commerce, and thus the "necessary and proper" clause authorizes regulation of that commerce even if there is also a purely intrastate noneconomic activity— overturning language in a California statute legalizing medical marijuana use.

What does this mean? It highlights the fact that the Supreme Court, much as the Founding Fathers desired, is the final arbiter of federalism. Sometimes the Court rules mostly in favor of Congress and the federal government, producing a strong national-level voice. Sometimes it rules in favor of states, providing a stronger balance of interest. There is some evidence that the Rehnquist Court rulings in the 1980s and 1990s were designed in part to help balance federal and state interests. Justice Antonin Scalia, among others, has noted the duty of the Supreme Court to maintain "a healthy balance of power between the states and federal government" (Conlan & De Chantal, 2001).

However, under Chief Justice John Roberts, who took over in 2005, the Court has taken a more muted position on federalism issues, particularly those limiting congressional power regarding the commerce clause and the Tenth Amendment. In 2007 the court did issue a ruling of practical federalism importance when it concluded that the federal Clean Air Act gave the EPA authority to regulate carbon dioxide and other greenhouse gases as pollutants. The case, *Massachusetts v. EPA*, was brought by twelve states and several cities to force the agency to enforce the act. This case was followed up by a similar lawsuit charging the EPA with failing to limit greenhouse gas emissions from oil refineries. When the Obama administration came into office in 2009, the EPA became more active in both areas. However, in another case in 2011, the Court ruled against states. In *American Electric Power Co. v. Connecticut*, eight states filed suit against the nation's five largest electric power companies, charging that the companies were a public nuisance by polluting the air and water. The Court threw out the suit, saying it should be decided by the EPA, not the Court (Savage, 2011).

The Court's decisions in 2009 and 2010 regarding the Second Amendment right to bear arms—striking down gun control laws in the District of Columbia and Chicago—were significant to public health and federalism. The 2010 case

(*McDonald v. Chicago*) affirmed that gun ownership is a fundamental right, like freedom of speech, but opponents on the Court feared that the decisions would lead to an "avalanche of litigation" testing whether variations of state and local gun laws would violate this right (Barnes & Eggen, 2010). The Roberts Court has also been strongly supportive of First Amendment rights of free speech in decisions that have an impact on states. In *Citizens United v. Federal Election Commission* (2010) the Court ruled that corporations have a First Amendment right to spend unlimited amounts of money on candidates in elections. Some argue that this opinion opens the floodgates on corporation spending, which was limited in a number of states. In another election-related case, *Arizona Free Enterprise v. Bennett,* the court struck down an Arizona law that provided escalating matching funds to candidates who accept public financing, arguing that the matching provisions adversely affected some candidates' freedom of speech (Liptak, 2011b). And in another First Amendment case in 2011, the Court struck down a California law restricting access of minors to violent video games, arguing that the law violated the free speech of the minors (Liptak, 2011a).

Seminal immigration and health care cases are even more directly related to federalism and the states. Regarding immigration, in 2011, the Court held that states have at least some role to play in the immigration arena, upholding by a 5-4 vote another Arizona law penalizing employers for hiring illegal immigrants. But in a more salient case, the Obama administration filed suit against a sweeping Arizona law that, among other things, permits police to verify a suspect's immigration status during an investigation of a possible criminal violation; police may detain that suspect if the person cannot provide verification of citizenship. The Obama administration has argued that such state actions usurp the federal prerogative to enforce immigration law (Kirkwood, 2011). However, several other states, including Georgia and Alabama, adopted similar immigration measures—arguing that in the absence of strong federal direction, states need to act.

But it was health policy that dominated the Supreme Court agenda in 2012 and would test the Roberts Court's federalism policy regarding the commerce clause. In *Florida v. HHS* (2011), 26 state attorneys general challenged the constitutionality of the individual-mandates component of the PPACA. The federal government argued that the individual mandate was a valid exercise of interstate commerce because health care is an economic activity and that, since everyone needs health care, everyone is engaged in that economy. The choice of citizens to not buy insurance is an individual decision merely to delay the date of health care purchase until care is needed. Therefore it is not "inactivity" as critics argue, and it affects interstate commerce and the market for health care. Opponents counter that Congress does not have the authority to regulate inactivity or to force individuals to buy insurance when they otherwise would choose not to. They say that the provision requiring every legal American resident (with limited exceptions) to acquire minimal adequate health insurance or pay an "exaction" exceeds Congress's enumerated powers. According to Joondeph (2011, 458), the states' capstone argument invokes the proverbial slippery slope: "If Congress could force individuals to purchase goods or services in a private market as a means of regulating interstate commerce, it could compel people to purchase GM cars to stimulate the U.S. auto industry, to join exercise clubs to reduce the nation's health care costs, or even to eat daily rations of broccoli. Its authority would effectively be unlimited, rendering the Constitution's enumeration of powers meaningless." As the Virginia attorney general put it, the PPACA suit "is not about health care, it's about our freedom and about standing up and calling on the federal government to follow the ultimate law of the land—the Constitution" (449).

Clearly, the rhetoric became heated and the issue pivotal. Meanwhile, some states, including Florida, refused to implement the PPACA, confident that the Supreme Court would see the case their way and invalidate the mandate provision and the sweeping bill that contains it. The mandate provision was also part of the political debate in the Republican presidential primary, which includes Mitt Romney, who was governor when Massachusetts adopted its major health reform—with an individual mandate. Although once an advocate, Governor Romney in 2011 stepped away from the innovation, calling on federalism language: he said the law was what Massachusetts wanted but not necessarily what was good for the United States. Given the toxic nature of individual mandates in the 2012 election, it is interesting to recall that they were originally a Republican idea supported by the conservative Heritage Foundation in the late 1980s and by Republican senator Orrin Hatch in 1993 as an alternative to President Clinton's ambitious health reform proposal (Canham, 2011).

Understanding the Difference between Federal and State Governments

The ways in which states differ from and resemble the federal government— and one another—affect their policymaking in health and other areas. States are similar to the federal government in their organization, structure, and policy-making processes. They are different in three key areas: budget constraints, direct democracy, and media coverage.

State government is structured and run much as the federal government is. Every state has a state constitution that contains a bill of rights and provisions setting forth the structure and function of the state and local governments. Every state has three branches of government, and all except one have two houses. Like Congress, state legislatures are organized by the dominant political party, and 49 states have bipartisan membership (only Nebraska is unicameral and nonpartisan). Every state has a governor with duties roughly analogous to those of the president, including administering state government and initiating a policy agenda. Like the president, governors appoint members of a cabinet, although in some states several important cabinet positions are elected or appointed by commission. Every state has a judiciary that includes both trial and appellate levels.

The duties of the three branches of government are nearly identical at the federal and state levels. In both, the legislature passes laws, provides appropriations, and oversees the executive branch. Federal and state legislatures are organized by parties, use committees as key decision makers, and have nearly identical flow charts illustrating "how a bill becomes a law." In both, the chief elected official of the executive branch sets the agenda, oversees the running of the government, and handles relationships outside the capitol. The judiciary at both levels of government determines the constitutionality of laws, adjudicates violations of law, and protects the well-being of individual citizens. Both levels of government are lobbied by interest groups and receive money from PACs. And, importantly, both types of government are sovereign and operate by virtue of the power of the people. Each citizen is subject to at least two governments, under which some rights are identical and some are very different.

States and the federal government differ in their revenue sources and their spending priorities. The big spending area for states has traditionally been education (both kindergarten through twelfth grade [K–12] and higher education). However, in 2010, Medicaid overtook K–12 spending as a percent of total state spending nationally (NASBO, 2010). Some 20 percent of the federal budget is for defense and security; 20 percent is for Social Security. Health expenditures—Medicare, Medicaid, and S-CHIP—account for 21 percent. Only 3 percent goes for education (Center on Budget and Policy Priorities, 2011).

Both states and the national government use the income tax as a major source of revenue. For the states, however, it is one of several lucrative taxes and is second to the sales tax in its revenue generation. Sales taxes (both general taxes and taxes on specific items, such as gasoline, cigarettes, and liquor) make up around 50 percent of the states' tax revenue; individual income taxes account for 40 percent. The states also obtain revenues from corporate income taxes, lotteries, motor vehicle and operators' licenses, gift and estate taxes, and document taxes (U.S. Census Bureau, 2011). The federal government relies overwhelmingly on the income tax, which accounts for about 43 percent of the total revenue (OMB, 2010a).

Other important differences relate to budget constraints, direct democracy, and media coverage.

Balancing the State Budget

One of the important things to understand about states is that, unlike the federal government, states cannot operate in a deficit. In 49 states, by constitution or statute, the state budget must be balanced at the end of each fiscal year (only Vermont allows a deficit by law, and it discourages it by custom). Most states have "rainy-day funds" that allow them to put away some small proportion of their revenues in good economic times to help them balance the budget in poor economic times. Beginning in 2007, states suffered bad economic times, during which states used up most if not all of their rainy-day funds in addition to cutting spending. Even with federal stimulus dollars helping to prop up state budgets in 2009 and 2010, state spending declined in both years—the first time in more than 20 years. During the FY 2008–10 period, state revenues decreased by nearly 12 percent (NASBO, 2010).

Figure 5.2 shows the allocation of state spending from 1987 to 2009. The figure highlights the dramatic growth in spending—in particular health spending, which grew at a much faster rate than any other item. In FY 2009, Medicaid made up over 21 percent of total state spending—only slightly behind elementary and secondary education, long a state spending stalwart, at 21.7 percent. The third-largest category was higher education, at 10.4 percent of total state spending. In FY 2010, with the addition of the enhanced federal match, the Medicaid percentage exceeded that of K–12 education. Not surprisingly, states differed in their Medicaid spending as a percentage of total state spending. The range in 2009 was from 7.0 percent in Wyoming to 32.4 percent in Missouri (NASBO, 2010).

Unlike the federal government, states have capital budgets for financing infrastructure projects such as roads and buildings. States also have many special accounts or trust funds, often funded with earmarked taxes, which can be used only for specific programs or functions. Most states are prohibited from

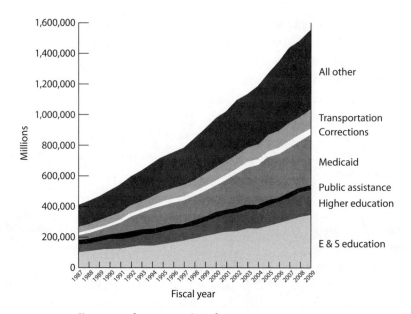

Figure 5.2. Allocation of state spending from 1987 to 2009. *Source:* NASBO, 2010. Used by permission.

borrowing money for operating expenses such as payrolls or benefit checks. This provision has caused difficulty for many states, particularly in times of economic downturn, but it has also forced them to make tough choices much earlier than their Washington counterparts must and to stay within limited resources in meeting their citizens' needs. If, midway through a fiscal year, state officials realize that the budget will not be balanced (that is, spending is exceeding expected revenues), they must either cut an existing program or enact a tax. (There are, of course, some stopgap measures such as delaying a payment to state employees and welfare recipients, but these delays usually raise little money and are often unpopular.) Having to choose between program cuts or tax increases is not popular, and legislators prefer to make careful choices in the initial budget to avoid getting into this unwelcome situation.

Finally, 30 states operate under some form of state tax or expenditure limit (TEL). A new era in state taxation began in 1976. Throughout the 1950s and early 1960s, citizens generally supported tax increases, which were often related to school financing. But by late in the 1960s, attitudes began to change as school bond initiatives failed in state after state. This growing antitax attitude culminated in 1976 in California with passage of a citizens' initiative labeled Proposition 13, which limited the growth in state property taxes and seemed to open the floodgates to tax or spending limitations in states across the country. There was also a second wave of state TELs, prompted in large measure by national antitax groups such as Americans for Tax Reform. These TELs not only limit tax collection and spending (or both) but often also include supermajority requirements (no tax or spending legislation may be enacted unless there is a greater-than-50% majority in the legislature) and voter approval requirements (voters must approve all new or increased taxes). While most TELs have been established by amending state constitutions, many are based in statutes and some represent both legislative and constitutional endorsement.

TELs and supermajorities constrain legislators' choices (as they are intended to do) and are not applied to the U.S. Congress. The most restrictive TEL was enacted in Colorado in 1992. In 2005, voters in that state, apparently alarmed by the decline in state services, suspended the limits for five years. However, in 2010, the amendment went back into effect. Even in a time of lowered state revenues, some officials still support TELs. The 2011 Florida legislature put a state-revenue-limit proposal to amend the state constitution on the 2012 ballot.

Eleven states with TELs require approval by a supermajority (usually two-thirds, three-fifths, or three-fourths) of the legislature (or of those elected) to raise taxes. South Dakota has no TEL but does require a two-thirds vote of the legislature to raise taxes. A few states require public approval as well. In Colorado, all tax increases must be approved by a vote of the people (NASBO, 2008).

Until recently, California was one of a small number of states requiring a two-thirds vote of the legislature to approve the annual budget. In November 2010, voters approved a repeal to that provision, although the two-thirds requirement for tax increases remains and now applies to fees as well (Initiative and Referendum Institute, 2010). An interesting component in the initiative was a provision docking legislators' pay if they did not enact the state budget on schedule. In 2011, the legislature did pass a budget on the day of the deadline, but it was vetoed by the governor. Legislators' pay was withheld—about $5,000 per legislator—until they passed a budget. It was the first time in five years that a budget was in place for the new year (Memmott, 2011).

Direct Democracy

Democracy is much more direct in many states than at the national level. In some states, citizens can initiate, endorse, or recall a law or an elected official.

In more than half the states, the people play a key role in ratifying or proposing legislation. Eighteen states have an initiative process that allows voters to propose constitutional amendments (constitutional initiatives). In 21 states, voters can propose statutory initiatives—which place the measure in law, not in the state constitution. Fourteen states offer both constitutional and statutory initiatives. In November 2010, voters considered 159 ballot propositions in 36 states; 42 were initiatives, proposed by the people and bypassing the state legislature. Of these, 43 percent passed. One of the most salient of them was a proposal legalizing marijuana in California that failed—46–54 percent. Medical marijuana measures were also defeated in Arizona, Oregon, and South Dakota. California voters turned down an initiative sponsored by two Texas oil companies to suspend a state law requiring reductions in greenhouse gas emissions. Washington voters repealed a temporary tax imposed on soft drinks through the initiative.

Twenty-four states use the popular referendum, whereby citizens can petition for a vote on statutes or ordinances that the legislature has passed and can, if they so vote, reject them. In 2011, voters in Ohio collected 231,000 signatures in 90 days to put on the ballot a referendum on a law limiting collective bargaining rights with public employees unions. Eighteen states have a recall provision that allows voters to remove an elected state official from office. Together, the three mechanisms—initiative, referendum, and recall—are referred to as direct democracy.

Direct democracy produces a type of accountability and responsiveness unmatched in Washington, D.C. It allows citizens to organize to support or oppose an issue or a person. Legislators and governors (and local officials) are aware of the latent power of the initiative, referendum, and recall and know they are accountable for individual decisions in a way a member of Congress is not. For example, in 1984, two Democratic members of the Michigan senate were recalled because they voted for a major tax increase (to balance a badly out-of-kilter, recession-affected state budget). Members of Congress might vote for a similar tax increase with the hope that two (or six) years hence voters will have forgotten the transgression or will wish to vote for them because of their positions on other issues.

Even if initiatives fail to garner the majority necessary for adoption, they may serve other purposes. The possibility of an initiative or referendum affects the kind of law proposed by the legislature. Unlike Congress, which has no public mechanism for citizens to express approval or disapproval of individual laws, a state legislator might see her long-sought law up for public approval, sometimes brought there by a petition-signing effort sponsored by interest groups defeated in the initial legislation. The possibility of such a reassessment, and of bringing up original bills, affects the design, strategy, and politics of state legislation, particularly in highly salient issue areas. Interest groups can send a message to legislators that the issue is important, and even if the initiative fails, it often lands on the legislative agenda following the election. Indeed, Elisabeth Gerber (1999) found that policies in states with initiatives reflect voter preferences more closely than do policies in states without and that this effect is greatest where access to the direct-legislation process is easiest. It is also interesting that the initiative can be used to directly curb legislative behavior. Most term-limit provisions and TELs are put in place through initiatives, not legislation.

Direct democracy was the idea of populists at the end of the twentieth century who wanted to reduce corruption in legislatures by giving the people a direct voice. Ironically, some believe that this idealistic notion has led to what Gerber (1999) called a populist paradox, where economic interests and citizen interests benefit from different aspects of the process. Economic groups are particularly successful at getting their initiatives on the ballot and blocking initiatives proposed by others. But citizen groups often see their proposals adopted by the voters.

Initiatives are very popular in states and are increasingly used for major environmental and health issues. Toxic cleanup, nuclear waste, gun control, AIDS-related issues, medicinal marijuana, Medicaid spending for abortions, health insurance reforms (including a single-payer system), and right-to-die laws—all have appeared on the ballot in states across the country. Citizens' groups tend to initiate and support environmental measures, whereas health measures are often launched by economic and professional interests.

Florida's long record of amending its state constitution with often trivial issues ended in 2004 with adoption of a requirement for a 60 percent majority to amend the constitution. Ironically, the amendment setting the higher vote standard was ratified by a simple majority of 50 percent plus one vote. Despite the higher standard, citizens and the legislature continue to place initiatives for constitutional change on the ballot, although fewer pass now. In 2010, only three of six constitutional proposals were adopted—two initiatives and one legislative referral.

The Press and the State Legislature

A major difference between most state legislatures and the U.S. Congress concerns media coverage. As discussed in chapter 1, members of Congress have become masters at manipulating the media by making clever pronouncements in 30-second sound bites and writing press releases and editorials that are often used verbatim in hometown newspapers. News coverage, especially local coverage, is widely available and highly useful to members of Congress. Press secretaries are important staffers, often highly influential in both formulating and packaging legislators' policy positions.

In states, the media coverage and press staffing are markedly different. Relatively few reporters cover the state capitol, and what coverage there is tends to be focused on the governor and a few legislative leaders and to highlight partisan bickering and embarrassing or ridiculous situations. Most state legislators do not have much access to public relations staffs, and even those who do are often unsuccessful in their efforts to make the six o'clock news. In "professional" state legislatures, press functions are often handled by party caucus staffs.

News directors and city editors often view state politics as dull and unappealing to viewers and readers. There are few exciting "photo opportunities," and the issues tend to be complex and not easily explained in a sound bite. Further, most state capitals are small towns relatively remote from the state's largest media centers. Thus, Albany, Sacramento, Lansing, Tallahassee, and Springfield may seem unimportant to the media—and the people they serve. Television coverage of state government is especially poor. Layton and Walton (1998, 45) called television reporters in state capitols "an endangered species, rarely glimpsed except for a major speech or press conference."

The loss of reporters covering state houses has been severe. Between 2003 and 2009, the number of state house newspaper reporters dropped by nearly one-third—from 524 in 2003 to 355 in 2009 (Dorroh, 2009). Some 44 percent of statehouses had fewer full-time reporters than they did six years earlier. In only two states were there more reporters than in 2003. The concern is that with fewer reporters there will be less scrutiny of politicians, and the public will not be as well informed on the operation of their government. The reporters that are in the statehouse are increasingly being called upon to report local stories, revolving around individual members rather than the policies they enact. Some newspapers, like the *St. Petersburg Times* and the *Miami Herald* in Florida, have combined their bureaus.

Newspaper statehouse coverage, like press coverage in general, is often undertaken by digital news outlets and blogs. Newspapers like the *Sacramento Bee* are providing video and breaking-news alerts, website updates, and blogging. Also coming into play are online journalists who report on state government in Connecticut, Texas, Louisiana, Colorado, and Michigan, among other states

(Dorroh, 2009). In Arizona and Florida, new outlets sell online subscriptions for in-depth coverage of state government.

Also noteworthy is the monitoring of media coverage of health issues funded in part by the Kaiser Family Foundation and the Pew Research Center's Project for Excellence in Journalism. There is an association of health care journalists who participate in periodic assessments of the state of health journalism in the United States (Schwitzer, 2009).

State house coverage—like all newspaper and media coverage—is in a state of flux. The possibility exists that 24-hour news cycles and new media outlets, including mobile devices such as cell phones or other wireless devices such as iPads, will bring about improvement in state house coverage so that citizens will be more attentive to activities in their state capitals. This would be a desirable change because an overall lack of media attention allows state policymaking to take place in a setting without widespread public input and feedback. Such a less visible process is dominated more by those with special interests and concerns than in Washington, not because of any real intent or differences in state legislative rules or procedures but rather because of the media coverage, or lack thereof. As one North Carolina legislator put it, "One of the first things I was told when I came to Raleigh was, 'You can vote any way you want to up here because the folks back home will never know'" (Layton & Walton, 1998, 54).

Interstate Differences

The similarities among the states are legion and unmistakable. A transplant from Rhode Island walking into the North Carolina state capitol would have little difficulty finding his way around or understanding the process, language, and operation of the legislative body. (Only in Nebraska would a visitor be confused: it has the country's only unicameral legislature.) Similarly, governors' offices, executive-branch agencies, and lobbies operate in roughly the same manner across the 50 states. However, it would be a mistake to think that state legislatures are identical from Maine to New Mexico. They differ in many ways, especially in what is known as their "professionalism."

Every state legislature in the country modernized to some extent in the 1970s, adding staff, increasing time in session, adopting procedures to expedite and streamline the legislative process, increasing salaries, and adding technology that links legislators to one another, to state agencies, and to the public. Many states reduced the size of their legislative institutions as a way to achieve more efficient organization and more effective policymaking. Reducing the size of the legislative body increases the number of citizens represented per member, affecting large states more dramatically than small states. For example, the average member of the California assembly represents 423,396 constituents. At the other extreme, the average New Hampshire house member represents only 3,089 persons. The range in state senates is similar. A California senator represents, on average, 846,791 persons; a North Dakota senator must report to 13,106 (NCSL, 2011). Is this fair? Certainly citizens of North Dakota and New Hampshire are more likely to know their representatives and participate more easily in the legislative process. For California and other large states that try to hold down the size of their legislative institutions so as to facilitate collective-action decisions, there is a tradeoff between efficiency and representation.

Not all states have made the same level of progress in modernization. Eight state legislatures can be referred to as professional—they have many specialized and personal staff, they are compensated at relatively generous levels, and the legislatures are in session nearly full-time. At the other end of the spectrum are 17 nonprofessional, or citizen, legislatures, which have few staff, low pay, and limited sessions. Twenty-five states are hybrids, having some of the characteristics of each (Kurtz, 1989).

Table 5.2 shows the range of professionalization of state legislatures, characterized by time in session, legislative salaries, and expenditures for staff services and operations. The level of professionalization reflects how closely each state legislature approximates Congress in the three areas of time, salaries, and staff spending. The measure used for each state is the mean of the percentage of the congressional standard the state achieves for each of the three areas. The table illustrates the enormous diversity of the states in their professionalization. California, the most professional state legislature, has a professionalization level of 63 percent (that is, 63% of Congress's level). At the other extreme, New Hampshire's legislature has a professionalization level of only 3 percent (Squire, 2007). The mean level for all states is 18 percent. Also noteworthy is the big gap between the most professional state—California—and the other professional states (the professionalization level of the second-place state, New York, is only 48%). Half of the states fall in the 10–19 percent category. Clearly, state legislatures retain their nonprofessional nature—at least compared with their national counterpart.

State legislatures also differ substantially in their levels of partisanship. Nebraska is the only state where legislators do not run on a party label. In other

Table 5.2. State levels of professionalism (in percentages), compared to Congress

>50 Percent	30–49 Percent		20–29 Percent		10–19 Percent		<10 Percent	
California 63	New York	48	Illinois	26	Connecticut	19	Maine	9
	Wisconsin	44	New Jersey	24	Maryland	19	Montana	8
	Massachusetts	39	Alaska	23	Oklahoma	19	Alabama	7
	Michigan	34	Arizona	23	Iowa	17	Utah	7
	Pennsylvania	34	Hawaii	23	Minnesota	17	South Dakota	6
	Ohio	30	Florida	22	Missouri	17	North Dakota	5
			Colorado	20	Nebraska	16	Wyoming	5
			N. Carolina	20	Oregon	16	New Hampshire	3
			Texas	20	Delaware	15		
			Washington	20	Kentucky	15		
					Idaho	14		
					Nevada	14		
					Vermont	14		
					Kansas	13		
					Louisiana	13		
					Rhode Island	13		
					Virginia	13		
					West Virginia	13		
					Georgia	12		
					S. Carolina	12		
					Tennessee	12		
					Arkansas	11		
					Mississippi	11		
					New Mexico	11		
					Indiana	10		

Source: Squire, 2007.

states, parties are important in identifying members to the electorate and in organizing legislative activities. The speaker or senate president is generally from the majority party, selected in caucus and then voted on by all members. But exceptions do occur—and more frequently than in the U.S. Congress. In 2005, a Democrat edged out a Republican for the top position (the speaker) in the Tennessee Senate, even though Republicans held the majority of seats in the senate. The losing Republican candidate became majority leader in an unusual bipartisan leadership arrangement (Locker, 2005). And there is generally at least one tied chamber in one state at any given time. In 2010 it was the Oregon House of Representatives and the Alaska Senate. For some of these chambers—such as Oregon's—the bipartisan accommodation that such a tie entails can lead to policymaking that is shared and productive (see Loepp, 1999, for one insider's view of sharing of power in Michigan).

Hawaii has long been one of the most Democratic legislatures, with only 1 of the 25 senators and 8 of the 51 house members Republicans in 2011. Massachusetts is also a Democratic stronghold, having only 4 of its 40 state senators and 32 of 160 house members in the Republican Party in 2011. At the other extreme, Idaho is highly Republican; in 2011 there were only 7 Democratic members in the 35-member senate and 13 Democrats in the 70-member House of Representatives. In other states, parties are more competitive. The 2009 Montana senate was split (23 Democrats and 27 Republicans), while the house was split 50-50. Shifts can occur quickly in state legislative elections. The 2010 election was a case in point. In 2009–10 there were 27 states where both houses were controlled by Democrats, 8 where both houses were in Republican hands, and 14 states where one party had the majority in the upper house and the other in the lower house (split states). In 2011–12, following the November 2010 election, the Republicans had control of 26 states (an increase of 16), Democrats had control of 15 (a loss of 12), and 8 were split.

Governors are important too, of course, and in November 2010 Republican governors came out on top. In 2011–12, 29 states have Republican governors, 20 have Democratic governors, and 1 state (Rhode Island) has an independent governor. In 2011–12, 21 states have united Republican leadership, with the governor and both chambers Republican. Democrats have control over both branches in 11 states, and 17 are split. The Republican dominance in the November 2010 election was especially important because in most states, the state legislature draws the lines for state legislative and congressional seats following the 2010 election. Given the importance of drawing lines—and potentially benefiting the party in control—the Democratic losses in 2010 were major indeed.

A final difference among state legislatures, one that has a large potential effect on state policymaking, is in term limits. Fifteen states now have term limits on their state legislators. Not all term limits are the same. The toughest provisions, in place in Arizona, California, and Michigan, limit service in the lower house to six years and in the senate to eight years, with a lifetime ban on further service. Louisiana's term limits allow 12 years in either the house or the senate (or a combination of the two). Nine states have consecutive-term limits, meaning a legislator could serve the limit of terms in the senate, stay out for a term, then return and start the term-limits clock again (NCSL, 2005). In six states, term limits have been repealed, in most cases by the state supreme court.

Term limits were expected to change legislative composition, behavior, and power balance. Supporters clearly wanted to get fresher ideas and to turn out legislators who had, perhaps, become too ingrained in the system and may not have been responsive to the electorate. Although the effects of term limits are not fully known (they went into effect in Louisiana only in 2007 and Nevada in 2010), there is little evidence that legislative composition is greatly changed. The number of women and minorities elected to the legislature has not changed substantially, and legislators tend to be similar in occupation, education, income, religion, and ideology to those they replace. Hispanics in California are one exception to this. Their number increased after term limits were imposed. Somewhat unexpectedly, legislators elected under term limits seem less inclined to be concerned about district needs and more concerned with statewide issues (perhaps because they are looking forward to their next race). They report spending less time keeping in touch with constituents than do non-term-limited legislators. But as yet there are no differences in the ability of the newly elected legislators to build coalitions or specialize in issues. Indeed, if congressional theory applies, one could speculate that an absence of trust might make deal-making harder to enforce, since members are likely to be term-limited out of the legislature before they can be punished by other members for breaking promises.

The greatest impact seems to be on power. In term-limited legislatures, governors and state agency officials now seem to be more powerful, party leadership less powerful (Carey, Niemi & Powell, 2000). Although some argue that interest groups are more influential in term-limited legislatures, others note that lobbyists have to work harder for their keep in these legislatures, because they have to make new friends each time members are replaced.

Gubernatorial power, too, varies across the 50 states. Term limits are more prevalent in states' chief executive offices than in legislatures. The majority of governors have some type of term limit imposed on them; most can serve only two terms. Governors' formal powers—those outlined specifically in state constitutions or statutes—include the length of the term, the possibility of serving multiple terms, and the governor's role in shaping the state's budget, authority to appoint cabinet members, and authority to reorganize state agencies. Some governors have relatively little formal power: limited to two terms, with few cabinet appointments, and without the power to revamp the state bureaucracy unless they have legislative approval. For example, the governor of Texas does not present an executive budget to the legislature and cannot reorganize departments without legislative approvals. Other governors can serve many terms, have a large slate of possible appointments, and can make changes in state agencies with minimal legislative interference. Forty-three governors have the line-item veto, and 37 can reduce the budget without legislative approval. Fourteen governors can even veto selected words in laws, and three can use a veto to change the meaning of words (NASBO, 2002).

State judiciaries differ in how they are selected. States use three methods of choosing judges, and some states use a combination of methods (that is, one process for supreme court justices and another for lower trial judges). Many state judges are elected by the citizens, usually on nonpartisan tickets. In some states, judges are appointed by the legislature or the governor or both. Nearly half of the states have adopted a modified merit approach, called the Missouri Plan, in which judges are initially appointed by the governor based on recommendations by a blue-ribbon committee, and then after a short period of time in service they must face the voters in an election.

State executive agencies also differ markedly, with some states having large professional bureaucracies dominated by civil service rules and others having fewer, more generalist officials who are not uniformly hired or protected by merit-based nonpartisan rules. State agencies in some states work closely with the legislature in drafting and producing legislation; agencies in other states might work in a more "arms-length" fashion, meeting only occasionally with legislative staff and others. Sparer (1996) found that differences in state agencies were key to understanding Medicaid programs in those states. In California, for example, officials implementing Medicaid enjoyed significant autonomy and were able to pursue the goal of cost containment. New York Medicaid officials, in contrast, operated in a fragmented, decentralized environment in which interest groups had an important role and agency goals had a secondary role.

Finally, the importance of lobbyists varies from state to state. Every state, like Washington, D.C., has seen the number of lobbyists increase over the past decades, but the style of lobbying and the effect of lobbying on the legislative product can vary considerably. In some states, interest groups are more influential than political parties in helping recruit and elect candidates as well as shape legislation. Especially in citizen legislatures, lobbyists serve to provide valuable information on both substance and political issues. Rules vary on who is considered a lobbyist and to what extent lobbyists must report their activities. In Iowa, lobbyists must register which bills they intend to support or oppose. In many states, multiclient lobby firms are the norm—a handful of lobbyists serve dozens of corporate and association clients (Rosenthal, 1993). In every state, economic and professional health interests are important policy players.

The variations in state process and policy are, of course, not random but depend on large differences in citizens' wealth and education, the states' businesses and industries, and state residents' expectations, ideologies, and views of government. A large body of political science research has considered the role of political and economic factors and measures of "need" in state policy choice and has found that all are important, but with differences across policy areas. The variables that successfully predict what makes a state generous in welfare or Medicaid payments or eligibility criteria are not necessarily good predictors of which state policies will be enacted on water pollution or education or health professions education. Political variables, in particular, seem to weigh more heavily in some kinds of policy choices than in others (Lambert & McGuire, 1990; Mueller, 1992; Weissert, Knott & Stieber, 1994).

Also important is the presence of a policy entrepreneur who sells an idea and continues to push it through innumerable hurdles and who has the standing to make things happen. Governors are often very effective policy entrepreneurs: they can put issues on the agenda, work with legislative leaders and interest groups to shape the plan, and obtain the public's backing for the plan (Paul-Sheehan, 1998; Sardell & Johnson, 1998). State attorneys general have also played the role of policy entrepreneurs in health policy—particularly in bringing high-profile litigation against tobacco companies (Spill, Licari & Ray, 2001).

Federal-State Health Programs

The state role in health goes back to long before the New Deal. Social legislation, particularly programs protecting the public's health and assisting persons who are poor or disabled, was initiated in many states in the early years of the twentieth century. States and localities were the traditional source of health care for poor people until World War II. States provided the money to build hospitals and adopted scores of public health measures. State regulation of health providers goes back to before the United States was established. The first law licensing physicians was enacted in 1639 in Virginia. State mental institutions trace their history to the early 1800s in Virginia and Kentucky; in the early 1950s, states began to establish departments of mental health. Following World War II, the federal role in health became more evident. Federal law permitted firms to deduct costs of employee health benefits, and in 1946 the Hill-Burton Act provided incentives for establishing new hospitals and for care of the indigent (Rich & White, 1996).

In the 1960s and 1970s, the federal government stepped up its spending in many health areas, including mental health, substance abuse, the environment, and public health. The biggest change in the national arena was the enactment of Medicare and Medicaid in 1965, which dramatically changed the nature of health care financing and services in the United States. Medicare and Medicaid put the federal government in the role of a major purchaser of health care and, as such, a shaper of the way in which care is delivered. The Bush administration's addition of prescription drug coverage to Medicare was a big change in Medicare program spending; it deprived states of the authority to battle drug firms over drug prices for many Medicaid patients—those also eligible for Medicare, a group that is typically the most expensive Medicaid population for states (Weissert & Miller, 2005). The 2010 Patient Protection and Affordable Care Act also made an impact on state health policy. Medicaid was dramatically expanded to include more of the near poor, the health insurance industry was brought to new standards of performance well above those of many state insurance regulations, and state health exchanges were established to offer private insurance plans to previously uninsured people.

Medicaid

Medicaid is the premier federal-state health program. It is large, important, and controversial. In FY 2010 Medicaid financed health care for 58 million low-income children, adults, seniors, and people with disabilities at a total cost of $367 billion (Kaiser Family Foundation, 2011c, 2011d). Medicaid makes up nearly one-fourth of all state spending (including federal grants) (NASBO, 2011). In the tough economic years of 2008–11, state officials were dismayed to see their Medicaid costs increase even as their revenues were stagnant. In 2011, states like Florida saw the share of their state spending devoted to Medicaid grow larger than their K–12 spending.

Medicaid is not one program but several, providing for different groups of recipients:

- low-income, uninsured children, some parents, and low-income pregnant women;

- people who are disabled, including elderly nursing home residents and people of all ages with developmental disability, mental retardation, and mental illness;
- people too poor to pay the premiums and copays required for Medicare, the federal program for elders;
- safety-net hospitals and community health centers that serve the poor; and,
- all otherwise uninsured U.S. citizens and resident aliens whose income is less than 133 percent of the poverty level, whether they have children or not and whether they are working or not (this group to be covered once the Patient Protection and Affordable Care Act of 2010 is fully phased in).

Medicaid (along with the much smaller S-CHIP program, mentioned earlier and described below) accounts for more than one-third (35%) of all federal outlays in health and of state health expenditures an even larger percentage (39%). Enrollments are cyclical and increase with a poor economy, which, unfortunately for the states, is also the very time when their revenues decline. The most troubling aspect of Medicaid is not its size but its rate of growth. Figure 5.3 illustrates the variation and annual growth of the program's enrollment, which brings substantial new expenditure demands. No wonder Medicaid is viewed as an 800-pound gorilla or a budget-eating monster by state and federal officials trying to control—or even predict—their outlays.

Several aspects of the Medicaid program entail policy choices that affect costs. The first is the number of persons eligible for the program—it is an entitlement program, which means that all eligible persons are provided for under the program. Also important is the scope and level of recipients' benefits. A third important component is the level of payment to providers of the health care service. There is a substantial federal match in Medicaid, based upon the states' income, ranging from 50 percent for 15 states, including Connecticut, New Jersey, California, and others, to 74 percent for Mississippi. In 2009 and 2011 the federal medical assistance percentage (FMAP) was made more generous as part of the economic stimulus package. But in July 2011 (the beginning of FY 2012), the usual FMAP percentages returned. The differences to states were dramatic. For example, Florida's 2011 FMAP should have been 55.5 percent; the enhanced FMAP in the first quarter of FY 2011 was 67.6 percent (Kaiser Family Foundation, 2011a).

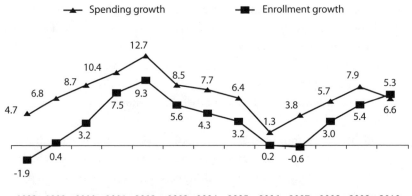

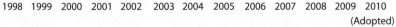

Figure 5.3. Percent change in total Medicaid spending and enrollment, FY 1998–2010. Note: Enrollment percentage changes are from June to June of each year. Spending growth percentage changes are based on the state fiscal year. *Source:* KCMU, 2011.

Federal law requires that certain groups of persons be covered and certain services be provided to them. However, states can expand eligibility to include persons who are "medically needy." In the early 1990s, the federal government mandated expanding the Medicaid program to cover all children up to age 6 in families with incomes between 100 and 133 percent of the federal poverty level and children aged 6 to 15 in families earning up to 100 percent of the federal poverty level. When the Patient Protection and Affordable Care Act is fully implemented, childless adults will qualify if they have incomes below 133 percent of the federal poverty level. All children on Medicaid get early and periodic screening, diagnosis, and treatment (EPSDT) services, and most Medicaid-eligible children also receive vision, hearing, and dental screening services. When states must reduce Medicaid, they can often reduce eligibility for near-poor children and near-poor pregnant women and eliminate or reduce their programs for the medically needy. However in 2010–11, states were prohibited from changing eligibility standards by a provision in PPACA that states accepting the enhanced Medicaid match must adhere to "maintenance of effort." Florida ran up against this provision by proposing enrollee copayments that were likely to discourage enrollment. Failure to maintain effort could result in loss of all federal Medicaid dollars.

Federal law requires that certain health services be provided to recipients, and states can offer additional services from a list of optional services provided in federal law. During times of state fiscal stress, states limit these optional services, such as dental care, podiatry, chiropractic services, eyeglasses, hearing aids, hospice services, nonemergency use of emergency rooms, and prescription drugs.

States have flexibility in determining the reimbursement policies for most providers. Federal rules set forth administrative requirements in such areas as the designation of a state plan, provider certification, timeliness of provider payments, and quality control. States must also pay the Medicare copayments of poor elderly people who are eligible for both Medicare and Medicaid. A 1997 federal law (the Balanced Budget Act, BBA) gave states more flexibility in negotiating reimbursement rates for health providers; this was achieved by repeal of the Boren Amendment, which had required states to reimburse hospitals and nursing homes at rates that were reasonable and adequate to meet the essential costs of efficiently and economically operated facilities. In a move typical of the give-and-take of federalism, the BBA also contained several mandates that "cost" the states more. The law restored Medicaid coverage for certain immigrants who lost their eligibility under the Personal Responsibility and Work Opportunity Reconciliation Act (PRWORA) and increased the Medicare Part B premiums that states pay for low-income beneficiaries (Tannenwald, 1998). In tight state budgets, states often freeze or cut reimbursement rates for physicians, pharmacies, hospitals, and managed care plans.

Medicaid also pays hospitals for uncompensated care; this is an important source of support for hospitals that function as the safety net for poor people, including those with mental illnesses admitted to state mental hospitals. These payments are called Disproportionate Share Hospital (DSH) payments and are directed to facilities that serve large numbers of Medicaid and uncompensated-care patients. Payments were about $11.3 billion in FY 2009, or about 5.2 percent of federal Medicaid spending for that year (National Health Policy Forum, 2009). DSH allotments were reduced in the PPACA and the secretary of HHS was directed to develop a methodology to distribute dollars to benefit states with the highest percentage of uninsured among other factors (Kaiser Family Foundation, 2011b).

Over the years, states have adopted a variety of innovations and administrative improvements in the Medicaid program, such as prior authorization (used primarily for prescription drugs—the physician must obtain the state's permission to prescribe a particular drug, typically an expensive brand-name drug), Medicaid Management Information Systems, provider profiles (the state examines physicians' practice patterns to identify any outliers on high-cost procedures such as surgeries), and computerized billing. Some states have established successful programs to control hospital costs, including rate-setting based on prospective payment. In the 1990s, the states moved thousands of Medicaid recipients into full-risk managed care arrangements—far ahead of the progress in enrolling Medicare patients in these entities. States, led by Arizona, have also adopted managed care arrangements for elderly long-term-care patients. A provision in the Medicare Modernization Act supports creation of "special needs plans" or managed care plans for specific groups. Maryland developed a special managed care plan for those who are eligible for both Medicare and Medicaid (Foxhall, 2005). In 2011, the Centers for Medicare and Medicaid Services funded 15 state demonstration projects to coordinate care for this dually eligible group. The PPACA set up a Center for Medicare and Medicaid Innovations within CMS to test innovative payment and service delivery models (CMS, 2011).

One way states have been able to innovate within the strictures of the federal guidelines on Medicaid is through Medicaid waivers. States can apply for a waiver from certain federal requirements to allow them to more efficiently operate the program. A key component of the waiver is a budget neutrality rule. Program spending under the waiver cannot exceed what it would have been without the waiver.

Several federal program waivers for Medicaid requirements are available to states:

—Section 1915(b) freedom-of-choice waivers allow states to waive statewideness, comparability of services, and freedom-of-choice provisions of the law. Many states have used this waiver to enroll beneficiaries in managed care programs, although a 1997 law allowed states to accomplish this via a state plan amendment. Others have used it to carve out a system for special populations or create programs that are not available statewide.

—Section 1915(c) home and community-based services waivers allow states to cover home and community-based services as an alternative to providing long-term care in institutional settings.

—Section 1115 research and demonstration waivers are more comprehensive, enabling states to deviate from standard Medicaid requirements to try out new approaches.

In the 1990s, states used these waivers, especially the broader Section 1115 waiver, to extend Medicaid coverage to previously uninsured groups, to expand the package of medical benefits available to program beneficiaries, and to mandate the enrollment of Medicaid recipients in managed care plans. The most famous pre-1990 waiver was the Arizona Health Care Cost Containment System (AHCCCS), a statewide managed care network, set up in 1982 to use the bidding process to select providers. For the first few years, AHCCCS delivered only acute care; in the early 1990s, it expanded to cover long-term care, home health care, and mental health care. In the mid-1990s, most Section 1115 waivers emphasized managed care.

Oregon used the Section 1115 waiver to provide a new system whereby all of its poor citizens would be provided with a set of health care benefits. Tennessee used the Section 1115 waiver to expand Medicaid to all poor persons in the state. In 2002, Utah used a 1115 waiver to launch its Primary Care Network. The state began to provide primary care to adults between the ages of 19 and 64, with or without children, who had not had health coverage for six months or more and who had annual family incomes of less than 150 percent of the federal poverty level. In order to expand coverage for this population, some services for Medicaid recipients were curtailed or eliminated, including hearing, vision, and dental services, nonemergency transportation, and mental health services. Newly covered recipients of Utah's program pay an annual enrollment fee as well as copayments (AcademyHealth, 2003).

A special subset of 1115 waivers is a pharmacy-plus demonstration, which allows states to provide prescription coverage to individuals not eligible for Medicaid whose income is at or below 200 percent of the federal poverty level.

Changes in Medicaid adopted in the 2005 federal budget reconciliation act obviated the need for many of these waivers, permitting states to add such innovations to their state plan as a covered service without need of special permission. Yet waiver authority remains and is likely to be used for innovations not yet adopted as typical Medicaid program features. For example, in 2011, New Jersey received a 1115 waiver to provide Medicaid-equivalent benefits to some 70,000 nonpregnant and childless adults who were poor and uninsured (CMS, 2011). Florida sought to expand a five-county pilot project testing Medicaid managed care statewide. But as noted earlier, copayment requirements for enrollees raised CMS concerns.

Complaints by state officials that Medicaid is bankrupting them and that its costs push out all other state initiatives are ubiquitous. Consequently, efforts to alter the program in ways that officials hope will cut costs are so frequent that the Kaiser Family Foundation's Statehealthfacts.org now reports changes in Medicaid program policies on a yearly basis. For FY 2011, 36 states changed provider payments, 30 added pharmacy controls, 13 reduced benefits, 1 cut eligibility, 5 imposed or increased copayments, none made changes to their application renewal requirements, and 10 put changes in place in hopes of reducing long-term-care expenditures. Ironically, even in bad times and despite cuts and complaints about growing costs, most states made policy choices that expanded access to their programs.

State Children's Health Insurance Program

A second important federal-state health program emerged in the late 1990s as the State Children's Health Insurance Program. S-CHIP is a block grant that allocates money to states based on the number of uninsured low-income children, adjusted for the state's average cost of health care. After modifications, the formula now also takes into account the number of all low-income children, covered or not, residing in the state. The program's matching-fund arrangement (the state's contribution) is more generous to states than is Medicaid's.

States have considerable leeway in designing their S-CHIP programs. Under the federal law, states can establish a new children's program, can fold the new program into their existing Medicaid programs, or do both. Some 23 states elected to expand Medicaid, 15 set up a separate S-CHIP program, and 18 both expanded Medicaid and set up a new S-CHIP program (GAO, 2000). States set eligibility standards limited only by federal ceilings of children living in families with incomes below 200 percent of the federal poverty level. However, states must deal with provisions in the federal law that stipulate minimum benefits, impose maintenance-of-effort requirements, limit use of premiums and copayments, and prohibit states from enrolling in S-CHIP any children who qualify for Medicaid.

For Congress, S-CHIP was for a time a popular issue for which both Republicans and Democrats could take credit. Democrats had long supported federally funded coverage for children. When the program passed in 1997, Republicans also viewed S-CHIP, along with welfare reform, as part of an ideological plan to devolve more authority to states, and the program was authorized for 10 years. By 2007, however, attitudes had changed. Democrats wanted the program expanded, but to Republicans the expansion translated to a back door to national health insurance. A Democratic Congress passed it, but President Bush vetoed it—twice. When a Democratic president and Congress took over Washington, D.C., in 2009, S-CHIP became one of their first orders of business, and it was reauthorized and expanded.

S-CHIP was also covered in the PPACA, which requires states to maintain current income eligibility levels for children in S-CHIP until 2019 and extends funding through 2015. In 2015, states will receive a 23 percentage point increase in the S-CHIP match rate (Kaiser Family Foundation, 2011b). S-CHIP in 2010 had a monthly enrollment of 5 million children and total annual spending of $10 billion.

Medicaid and S-CHIP, though important, are not the only health programs in states or the only areas where innovations have occurred. State-supported health programs range from state mental health institutions to professional licensure and a wide range of health education, data collection, environmental, and health care delivery programs, many run through county health departments. Typically, spending for these programs costs states far less than their spending on Medicaid.

State Innovations in Health

Innovations in health and other key areas at the state level are very useful in that they can serve as test cases, working out problems and highlighting consequences before being implemented nationally. The use of the states as "laboratories of democracy" has a long history in the United States. The 1921 Sheppard-Towner Act, providing social and medical assistance to pregnant women and babies, was copied from a Connecticut law, and states provided models for the 1935 Social Security Act, the 1973 Supplemental Security Income programs, and dozens of health measures. Medicare's DRG payment system was based on a program in New Jersey. S-CHIP was based on existing state programs, and federal patients'-bill-of-rights legislation was patterned on state enactments. New York governor Nelson Rockefeller once noted that "those elements of the New Deal which failed were largely in areas not tested by prior experience at the state level" (Silver, 1991, 445).

States have the resources, the infrastructure, and the desire to make health system changes that positively affect their citizens. Sometimes these changes are copied by other states and the policy "diffuses" throughout the nation. State efforts to regulate managed care organizations are one example. Over a period of three to five years, legislation on managed care was introduced in every state, and 40 states enacted new restrictions on managed care organizations (Hackey, 2001).

States often act when political difficulties prevent national action. Massachusetts was able to design, legislate, and implement a health reform initiative that became the model for the Patient Protection and Affordable Care Act of 2010. When Washington could not or would not act, states acted to reduce greenhouse gas emissions (California), allow assisted suicide (Oregon) and allow the use of marijuana for medical purposes (16 states)—to name a few innovations.

States can also act quickly when issues arise that engage or outrage constituencies. When a young Washington state high school student suffered a brain injury playing football, the state legislature quickly crafted legislation mandating education for coaches and imposing new rules requiring removal from the game of head-injured players. Other states and Congress rapidly took up the cause as well, using the Washington law as a model for their hearings.

States learn and pick up ideas from other states. Sometimes policies spread quickly from one state to another. Many groups help states in their policymaking. National interest groups with local affiliates often promote state legislation that they like. For example, the national organizations of nonprofit hospitals and other interests were active in promoting state legislation that prescribed how mergers and acquisitions of nonprofit hospitals were to be accomplished. The diffusion of state policies has long been of interest to political scientists. Early research indicated that diffusion was largely regional, as states within a region looked to "leader" states for guidance in handling similar problems (Walker, 1969).

With improved technology and the expansion of sources of information and networking, states now tend to reach farther afield for their ideas, often to try out an idea of a state unlike their own in population, wealth, and ideology. Many state legislative staffs communicate with one another, and organizations such as the National Conference of State Legislatures and the National Governors Association provide opportunities for face-to-face meetings with counterparts across the country to obtain up-to-date information about what other states are doing, including legislative language and technical assessments. Balla (2001) showed that the National Association of Insurance Commissioners played an important role in helping model HMO rules diffuse. States of members who had served on committees that acted on the model law were more likely than other states to adopt them.

Texas governor Rick Perry (R) told National Public Radio's *Morning Edition* reporters that states should be allowed to compete in designing a health reform package, not forced to buy from a "Washington-devised program." "You let California, New Mexico, New York, Texas and Florida compete against one another, and they'll be laboratories of innovation . . . They will come up with the best way to deliver health care" (NPR Staff, 2010, para 12).

Not all states want to be laboratories, however. Some states pride themselves on being more innovative than others. These are states with policy cultures or legacies that are conducive to major innovation. One observer of intergovernmental affairs, John Shannon of the Urban Institute, likened states to convoys. No state wants to be too far ahead of the pack, and no state wants to be in a vulnerable position in the rear. But some like to be among the first to try new programs. Maine, Vermont, Minnesota, and Oregon have often led the way in new approaches to dealing with problems in health, the environment, criminal justice, and other areas. Virginia, by contrast, is more comfortable letting other states try out ideas and work out the problems. There are some noteworthy exceptions, however. In 1993, Tennessee, generally comfortable in the middle of the convoy, launched its innovative TennCare program, which was examined and watched closely by states across the country. And innovative states are often not innovative in all areas. In one study of health professions education, for example, Maine, Massachusetts, and New Jersey, often innovative, were not among the innovators in this area (Weissert, Knott & Stieber, 1994).

While some innovations are more associated with Democratic governors and legislatures—efforts at universal health care coverage for example—others are not. For example, Republican state officials have innovated in the development of health savings accounts and managed care. In the mid-1990s, medical savings accounts were launched in seven states including Arizona, Colorado, Idaho, and Missouri—prior to a federal pilot program in 1996 and a federal law establishing health savings accounts in 2006 (NCSL, 2011). Similarly, Republican states have typically endorsed Medicaid managed care. In 2011, Florida—led by a Republican governor and extraordinary majorities of Republicans in both houses—launched an ambitious Medicaid managed care program including both the disabled and elderly recipients.

In 2011, there was a rash of anti-abortion laws adopted—at least 64 according to one count (Bazelon, 2011). The new laws require women to view ultrasounds, impose additional waiting periods, cut funds for clinics, and ban abortions at the 20th week after conception—the latter a provision that seemingly is in direct conflict with the threshold set by the U.S. Supreme Court (Eckholm, 2011).

Conclusion

Few would question the role of state governments as key factors in health care in the United States. They serve as the providers, financiers, administrators, initiators, and regulators of health care delivery. Their reach cuts across traditional health providers, insurers, businesses, educational institutions, and, of course, citizens. State governments are capable of adequately performing all their roles and representing all the groups and citizens they serve. They are the innovators and creators of many of the most promising ideas considered in the nation's capital and elsewhere. They are probably the most pivotal government actor in health care, since they implement and help define federal policies, define and implement their own policies, and define and oversee local health-related activities.

States and their local governments were the primary makers of health policy for the first 150 years or so of this country's history. States made laws dealing with public health, provided services for the mentally ill and the elderly, and even considered comprehensive health insurance.

Before World War I, there was intense interest in many states in adopting a compulsory health insurance program funded by employers, employees, and the public. At least 16 states introduced health insurance bills based on a model bill prepared by the American Association for Labor Legislation, a group that had led the successful drive for workers' compensation (Anderson, 1990). In the 1930s through the 1960s, the states provided essential health services but were generally not leaders in innovation or responsiveness to the public. A key turning point was the adoption of the Medicare and Medicaid programs, which developed into the major public health safety net for the elderly and the poor.

The 1970s and 1980s witnessed a spurt of innovation and activity in the states. In health care, innovations in financing, new forms of delivery, and systems allowing citizens to make tough "rationing" choices were developed at the state level, and in the early 1990s the states developed the ideas of managed competition, global budgets, and major insurance reforms—ideas only talked about in Washington, D.C. In the rest of the decade, states led the way in the use of managed care in Medicaid programs and in regulation on behalf of citizens in public and private managed care systems, in providing prescription drugs to those unable to pay, and in controlling costs for public programs. States dealt with legal protections, accountability, and health access and quality—issues that stymied congressional attempts to enact national laws. In the early years of the twenty-first century, the states expressed renewed interest in universal health coverage.

Nevertheless, state actions are stymied by fiscal constraints such as federal law (ERISA), the necessity to balance their budgets, and limits on revenues and expenditures that are not in place at the national level. States that enact broad health care reforms (Tennessee, Minnesota, and Washington) can be forced to abandon the reforms when the needs of citizens swamp the resources of the state to deal with the costs. States that lead the way in controversial areas such as limiting minors' access to violent games may see their actions nullified in federal court. States that enact incremental reforms are often criticized for being cautious and masking the failures of the private market (Beamer, 2004). These reforms also illustrate what Paul Peterson (1995) calls the "price" of federalism— inequity. Citizens' eligibility for and benefits from health services in a progressive state may differ from those in another state. Critics argue that only the federal government can successfully reform the many faults of the current health care system. But the truth is that it hasn't done so.

The limited, yet highly controversial 2010 effort of the national government to deal with comprehensive health care reform finds itself mirrored in state efforts. Backlash against the federal effort led in part to a Republican sweep of the 2010 elections and the determination by those newly elected to roll back the reform. Gray and colleagues (2009) showed that similar patterns prevail in the states: reforms tend to be incremental and tend to pass only in states dominated by Democrats. Some states have even seen legislation adopted by a Democratic legislature rolled back by the next more conservative legislature, so that the same staff that drafted the reform law is told to draft the repeal. Many—though clearly not Governor Perry of Texas and probably others—believe that a national system of health care access cannot be dominated by states, which simply lack the resources and constitutional scope to run a national health care system. Some commentators continue to bemoan the lack of a national system and the impossibility of a decentralized health care system. However, states can and do dominate in designing effective policy for their own citizens.

The U.S. health system is neither a decentralized health market nor a centralized health system. Rather, health is a combined federal-state responsibility with substantial federal oversight and funding, imbued with state innovation and implementation. The system may be confused and confusing and may always function amid a cacophony of noisy arguments over the proper roles and responsibilities of the levels of government, but it seems to work. If not all that efficiently and well, at least well enough for enough people that it's very hard to get a consensus to make major nationwide reform, regardless of the role of states.

PART II / Health and the Policy Process

CHAPTER SIX

The Policy Process

One sister, Rosa, moved a few years ago to a beach town halfway down the long eastern coast of Florida. Unaccustomed to managed care and aware of its bad reputation among older people, Rosa initially opted to continue her fee-for-service Medicare coverage. After some persuasion from a friend in her bridge club, she and her husband agreed to call one of the local Medicare managed care firms and hear its pitch. They were amazed to find that the plan would charge no monthly premium, cover drug costs of up to $800 a month, and cover stays at either of the two nearby hospitals in their beach community. Clearly, coverage in the same federal program differed between fee-for-service and managed care, and it might be still different at a managed care firm other than the one Rosa and her husband chose.

When she had a small stroke a few days after joining the managed care plan, Rosa was very pleasantly surprised at the range of specialists who were quickly assigned to her case: a neurologist, a neurosurgeon, internists, and a physical therapist. After her first night in the hospital, she was visited by the managed care firm's medical director, who was taking a special interest in management of her potentially high-cost case. Had she remained in her fee-for-service plan, or had her stroke occurred a week earlier, before she'd made the switch, Rosa would have been worse off in several ways. She would have faced a one-day cost-of-hospital-care deductible, a daily copayment, a 25 percent copayment for drugs, a major gap in her drug coverage once she'd spent the limits of her coverage a few months after her stroke, and substantial copayments for ambulatory care visits to her physicians after leaving the hospital. She would have had a broader choice of physicians—not just those who were members of her plan—but the ones she had seemed fine and she liked the lower costs and referrals to specialists without searching for one herself.

Medicare notified Rosa and her husband a few months later that their managed care firm was losing its Medicare contract over some compliance issues.

She and her husband went through another round of managed care plan visits and chose another one, and for the most part they were again satisfied, except with their primary care doctor. At the next open enrollment period a year later, they switched plans again in order to get a different primary care doctor. Luckily, she was assigned to a female internist whom she really liked. When she was again hospitalized, with lung cancer, she was attended by two hospitalists (specialists who practice only in the hospital, not in the community), a pulmonologist and a rehabilitation specialist. Managed care firms prefer hospitalists to manage their inpatient care to make sure things go well and don't become unnecessarily expensive. The two hospitalists managed all her hospital care, were very responsive to questions, went by their first names, and seemed to take a real interest in her personally. Ultimately, she did not opt for care by an oncologist because her cancer was too advanced for such care to do much good. She had been a lifelong smoker, and she failed to comply when her internists asked her to get an x-ray, but it was not for lack of excellent care. She did not have an excellent life style, of course, at least with respect to protecting her health.

Meanwhile, across the state, her sister Mae, not yet 65 and working for one of the thousands of service industry firms in Florida, needed back surgery—or at least was told she did, despite government warnings (based on government-sponsored research studies) that back surgery is often not very effective. With no health insurance and an income not close enough to poverty to qualify for Medicaid, Mae and her husband would not be able to pay for her hospital care or for the doctors who would do the surgery.

Were she to collapse at work, Mae might be able to claim workers' compensation coverage. If she were in a car accident and further injured her back, she might be able to get some of her medical expenses covered by the mandatory medical injury coverage that many states, including Florida, require auto insurance companies to include in their policies. Or if she were rushed to a hospital emergency department after such an accident, the federal EMTALA (Emergency Medical Treatment and Active Labor Act) law would require that her condition be diagnosed and stabilized by physicians and staff before they could send her home, but with no plans or obligations related to follow-up care that she might need. The EMTALA law doesn't cover that.

Of course, EMTALA would not stop the hospital from turning over the bill to a collection agency, which would dun Mae repeatedly and quite likely try to garnishee her wages to force her to pay the bill. In fact, Medicare and Medicaid agreements signed by the hospital would require it to go after her for payment—

unless the hospital management wanted to adopt a policy of going after nobody who owed them money; Medicare and Medicaid want to be assured that their patients are not singled out for extra charges.

Mae's congressman heard about the problem of the bad-debt collection policies of hospitals and was concerned that poor people were getting worse care than the nonpoor. She asked the administrator of the Centers for Medicare and Medicaid Services to testify before her House committee to explain how Medicare and Medicaid policies affected bad-debt collection by hospitals. The CMS administrator answered the committee's questions, many of which were written for the committee members by congressional staff who had read a report on the subject—most likely prepared by the Government Accountability Office, the Congressional Budget Office, or the Medicare Payment Advisory Commission.

For their research in preparing a report of this type, any or all of these agencies or individuals quite likely made use of the extensive Medicare and Medicaid data on use and cost provided by the hospitals, as well as cost reports covering all patients and all expenses and bad debts that hospitals must file regularly if they want to participate in Medicare or Medicaid. Or the researchers might have used one of the many surveys of hospital admissions, discharges, payment sources, and other features paid for with public funds.

If Rosa, the sister with Medicare coverage, had been discharged to a nursing home, Medicare might have paid for a few days' stay. A longer stay would have had to be paid for out of her own pocket, until she was poor enough to qualify for Medicaid to cover that portion of the bill that her Social Security and other funds could not pay each month. If either sister died during her hospital stay, state law would dictate whether the case had to be counted in some kind of published hospital mortality index, since the federal mandatory hospital death index was repealed some years ago and replaced in only a few cases, including Florida, by state law. (The new Obama health reform act contains another version of the death index.) And the federal Centers for Disease Control and Prevention would, of course, want to know about the death from a death certificate, so that mortality rates by cause of death and by state and county could be reported. The death might not result in an autopsy, since state laws vary on whether an autopsy is required in routine cases. Florida leaves the decision to the discretion of the state attorney, if that official thinks a crime may have been committed.

But the hospital might do an autopsy anyway, if it had the permission of the family, because the Joint Commission on Accreditation of Healthcare Organizations (JCAHO), a private group operated by hospitals, is a strong proponent of autopsies, and the hospital would not want to risk its state and local licenses to operate as a hospital, or lose its Medicare and Medicaid certification, by becoming careless and losing its JCAHO accreditation. Licensure and certification often require accreditation as one condition among many others. Furthermore, some states might require, as Florida does, that the deceased be transported from the hospital to a burial site under the direction of a funeral director, since the funeral industry has been successful in some states in lobbying the legislature to make it illegal to transport a corpse without involvement of a funeral director.

If neither sister died, after recovering at home they might go out and celebrate, vowing to give up smoking and go on a diet, especially after reading the antismoking, diet, exercise, and other health promotion materials prepared by the CDC and state public health agencies that their husbands had picked up for them in the hospital cafeteria. Driving home from the celebration, whoever was driving would want to be quite sober to avoid violating state driving laws aimed at preventing motor vehicle–related morbidity and mortality.

This is health care policy in the United States: who is and is not eligible to receive subsidized care; what share the individual pays; which types of health care and which services and procedures are covered; who can render care and get paid for rendering it; what government does and does not do when a person needs care but does not have the money to pay for it; who gets financial help with medical care training; what nurses can and cannot do for patients; how wide the doorways of hospital bathrooms should be; what data must be supplied to the federal and state governments; how federal tax policy and workers' protection laws interact with various health care laws; how federal agencies translate congressional intent into regulations affecting health care providers and patients; what records must be kept, how they must be kept, whom they can be shared with, and whom they must be shared with; what kinds of educational materials about healthy living are distributed and which behaviors are restricted or encouraged in the interests of improved health status—and much, much more.

Health care policies are not unique to government. Hospitals have their own private policies: some will not perform abortions; many operate as not-for-profits, while others operate for profit, many of them part of a chain of hospitals owned by investors; some have strong data system firewalls that protect medical records from unauthorized access, others weaker ones; bad debts are absorbed graciously or collected aggressively; infants under a certain weight at birth must be kept in the hospital until they gain weight at some hospitals but not others; one hospital does not operate a drug detoxification center, another does. Insurance companies, in the interest of reducing liability, may require of their nursing home clients that all residents be accompanied to the bathroom whether they need help or not. These private policies share many characteristics with public policies. They differ in that they do not usually have an explicit public purpose and are not compelled by public authority. People do not go to jail for violating a corporate policy (but they may be fired—for example, for violating corporate policy that forbids one worker to tell another worker his pay rate). The real difference, however, is that government policies are made by government and, as such, are the product of a political process in which public elections are a key determinant of who gets to make policy.

The Ambiguity of Public Policy

It would be naive to think that the purpose of health care or other public policy is always obvious. Policy is formed by compromise. In chapter 1 we described how Congress forms an enacting coalition—a specific group of members willing to vote for a specific proposal at a specific time—with a majority large enough to pass a proposal, sometimes just barely. Things are left deliberately vague so that many people with different perspectives can see their views represented in the same ambiguity. More detail might lose a vote. For this reason (and also because of incompetence, uncertainty, time pressures, and bad writing), even though policy always has a purpose, that purpose may not always be easy to figure out. Indeed, the members of Congress who voted for a policy may have many different purposes in mind. Program evaluators find this out early, for health care and every other type of program. Asked to evaluate how well a program is achieving its goals, more often than not the evaluators discover the program does not seem to have any goals. Sometimes it has too many, often conflicting, goals. That a program has been running for several months or years on some vaguely worded rationale may be disturbing to evaluators, but this rarely seems to get in the way of the actors. So an evaluator quickly learns that while no one has articulated goals for the organization, those who work there seem to have some in mind.

At other times, ambiguity can be more troubling. Laboratory administrators serving doctors or hospitals in different states complain about the contradictions and administrative burden of interstate variations. The same firm must adopt different procedures for different states and, in some cases, for counties or regions within a state.

The (Unintended) Consequences of Public Policy

Policy action in health care and other fields frequently differs, sometimes painfully, from intention. As we noted in chapter 1, policymakers vote only on policies, not on outcomes. Their committee specialists tell them what is likely to work, but they may not be right. When health care policymakers wrote new standards for participation in the Medicaid program in the late 1980s and 1990s, they intended to improve the quality of nursing home care for publicly subsidized patients. Although that purpose was accomplished for many patients, for others—low-income, privately paying patients living in facilities too poor to meet the new standards—life was probably made worse when nursing homes dropped out of Medicaid because they could not afford to comply with the new standards. Similar dilemmas face those who wish to upgrade fire and sanitation standards for inner-city apartment buildings and hotels (flop houses) and for assisted living facilities serving people who are elderly and disabled. Tenants too poor to pay the higher rent that accompanies the improvements demanded by new regulations have to move to settings worse than those they inhabited before the government decided to help them. Indeed, in health care policy, much of the problem lies in trying to resolve the inherent tension between reform efforts aimed at improving quality and their unintended consequences for poor people's access to care, or between cost-containment strategies and reduced quality or access. Every time premiums rise, some people drop their insurance. And if one state's regulations become too onerous, corporations and small businesses may choose not to set up shop in that state, moving instead to one with more lenient rules.

The Evolution of Public Policy and Policy Legacies

Policies evolve. Ask any nursing home operator about Medicaid's policy on the quality of care in general, or on the prevention and treatment of decubitus ulcers in particular, and you will most likely get a puzzled look followed by a long-winded answer. As she winds down, the operator will probably have worked herself into a bit of a pique and may finish by saying, "You tell me" or "Do you mean this week or next?" Policy is not written in stone. It is dynamic, a potpourri of laws (often vague), regulations (often late, ambiguous, changing), government officials' interpretations (often conflicting, sometimes wrong), court decisions (sometimes bizarre), and, in the final analysis, the level of compliance by providers, fiscal intermediaries, and patients themselves—who sometimes find ways to systematically alter policy by, for example, giving away their assets instead of spending them for care in lieu of public subsidy. Policies evolve and change because they reflect the negotiated preferences of many parties over differing periods of time. They change because the world changes and the policies must reflect the private sector and the everyday activities of consumers. They change and evolve because they must, so as to be effective and reflect changing demands.

The evolution of public policies builds in part on what is called policy legacies or path dependence. Initial decisions, particularly those affecting institutional choice, become self-reinforcing and develop networks of individuals and groups that benefit from the status quo. As Pierson (2000) put it, earlier actions may "lock in" options that actors would not now choose to initiate. Thus future decisions are path dependent on past policy decisions. In health policy, the current system of employer-based health care, which flows from a decision of a half century ago, tends to curtail the reform options that are considered. While the system could be drastically changed (through a single-payer system, for example), in fact, most policy options to improve access in the intervening years—and there have been many—have built on this employer-based system.

Demands for Health Care Policy Change

In health care, as in every other field, policies come from demands for action or for deliberate inaction. Poor people want access to care. Physicians want a new procedure paid for by Medicare. Hospitals want a place to send discharged patients who cannot find a bed in a Medicaid nursing home, or they want relief from antitrust enforcement, which makes it risky to talk about mergers with other providers. Nursing homes want fewer visits from federal quality-of-care surveyors; the Citizens Coalition for Better Long-Term Care, a patient advocacy group, wants more such visits. Demands may be general or specific: demand that something be done or that something very specific be done. The demand may inspire new health care policy or give existing policy content, direction, or interpretation. The form of the policy may be a new law, a change in an existing law, a regulation, a court decision, or a supervisor's memo interpreting policy to the field staff.

Whatever the genesis, the demand is important to the success of any public policy. Who participates, what resources that person or group possesses, and how that group translates its resources into influence are all important elements of policy development (Hayes, 1992). In addition to the important role of interest groups (see chapter 3), informal groupings of experts in academia, think tanks, and agencies can also play an important role in helping policymakers understand issues and come up with reasonable solutions. These actors, part of what Kingdon (1995) called the policy community, constitute their own attentive public, which can actively aid the progress of an idea. When this community is integrated and in agreement on the nature of the problem and its optimal solution, it can play a major role in policy development. If it is fragmented, or if multiple groups claim community standing, its influence is diminished and the likelihood of developing successful comprehensive policies is lessened.

An important distinction in public policy is that it reflects the public's concerns. Members of Congress and the president (and their counterparts in the 50 states) do not make policy in a vacuum. They listen to their constituents, interest groups, and colleagues and (increasingly) rely on polls and focus groups for policy guidance in answering crucial questions. Are the prescription drug costs of Medicare patients too high? Should guns be more tightly controlled? Is food safety a real concern? Experts in think tanks, universities, and the bureaucracy can help answer these questions, but expert advice alone is not the key to policy initiation. The public must perceive a crisis—and for health care coverage, for a while in 1994 and again in 2009, it did. But in each case, after a few months had passed, the crisis seemed to have abated and attention turned to concerns about too much federal spending.

The pattern of public support for health care reform closely follows what Downs (1972) called the issue attention cycle: the public becomes interested in an issue (or problem) and, for a while, its attention grows as the issue gains salience, is covered by the media, and is the focus of congressional hearings and presidential speeches. At some point, however, it becomes clear that the problem cannot easily be solved, that it will likely involve great expense, and that some groups will be hurt by proposed solutions. The public may now begin to lose interest, and policymakers may lose support for making tough decisions to solve the problem. The public, fickle in its attention, may switch its concerns to another issue. So Congress moves on as well. The 1993–94 debate on national health care reform seemed to fit this pattern. In the spring of 1994, health was the top concern of the public; a few months later, it had been replaced by crime. One thing that pushed health care reform off the agenda was widespread concern that it would raise the insurance premiums of the middle class. In 2005, health care reform was again a focus for several national foundations and a new coalition of business groups and nonprofits interested in alleviating the growing numbers of uninsured while holding down health care costs. In 2009–10 support was so strong for health reform that it finally passed Congress and was signed into law. But within months, Republicans were overwhelmingly elected to formerly Democratic congressional seats on a promise to "repeal and replace" the reforms that had passed.

Downs's model, then, is pessimistic about the possibility of major reforms. But others believe that actions can be taken within the attention cycle to perpetuate the interest and promote long-term reform. Baumgartner and Jones (1993, 87) argued that "even [a] short-lived spurt of [public] interest may leave an institutional legacy" such as an office, group, or staff committed to the issue.

The public is very susceptible to symbolism, and politicians are often successful at manipulating such value-laden issues as patriotism or universal health care coverage to seek public support. When President Clinton promoted national health care reform as "health security" for everybody—ensuring portability from job to job and coverage of existing conditions—rather than focusing on the problem of the uninsured, he was, in Schattschneider's term (1960), trying to "widen the scope of conflict." He wanted to make average Americans feel they had something to lose if health care policy was not reformed. The public likes symbols that oversimplify and often finds comfort in their use (Edelman, 1964). A more recent explanation of public opinion and health policy deals with the idea of policy metaphors, or the combination of norms, practices, and organizational arrangements that shape the public's interpretation of a given policy. Schlesinger and Lau (2000) argued that public opinion is based on policy metaphors rather than details of policy or the workings of U.S. politics. In health, they identified five policy metaphors: health care can be viewed as a community obligation, a marketable commodity, a societal right, an employer responsibility, or an issue under professional control.

Categories of Public Policy

Policies can be categorized in a variety of ways. They can be grouped by issue (say, the health care workforce) or by target audience (Medicare beneficiaries or vulnerable populations or people with disabilities). Policies change over time and so may also be categorized by period: as New Deal policies, or Clinton-era policy, or current policy. Some policies emanate from the states, others from the federal government, others from the 82,000 or more local jurisdictions making policy on everything from screening for HIV to water quality. Campbell (1992), writing about health policymaking in Japan, classified policies in a matrix: big or small, old or new. Old, small policy ideas, he noted, are easiest to pass.

Policies are either substantive or procedural. Substantive policies do things like improve health care, protect the environment, or regulate employment practices. Procedural policies are concerned with *how* the government is doing things. The Administrative Procedures Act of 1946 is the quintessence of a procedural policy, or set of procedural policies. It requires that government regulatory and administrative actions be taken only after notice of proposed rulemaking, opportunity for comment, and publication before becoming effective; and it sets forth explicit procedures for relief and appeal. The National Environmental Policy Act requires environmental impact statements before government agencies can act. Title XIX of the Social Security Act (Medicaid) requires states to adopt a state plan for Medicaid participation and seek approval of any changes in its plan from the CMS, which manages the Medicaid program for the federal government and pays states the federal share of costs.

Environmental policy is fraught with opportunities for both sides to call in their attorneys to argue that proper procedures were not followed. Often the effect (and the intent) is to slow things down, delay, and wait for a better deal or make time for negotiation. Cynics have called the Administrative Procedures Act the "Lawyers Relief Act," but every day this act protects many citizens from arbitrary action by a civil servant. Changes in abortion policy are often sought through procedural requirements. Michigan prochoice supporters argued that a state legislative proposal requiring that women seeking an abortion must be advised of the risks of abortion was a substantive policy masquerading as a procedure. They were particularly outraged by the requirement that the information be provided only by state officials.

Politics shapes policies, but policies also determine politics. Policies can be viewed as distributive, regulatory, or redistributive. Distributive policies often concentrate benefits on hospital corporations, medical schools, or other such beneficiaries, whereas costs are diffused among taxpayers at large and concentrated on no one specific group. So the winners have a big stake in the policy and actively support its passage, while the losers do not lose much and pay little attention. A typical distributive program would be one that sets up federal scholarships for nurse practitioners who agree to practice in medically underserved areas of the state. The witnesses before Congress would likely be nurse practitioner groups, nursing school deans, and spokespersons from hospitals in rural areas that would benefit from the program. There would be few, if any, witnesses speaking against the program. The only possible opposition might come from physicians' assistants or other providers who might think they should have similar programs. Overall, it would be a "love fest," to be repeated in the other house and passed with little fanfare some weeks later. Office of Management and Budget representatives or the Congressional Budget Office might point out that the program would be expensive and ask how it was going to be funded. Only to the extent that the nurse practitioner program would be in competition with programs for physicians, pharmacists, or community housing advocates, would the politics of distributive programs become conflictual. (The impact of the federal budgetary constraint on policymaking is described in chapter 1.)

Regulatory policies restrict the behavior of private and government actors. In health policy the actors are hospitals, physicians, nurses, and graduates of foreign medical schools who want to practice in the United States; drug manufacturers, medical laboratories, and home health agencies; hospital janitors in charge of disposing of medical waste; dentists, who must wash their hands, change gloves, and wear masks to prevent transmission of infections; nuclear power plants, auto manufacturers, farmers, food processors, restaurateurs, and hospital CEOs who want to take over the competition. Continuing the nurse-practitioner example, regulatory policies would be state laws requiring that nurse practitioners practice only under the guidance of physicians. There are clear winners and losers in regulatory policies, and although the losses may be limited (nobody gets killed), they can also be substantial—the opportunity to earn millions or even billions of dollars. Generally speaking, regulatory policies are more controversial than distributive policies, and they are often fought out on the congressional floor and in committee markup sessions. Many are salient and can easily arouse the ire of the group to be regulated. Sometimes the group is state or federal government, as in the case of federal restrictions on state regulation of self-insured managed care firms under the federal Employee Retirement Income Security Act of 1974 or more recent laws to prohibit liability suits against gun makers.

Some regulatory policies—a substantial number in the health care field—are "self-regulatory." Physicians set the standards of practice for physicians, hospitals accredit themselves based on standards set by their own organization (the JCAHO), and schools of public health decide what courses will be required of graduating students in order for them to receive the imprimatur of their association (the Council on Education for Public Health). Government often devolves authority to these self-regulating bodies, taking their seal of approval as evidence that minimal standards have been met and removing some of the political heat—and the cost of enforcement—from government actors.

Redistributive policies take money or power from some and give it to others. In health care policy, redistribution translates to taxing persons with higher incomes to pay for health services for those with lower incomes. The U.S. income tax system is progressive, taking taxes at a higher rate as income rises, because it is believed that those who have the ability to pay are the ones who should pay. Economists argue that extra or marginal units of almost any good are of less value to the recipient than the first units. Following that logic, a little money to a poor person has a lot more social utility than a little more money to a rich person. Religious teachings make a similar point in parables: for example, the New Testament story of the poor widow whose small gift was valued more highly than the larger gift of the rich man.

Medicaid is a redistributive program, taking tax dollars from the middle and upper classes to pay for health care for the very poor and the near poor. Minority hiring policies redistribute job opportunities from white middle-class men to women, persons of color, and members of other minority groups. Many expensive public programs are not very redistributive, and many of those that are redistributive are rather small. Medicaid is an exception. It is large, growing, and very efficiently targeted: three of every four dollars spent by Medicaid goes to people who were poor before they received the services paid for by these funds.

Redistributive policies produce fierce politics. These policies are combative, controversial, constantly under attack, hard to obtain, and hard to retain. When the Reagan administration ushered in its program of government spending cuts, which health care program was the first to be cut? Was it Medicare, the (then) nearly $100 billion program serving all elderly Americans, a group that is mainly middle class and has a poverty rate lower than that of the population in general and roughly half that of children? Or was it Medicaid, a program for the very poor or needy and those who must "spend down" everything they own to a few dollars per month of personal money before they can qualify for benefits? Of course, it was the latter. Because many people wrongly think that Medicaid is more or less exclusively a welfare program aimed at unwed mothers and their children, many of whom are members of a minority group, this is never a popular program with the majority of voters.

Most policies are economic in nature: someone or some group wins, and another loses. Someone pays—although the payment may be spread over so many individuals that little notice is taken. Some scholars have focused on policies with clearly identified losers. The loss might be experienced by a group (dropping those who are medically needy from Medicaid), a geographic area (allowing oil drilling off the Florida Gulf Coast), or a business (cutting hospital reimbursement in Medicare). What is interesting in this line of inquiry is the strategies available to policymakers who must act but who do not want to offend any potential voters. Pal and Weaver (2003) noted the available choices:

—manipulate procedures: delegate responsibilities to bureaucrats or advisory bodies, bury the policy choice in a reconciliation bill or omnibus bill where it might "get lost," or shift venue to the states or the courts;

—manipulate perceptions: use technical language or changes to lower visibility and find a scapegoat (globalization, for example); or

—manipulate payoffs: delay or phase in implementation of the policy or provide some benefits along with the pain.

A nonmonetary loss can also be incurred, something Pal and Weaver (2003) categorize as a symbolic loss. Such a loss is often in the area dubbed "morality" policies, a subset of noneconomic public policies. Several health issues fall into this category, including abortion, the "morning-after" pill, the right to die, and gun control. These issues address social relationships and are associated with "values" rather than facts. Morality issues tend to be highly salient and very controversial in a way that sets their development and implementation apart from other issues. Morality issues tend to be seen as absolutes by those who care about them, making it difficult for politicians to take a middle ground or for compromise to occur (Mooney, 2001). Morality policies are generally technically simpler than most other types of policy; everyone can be reasonably well informed on an issue and have an opinion. In abortion policy, for example, the issue is well understood and individuals have staked out a position. In one national survey, only five respondents—0.3 percent of the sample—had no opinion on the abortion question (Norrander & Wilcox, 2001). Morality issues also generally involve grassroots organization and mobilization. Given the political difficulty with morality issues, legislative bodies often avoid making decisions in these areas—and judicial action frequently is the result (McFarlane & Meier, 2001).

The Extent of Policy Change

Not all policy changes are equal in their scope, range, and depth. Some changes are clearly monumental, generally reflecting a value change in society, often leading to institutional changes and pointing policy in a new direction. One example was the enactment of Medicare in 1965, the first major federal health program guaranteeing health care for a large targeted population. But most public policies are not comprehensive. Rather, they are incremental: they build on earlier policies, are implemented by existing agencies and departments, and generally follow the policy direction of earlier policies. The 2010 Patient Protection and Affordable Care Act expanded access by expanding Medicaid and providing subsidies to small businesses and poor and near-poor individuals. It did relatively few things to cut costs, and to improve quality it did little more than authorize demonstration and pilot programs. It did not remove the tax deductibility of employer-sponsored health insurance, and it did not enact an all-payer system or expand Medicare as a single payer system to replace private health insurance. It was incremental. Yet it incurred great wrath among conservatives as going too far in expansion of the government role in health care (Weissert & Weissert, 2010).

The politics of the two types of policies—comprehensive and incremental—are quite different. Comprehensive policies flow from major changes in public attitudes, often expressed through election results. Hayes (1992) argued that these nonincremental policies can be adopted only when values are agreed upon and when there is an adequate knowledge base. Even with these two criteria in place, the environment must be right for change—usually a turbulent environment characterized by a dramatic shift in the political world or public opinion. Public support is crucial to successful adoption of comprehensive change. Support by "elites," those who are influential in the thinking of policymakers and the president, is important as well. It also helps if leaders are willing to take a chance and opponents are unable to defend their position. But as Hayes noted, nonincremental change is simply impossible for many issues. Incremental policies are most likely to emerge from situations in which there is not much information and no national agreement on values. Incremental policies pit interests against interests, sometimes in a situation where public attention is low and interest groups, federal agencies, congressional committees, and other interested parties grapple with the problems and their possible solution quietly and without public fanfare. In the case of national health insurance, lack of consensus on the role of government often divides the parties and the country, so that what emerges is a compromise struck between interest groups and the majority party, with little participation by the minority party—resulting in incremental change.

Some argue that the distinction between incremental and comprehensive change is extremely vague and may reside in the eye of the beholder. And, in fact, a series of what one sees as incremental changes can have the combined power of major change, and seemingly comprehensive change may be simply an amalgamation of incremental steps. For example, changes in federal reimbursement systems encompassed in the Medicare Prospective Payment System in the 1980s led to a redefinition of health care delivery by hospitals and other providers. Yet the changes were accomplished across several years and several decisions and are hard to view as a single comprehensive change. The Medicare Modernization Act of 2003 was a major change in Medicare—offering for the first time selective coverage of prescription drugs. But other aspects of the law, such as expansion of health savings accounts, were clearly incremental.

Incrementalism is often an easier sell to the voting public and Congress, because most people are averse to risk. They are reluctant to make large and risky changes because the consequences and costs are hard to predict and unintended consequences can be costly. Many have observed that savvy politicians use this understanding of the policy process to select a strategy for creating policy change. No one was a greater master of this incrementalist strategy than the very liberal Henry Waxman (D-CA), former House health and environment subcommittee chair. "He sets such ambitious policy aims that colleagues might consider him a pie-in-the-sky fool if they were not by now so familiar with his technique of taking a small slice at a time until years later he is holding the whole pie—even in the face of spending retrenchment. Persistence and patience are his strengths" (Duncan, 1993, 188). Others call this strategy "the nose of the camel under the tent." Once the nose is in, it is hard to keep the rest of the camel out.

Kingdon (1995, 83) quoted one of his sources as saying, "These things proceed in small, incremental steps. Something is enacted, everybody concludes that it's not so bad, and that gets people ready for the next bite." Aware of the higher likelihood of success with incremental than with comprehensive approaches, national health reformers have battled for 40 years over which approach would produce more success.

Despite the failures of most previous presidents who sought major change in health policy, President Clinton rejected a narrowly focused plan addressing only catastrophic care costs, in favor of a broad plan that covered everyone, expanded benefits, reduced copayments, and mandated businesses to pay three-quarters of the cost of premiums. Political and health policy advisers urged him to focus on the vision of major change that he had promised in the campaign and that, they argued, the American people demanded and expected. Economic advisers, sensing Clinton's preference for this visionary approach and swallowing their reservations, couched their support in conditional language that took advantage of the fact that the choice between broad and narrow reform was being made without the benefit of cost projections (Woodward, 1994).

The post mortems would suggest that in addition to ignoring and then badly underestimating the costs, the boosters of comprehensive change had misread the voters. What the voters meant by major change was a guarantee of portability—an assurance that insurance would not be lost or priced out of their reach when workers changed jobs or lost employment. But to the Clinton administration and its potentially most ardent supporters—AARP, labor, and other beneficiary-group lobbies—this type of paltry change was the worst kind of incrementalism. Two years after delivering a crushing defeat to Clinton's comprehensive approach, Congress passed legislation guaranteeing portability of health care coverage for up to 18 months after job loss or change; this development suggested that it was indeed an incremental change that voters wanted.

Clinton was not the only president to succumb to the siren song of comprehensive change. President Jimmy Carter ridiculed incremental efforts, saying that "most of the controversial issues that are not routinely well-addressed can only respond to a comprehensive approach" (Wildavsky, 1979, 242). He thought incremental efforts were doomed because of interest groups' opposition and that with strong public support, comprehensive change could be implemented. Carter, like Clinton after him, found mobilizing and maintaining such public support difficult indeed. President Obama sold his plan as comprehensive, found himself barely able to pass it because not one Republican would support it, and ultimately signed into law an important improvement in poor people's access to care but by no means a comprehensive reform of the perverse and runaway payment system or the uneven quality it pays for.

The Policy Process Framework

The public policy process is too complicated, mutable, and variable for easy understanding, much less prediction. There are simply too many variables, and many of them are contingent on other variables and contexts. Institutions, rules, policy legacies, temporal conditions, electoral preferences, catastrophes, economic conditions, technology—all play a role in policymaking. Individual behavior is also key: lawmakers' preferences are contingent on many of the aforementioned factors plus their own personal views on the issue, their perceptions of voters and groups in their district, their relationship to party leaders, their electoral popularity, and on and on. And these are only the variables predicting policy adoption. There is an entire other aspect of policy, related to implementation, that involves a different, though sometimes overlapping, cast of characters and incentives.

Then there are the theoretical mechanisms for understanding the process. Elinor Ostrom (1999) (2010 Nobel Prize winner for her body of work) has helped us by categorizing the levels of analysis into frameworks, theories, and models. Frameworks are the most general and help us identify the elements and relationships among the variables that should be considered. Theories go a step further to include specification of which elements in the framework are particularly relevant to which questions and to make assumptions about the relationship. Models are the most specific and set forth precise assumptions leading to outcomes in ways that can be tested.

Using the framework approach, we can talk about the components that make up the policy process. One elementary, yet instructive, framework is the progression that public policies follow: (1) a problem is recognized and defined, (2) a public policy is developed to deal with the problem, (3) the public policy becomes law or is otherwise put in place, and (4) the public policy is implemented. The story does not end with policy implementation, however. During implementation, the lessons learned are applied to revising or improving the policy in an important feedback mechanism. But here we concentrate on the definition of the problem, the formulation of policy, its legitimation, and its implementation.

Problem Definition

One point on which all models and most students of the policy process agree is the importance of defining the problem. It is certainly true that policies sometimes begin with someone pushing a favorite solution, but these must ultimately be coupled to a problem or they do not become law. Problems are essential. Reich (1988, 5) asserted that "the most important aspect of political discourse is not the appraisal of alternative solutions to our problems, but the definition of the problems themselves." According to Baumgartner and Jones (1993), problem definition is the very engine of change because it is the essence of power. Problems are inherently political, because they are not simply out there waiting to be solved; they must be formulated and defined, using political skill to mobilize support for the desired position.

Definitions of problems are chosen strategically, "designed to call in reinforcements for one's own side in a conflict" (Stone, 1988, 122). Is it more accurate to describe a procedure to terminate a pregnancy as dilation and extraction or as partial birth abortion, and which will be more effective in arousing the ire of anti-abortion groups? Is requiring an HMO physician to use one brand of medication rather than another interference with medical decision making by faceless bureaucrats, or is it cost control? Should the focus be placed on medical errors or patient safety? Is smoking a choice made by adults or an addiction perpetrated on children by tobacco company advertising? The definition of a problem sets the parameters for discussion and lends legitimacy to an issue. The definition flows from the choice of values (Dery, 1984) and can also determine whether the problem demands public policy action. Not all problems are candidates for public policy. Some may be viewed as either intractable or not in the government domain. Eyestone (1978) provided three prerequisites for governments' recognition of a policy problem: governments must correctly identify a social problem or issue, governments must have the capacity to respond, and politicians must be persuaded that they should respond.

There is a strong pragmatic streak in problem definition. Policymakers tend to select for consideration those problems that can be solved. As Wildavsky (1979, 42) put it, "A difficulty is a problem only if something can be done about it." Problems that tend to defy solution, according to Downs (1972), are those for which one or more of the following conditions hold:

—A numerical minority (not necessarily ethnic) is suffering from the
  problem.
—Suffering is caused by social arrangements that provide benefits to the
  majority or a powerful minority of the population.
—The problem has no exciting qualities (or is no longer seen as exciting).

These qualities seem to fit the plight of the uninsured pretty well.

Consumed as entertainment, the news must stay lively to retain its readers and viewers. If the problem is of national scope and is, objectively, a major concern, it may sporadically recapture interest or attach itself to another problem that takes center stage. When it does so, it will usually receive a higher level of attention, effort, and concern than problems still in the prediscovery stage. As Schon (1971, 42) put it, "Old questions are not answered—they only go out of fashion." The uninsured are a sad example: important in 1965; back on the agenda and even more important in the early 1980s and again in the 1990s; rarely mentioned in the early 2000s, despite their growing numbers; and focus of the most spending in the 2010 reform, although the bill was sold more as a solution to costs (which it wasn't) than to access by the poor (which it was).

In health, the definition of a problem is crucial. Is the problem an unequal system of health care delivery, costs that are rising too rapidly, or the quality of the care provided? Is the problem excessive paperwork or waste, profiteering insurance companies, greedy doctors, or a third-party payer system that encourages inefficiencies? Or is it all these things, as President Clinton proclaimed in his health address before Congress in September 1993? Part of Clinton's task, as defined by Eyestone (1978), was accomplished: identifying the problem. But his harder task, persuading politicians and the country to respond, was only beginning. President George W. Bush decided that the problem was costs, so he proposed consumer-driven, high-deductible health savings accounts in his 2006 State of the Union address (Lee, 2006).

Where Problems Come From

Problems do not just emerge. Citizens, leaders, organizations, interest groups, and government agencies create them in the minds of their fellow citizens. Problems come to what Cobb and Elder (1972) called the systemic or public agenda. Problems originate when people perceive bias, groups seek advancement or assistance, or groups seek (their view of) the public good. The triggering device for a problem can be a natural catastrophe, an unanticipated human event, ecological change, or technological change. If it sufficiently affects many people, a problem can enter the formal or institutional agenda, where policymakers will recognize and consider the matter. Problems can also reach the institutional agenda through interest-group lobbying, congressional staffers, bureaucrats, constituents, or members of Congress themselves who discover a problem and wish to "solve" it with government action.

Measuring and Framing Problems

Problems are usually ill defined and, more often than not, exaggerated. Advocates often approximate prevalence and severity in congressional testimony and press reports. Their goal is to dramatize the problem and create a sense of urgency. They want to make people feel the problem is so widespread that they could be its next victims. Advocates must "oversell" their positions to avoid losing their audience, Kingdon (1995) contended. Some recent examples make his point.

Jon Kyl (R-AZ) was one of many voices claiming, "Almost everybody agrees that we can save between $100 billion and $200 billion if we had effective medical malpractice reform" (Hart, 2009). Yet the nonpartisan Congressional Budget

Office, after synthesizing all major studies of malpractice reform's effects where changes have been made, concluded that savings would be about one-half percent, or about $11 billion (CBO, 2009a).

Estimates of the prevalence of mental health problems in the U.S. adult population were also probably substantially overestimated by the long-regarded authoritative studies done by the National Institute of Mental Health. More recent researchers corrected the estimates by replacing simple self-report of problems with questions to determine whether treatment was being used, including drugs; whether a professional was being seen; and whether individuals experienced symptoms that interfered with their lives. Using these more behavioral indicators dropped estimates from 30 percent suffering mental illness and 50 percent needing help to 18.5 percent showing a disorder (Estimates of Mentally Ill, 2002).

Other examples include exaggerated claims of the number of battered women, the number of children abducted by strangers, the rate of infection with HIV among women, and the risk of HIV infection among children. The policymaking process must sort out the validity of the demands and decide whether a public policy solution is warranted or whether, for example, hospitals should be left to solve their own problems.

Finally, problems can be "framed" in ways that lead to very different solutions. The framing of problems can also be crucial in engendering public support for the problem—and its subsequent solution. One example of the importance of framing in understanding policy is in the area of assisted suicide. Proponents of assisted suicide framed the issue as one of individual rights and personal empowerment, emphasizing patients' dignity, individual rights, and autonomy. Opponents of assisted suicide framed the issue as contrary to the healing mission of physicians. A Michigan physician, Dr. Kevorkian, helped personify this notion of a physician gone amok (Glick & Hutchinson, 2001).

Attributing Causes

For years, airplane crashes were invariably attributed to pilot error. Manufacturers did not take kindly to having their aircraft designs and construction blamed, and flight controllers were not willing to accept blame when a plane missed the runway or two planes had a close encounter. Mechanical failures or accepting bad landing instructions became the pilot's fault: he was blamed for not doing a better job of inspecting his aircraft before takeoff or not figuring out that another plane was already using the runway to which he had been directed. As the aircraft industry improved, as air traffic controllers realized they were unlikely to get better pay and lighter workloads unless they admitted mistakes and reported near misses, as terrorism became a competing cause of aircraft failures, and as National Transportation Safety Board bureaucrats got better at their jobs, we began to hear more candid representations of the facts—though still typically couched in the most careful, caveat-ridden technical language, because powerful interests have a stake in the causes to which bad outcomes are attributed.

So, too, in health care: much of framing the problem involves linking the problem to its root cause. And different causes lead to different solutions. For the first half of the twentieth century, tobacco companies claimed that smoking did not cause health problems. When the data had mounted to the point of undeniability, the companies' lawyers worked to put the blame on the smokers themselves, who should have known better. Finally, by the late 1990s, blame for smokers' deaths had shifted from individual smokers to cigarette manufacturers and their advertising and marketing campaigns, especially those targeted at children. Policy shifted with each new perspective on the problem: from the federal government's including cigarettes in military box lunches until as late as the mid-1960s, to government warnings about adverse health effects printed on cigarette packs from the late 1960s, to restrictions on tobacco companies' marketing techniques, especially those directed at youngsters, in the 1990s. When bartenders who sold drinks to obviously intoxicated customers began to be seen as part of the problem of drunk driving, dram laws were passed in state after state. The malpractice debate often turns upon whether bad quality of medical practice, trivial lawsuits, runaway juries, or insurance company business practices are the root cause, a contributing factor, or not very important.

The linkage between cause and effect is crucial to policy choice. In fact, Deborah Stone (1989) claimed that people choose causal linkages not only to shift blame but also to create the idea that they can remedy the problem. The focus on "deadbeat dads," for example, is ideal for a quick and popular legislative initiative: track them down and garnishee their wages or throw them in jail for nonpayment of child support. Fair enough, but this is hardly a solution to the intractable and complex problem of out-of-wedlock teen pregnancies or even its enormous and intergenerational costs and consequences.

Formulating Public Policy Options

Not all problems are public problems; many can be solved in the private sector or simply will not be solved at all. Determining what is a public problem—to be solved by government—is not always easy. And it varies from generation to generation. In recent years, what once might have been public problems have been more and more relegated to the market. Other issues are also important in this formulation stage, including equity issues and the cost of the endeavor.

Is It a Public Problem?

American culture is built around core beliefs concerning individual liberty—defined as freedom from government constraints—that have a powerful effect on how people perceive the meaning of *public problems* (Bosso, 1994). In health care, as in other areas, the criterion for defining public involvement is this: is the problem better settled by the public than by the private sector? Policies on issues as disparate as airline industry regulation, sexual harassment, job training, international trade, and needle-exchange programs have all had to meet this "public role" criterion before government intervention could be justified (Rochefort & Cobb, 1994).

The meaning of *public*, however, is in the eye—or rather the ideology—of the beholder. People (including policymakers) differ in their views on the proper role of government. One recent issue illustrating this point is obesity. Many people in public health think the increasing incidence of obesity in the United States, particularly among children, is a public problem, but most of the public does not agree. For example, a 2003 survey of Michigan residents found that only 28 percent thought being overweight was a public concern (Ford, Olson & Baumer, 2004). While much attention has been focused on this issue, several barriers needed to be overcome before it could be justified as a public problem, including broad-based social disapproval, definitive research linking obesity with adverse health effects, emergence of a self-help movement, the "demonizing" of the relevant industry, organization of a mass movement, and interest-group action (Kersh & Morone, 2002). One step in that direction is *The Botany of Desire: A Plant's-Eye View of the World,* by Michael Pollan (2002). In this book the author attributes much of America's obesity problem to federal farm subsidies that make corn cheap, encouraging the oversupply and overconsumption of corn syrup, a high-calorie substance found in most fast food and soft drink products. It quickly became a best seller.

For many, markets are the preferred solution: government should be limited to instances of market failure. But does this simplify things? Not really, because claims of market failure do little more than open a debate about whether the market has failed. Is health care a well-functioning market? Or is it plagued by market failures because of several distinctive characteristics, including, for example, information asymmetry: patients as buyers and health care professionals as sellers are not equal players. Professionals use enormous amounts of technical knowledge to judge whether their patients need the care they prescribe. Most patients are completely or almost completely ignorant of the science underlying clinical decision making. This information asymmetry distorts the principle of consumer sovereignty and, to many, justifies public action to at least license professionals so as to weed out unqualified providers. Others would go further. Given that the physician has the power to influence the patient's decisions about how much of a product to buy, they advocate regulating physicians' fees and reviewing the appropriateness of prescribed care. Physicians strongly objected to the 2010 PPACA provisions empowering Medicare to reward physicians who used only care deemed effective by national standards and allowing the program to eventually decline payment for care deemed ineffective. "We do not need centralized government medicine," Dr. Lawrence Gorfine, president of the Palm Beach County Medical Society told the *Orlando Sentinel* (Gibson & LaMendola, 2010).

Externalities—costs or benefits falling on others—are also a concern in health care policy. Some health care problems affect more than the individual; infectious diseases are the principal case in point. Because of the risks involved in the spread of diseases, government must take responsibility for ensuring that everyone is vaccinated and, under some circumstances, evaluated for the presence of disease. Public health and sanitation laws and enforcement are justified on this principle. "Free riders" are another problem sometimes necessitating public action. Young healthy workers who decline to buy insurance are counting on the rest of us to pay for emergency rooms to care for them if they get sick or have an accident. They are free riders on an expensive health care system maintained by the insurance premiums paid by the rest of society.

Ideological differences about the role of government action help policymakers pick sides in the debate over whether government action is needed. Party affiliation helps people make up their minds. While Republicans are often quite willing to use government to restrict behavior related to moral issues, they tend to favor minimal government for solving domestic problems. They want the market to solve such problems, unless there is strong evidence that this approach is not working and cannot be fixed. Republicans strongly support market-based approaches, including improving competition, imposing substantial copayments, prohibiting the government from setting national drug prices, and instead setting up health savings accounts to encourage consumers to pay their own health care bills. Democrats, particularly liberal Democrats, are quicker to give up on the market and seek government intervention, and more of it. The 2010 Patient Protection and Affordable Care Act was an example. Democrats wanted to expand Medicaid and provide subsidies to poor and near-poor individuals and small businesses and to restrict or prohibit well-known insurance industry abuses, including rescissions of coverage, refusal to sell coverage, substantial rate hikes for policy renewal, and large rate differences between young and old, sick and well. Republicans preferred health savings accounts and tax credits to permit people to buy their own insurance, breaking out of the hammerlock of employer-sponsored insurance.

This tension between the parties over the role of government is predictable for many issues, as pointed out by Eyestone (1978). He noted that most social questions are not neutral with respect to the issue of government involvement. For any two competing issues, he said, one will almost certainly call for more government involvement than the other, and the contrast will invoke the government role to some degree. Further, he noted, the appeal against bloated government is often a conscious political strategy—a charge also made by Democrats when Republicans criticized President Clinton's proposed health insurance purchasing alliances.

The public, too, is often skeptical about government intervention and evaluates a proposal by whether or not its extension of government power will directly affect the public. Public skepticism has a long history in health policy and has played a major role in stymieing the development of national health insurance. The arguments used in 1964 and 1994 regarding freedom to choose a physician, quality of treatment, and the possibility of bureaucratic medicine were nearly identical. And both times, they were effective. When a poll asked people to choose between reliance on a government or a private-oriented approach, a majority chose the private approach (Jacobs, 1993). Further, although Democrats are more likely than Republicans to support a tax-financed national health plan, even liberal support is "tempered by concern over the problems of bureaucracy and the practical limits to what government can accomplish" (634).

Appropriateness of the government role is an equally critical standard of acceptability for health care policies—that is, for solutions. This criterion is easier to meet at some times than at others. During more liberal times, a significant block of voters moves from serious distrust of government's ability to solve problems to a willingness to suspend disbelief long enough to try out a new set of reforms. The Great Depression was a time when the private market had clearly failed many Americans, and they were willing to turn to government for help.

Again during the Johnson years, Americans seemed willing to experiment with public approaches to meeting a pent-up demand for solutions to a host of social concerns. Values seem to oscillate between relatively more liberal and relatively more conservative positions; these cycles are difficult to predict but at times seem to span three decades or so. In 2003 pharmaceutical companies were greatly concerned that Medicare price setting would stifle innovation and discourage new cures. Congress responded by passing a law that essentially guarantees that drugmakers will have their prices set by the market rather than by government, even though government was already a large purchaser of drugs and, through Medicare, is becoming a much larger one.

Even in more liberal times, a high level of distrust of government remains, making some proposals unacceptable. One such proposal is mandatory participation in government health insurance programs: the individual mandate in the 2010 PPACA. To many liberals, mandatory participation is the only effective solution to the free-rider problem—people at low risk avoid insurance, producing adverse selection as the sick seek insurance and premium costs increase, thus inducing more dropouts, more uninsured individuals, more adverse selection, and so forth; it is sometimes called a "death spiral." Insurance companies will not agree to admit patients with preexisting conditions if they can't also be assured that all people without illnesses will also be required to buy their insurance products. Yet little seems to enrage conservatives more than mandatory participation in a public program they do not support. This is particularly true when the problem is, as Downs (1972) suggested, one that does not affect most members of society. National health insurance proposals involve significant dislocations and costs for all those who feel they are already well served in the private market. With premiums for nonelderly people substantially paid by employers and care for the elderly and many people with disabilities paid for by Medicare and Medicaid, most people fall into this category. Either they have insurance or they think they do not need it. The exceptions are the poor and the near poor: they need it and want it but cannot afford it.

Over time, for some kinds of solutions, attitudes soften and ideas that were once anathemas gain support and can be adopted. Mandatory use of seat belts, initially strongly opposed as government intrusion into private lives, was later grudgingly tolerated and eventually welcomed as a necessary safety device effective against real harm. By 2000, some 30 years after the use of seat belts was first required and resisted, laws were being passed (with little opposition) allowing police to stop drivers for seat belt violations alone.

Requisites for changes in attitudes are the passage of time and accumulation of overwhelming evidence that benefits justify government intrusion. Kingdon (1995) noted that "softening up" occurs while time is passing. Promoters talk about their proposal and make people more familiar with it. They may also change it enough to make it more acceptable. As a result, ideas that failed the appropriateness test when first introduced tend to be introduced again and again; they become better understood, more familiar, and easier to accept as time goes by. Prospective payments to hospitals are a case in point.

Unfortunately, the time required for softening up is unpredictable; for some proposals in some places, more than a half century has not been sufficient. For example, drinking water has been fluoridated in this country since the mid-1940s, and fluoridation became official public health policy in the 1950s. To the experts at the American Dental Association, it has long been a settled issue. Their official position is this: "Studies prove water fluoridation continues to be effective in reducing tooth decay by 20–40 percent, even in an era with widespread availability of fluoride from other sources, such as fluoride toothpaste. Fluoridation is one public health program that actually saves money. An individual can have a lifetime of fluoridated water for less than the cost of one dental filling" (ADA, 2011). Yet fluoridation continues to be controversial in some communities. As of November 2011, nearly 30 counties, cities, and towns, inhabited by 2,571,500 people, had recently voted to stop fluoridating their water, according to an advocacy website that reports success of the stop-fluoridation movement (Fluoridation Action Network, 2011).

Explicit rationing of health care to control costs is still unacceptable to most Americans, but the idea began creeping into public policy discourse in the 1990s (Lamm, 1990) and was adopted for Oregon's poor residents early in that decade— although, in response to fierce objections, its most controversial provisions were watered down. Some solutions grow less acceptable with time. Forced screening for various infectious or inherited diseases, particularly those that uniquely affect a minority group, is not a publicly acceptable method of disease control or cost control and shows few signs of becoming acceptable, even though quarantine for infection was once more or less routine.

Equity

The reliability of government as a problem solver is not all that is at stake in the debate over the government's role. Often lurking behind the symbols is the real point of departure between conservatives and liberals: income equality, or re-distribution. Liberals typically want to use government intervention as a means of redistributing power and wealth to the poor and disenfranchised. Deborah Stone (1993) even pushed for such an outcome from the private sector on the is-sue of pooling health insurance risk. Arguing that the nation is a community, she rejected an insurance company's definition of actuarial fairness: "the lower your risk, the lower your premium" (288). On the contrary, she argued, each person paying for his own risk, when taken to its extreme, would mean every person's premium would be based on a perfect prediction of the person's health care costs. The result would be the end of insurance, since all who could afford to would simply put the money in the bank to avoid insurance company profits and administrative costs. She called actuarial fairness "anti-redistributive ideology" (294). In contrast, she argued, "Social insurance operates by the logic of 'solidar-ity.' Its purpose is to guarantee that certain agreed-upon individual needs will be paid for by a community or group . . . In the health area, the argument for fi-nancing medical care through social insurance rests on the prior assumption that medical care should be distributed according to medical need or the ability of the individual to benefit from medical care" (290).

Harvard philosopher John Rawls (1971) would most probably agree. Most peo-ple are risk averse; in situations in which their future status is unpredictable (they wear a "veil of ignorance"), they tend to adopt policies that raise the position of the least advantaged. Fearing that they could become part of the minority, they adopt redistributive policies that lead to greater equality of outcomes.

In voluntary insurance plans, the sickest people buy insurance, well people (es-pecially young people) wait until they get sick, and premiums rise over time, exac-erbating the problem. Insurance companies find it in their interest to sell insur-ance only to people who are not likely to use it, excluding in any way they can those who are likely to get sick. The means companies resort to include physical exams, exclusion of preexisting conditions, long waiting periods, and high and rising pre-miums for those who present an elevated risk, especially when "experience" shows that an individual has a tendency to use substantial care. Information about risk indicators and health care utilization is often accessed at the time an individual applies for a new job that includes health insurance. The result is that people with elevated risk may be unable to change jobs without becoming uninsurable or fac-ing prohibitive premiums. Sometimes the health insurance policies of an entire small firm face cancellation owing to the risks or costs of one unlucky individual.

Mandatory national health insurance covering the young and old, sick and well, and those who have no health problems today but may have them tomorrow is offered as one way to increase the size of the risk pool and distribute the costs of high-risk individuals among all policy holders. This raises the premiums of well people above what they would pay in an experience-rated plan and lowers the premiums of sick people. It may also require an expansion of the benefit package to meet the needs of enrollees with special problems; high limits on prescription drugs, coverage of experimental treatments, adaptive housing, transportation, special communications aids, and personal care for chronically ill patients may be needed. Because these are typically limited in the benefit packages and premium calculations of private plans, they may further increase premiums above those for private, experience-rated plans. The result tends to be premiums that redistribute wealth from some premium payers to others and expansion of the role of government into new sectors of the economy as it referees disputes among beneficiary subgroups over what services should be covered. The side one chooses in this perennial debate reflects one's values and typically involves a trade-off between greater efficiency and greater fairness in solving problems.

Reliance on the market to distribute income, wealth, and equity of access to health care may produce particular problems for minority groups. Even a quick review of the data shows that the market has not worked very well to remove differences in health status between minority and nonminority Americans. Members of minorities live sicker and die sooner from a wide variety of acute and chronic conditions. African Americans experience the poorest health outcomes of all racial or ethnic groups in the United States. Minorities account for half of all the uninsured in the United States. Even when they are insured, minorities are less likely to receive adequate care (Kennedy, 2005). African Americans and other minorities also confront significant treatment disparities. Socioeconomic status is a powerful determinant of both health and mortality (Fiscella, 2003).

Nevertheless, advocates of market-oriented solutions to health care problems do not see racial barriers as a problem. Free-market advocates argue that firms that discriminate will lose business to those that don't. But failure to confront the reality that poverty is highly correlated with minority racial status in the United States means that the special needs of minorities may not be met by the market, at least not in a kindly fashion. Likewise, policies that require poor individuals to pass through invasive and demeaning eligibility screenings to prove they are poor enough to receive benefits, as well as requiring them to accept care from providers willing to work for the invariably lower prices paid by government, are an affront to many advocates for the poor: these policies produce "two-tiered" care, the lower tier disproportionately provided to minority-group members. Policies since roughly 2005 have highlighted the need for an infrastructure for monitoring and tracking disparities, including the congressionally mandated National Healthcare Disparities Report, which has developed consistent definitions and tracks changes in quality of care over time (Moy, Dayton & Clancy, 2005).

Means Testing and Redistribution

Liberals and conservatives often part company over means testing as a way of limiting public subsidies and the scope of the public role. The two major political parties subscribe to different philosophies of how best to improve the lot of the poor. Conservatives fear creating dependency among those given free care, and they worry that further taxing the well-off will stifle investment and that the inevitable standards that accompany subsidies will discourage innovation. They prefer to restrict free care to the poorest of the poor and count on a growing and innovative economy to provide more income for everyone and more efficient production than a highly regulated economy can offer. Physicians tend to side with the conservatives on this issue, because they prefer to earn their incomes from middle-class, privately paying patients, restricting government health care programs to those who cannot pay on their own. Their fear is that with government subsidies will come fee schedules and other controls, eroding their income and freedom. Liberals prefer to use progressive taxation to raise revenues and provide the health care benefit free to all, removing the stigma attached to "charity" care and mitigating the temptation to render poor care to poor people (although this is hard to avoid if the poor and the middle class use different providers, as they often do because they live in different parts of town). Means testing is an approach to limiting government's role and making proposals more affordable. Even some liberal U.S. senators have supported it, based on cost concerns, when Republicans have made it a part of many of their own health reforms, including the 2003 Medicare Modernization Act, which charges higher drug coverage premiums for wealthier Medicare beneficiaries. Ironically, the private sector may also have moved to means testing in a serious way by beginning to charge more for health insurance to high-income employees than to secretaries and mail-room clerks (Abelson, 2010).

These differences in perspective between what are loosely referred to as liberal and conservative views reflect fundamental differences in social priorities and in notions about the efficacy of government as a solution to social problems. For these reasons, merely pointing out that a problem exists in no way ensures a consensus on the need for government action. In defining health care problems for public policy intervention, technical arguments must take shape within an ideological context. Values are often at least as important as data.

Who Will Pay the Costs?

When policy analysts think of costs, they think in terms of efficiency: the amount of output for each unit of input. Often they are concerned with cost-effectiveness or cost-benefit ratios: the marginal benefit for a marginal expenditure. Politicians make a similar but slightly different calculation. They are worried about how to pay the political costs—dollars, disruption, administrative burden—and whether the juice is worth the squeeze. Proposals that are very costly and of dubious effectiveness are dead letters.

National health insurance is a case in point. In most proposals, costs typically fall on one of two groups: businesses (through a government mandate or some other form of taxation) or taxpayers in general (usually through a payroll tax such as Medicare, supplemented by "sin taxes" or through taxation of employer-provided health insurance premiums). In an important if ill-fated variation in the 1980s, a catastrophic health insurance plan for elderly people tried a third approach: it taxed wealthy beneficiaries of the program to pay some of the costs for poorer beneficiaries. The law was repealed the following year as those who were targeted to pay complained about the cost for the value received. In 2010 Republicans hoped to use that earlier repeal as a model for gutting or repealing the Obama health reform.

Taxation of health insurance premiums paid by employers (Calmes, 2010) or taxes on policies with premiums above some threshold premium value ("Cadillac policies," as they were called when included in the 2010 PPACA) are appealing economically because, in addition to raising money, these kinds of taxes can make consumers more aware of their health care costs in a way that might help restrain spending or at least ensure receiving value for price. But, of course, they have one very great drawback. The benefits are diffused among the entire beneficiary population, many of whom are poor and most of whom are not well organized around the health insurance issue—so the latter group aren't likely to rally around such tax plans and encourage supporters. But the costs are heavily concentrated on employers and on insurance companies, which may lose lucrative business. Proposals that concentrate costs on powerful interests such as business are sure to be met by well-financed, well-organized resistance. Even though many economists have argued that costs of health insurance are shifted ultimately to employees, employers tend to see themselves as paying the bill. Hence, from their perspective, employer mandates put the burden on business, especially small businesses not currently offering coverage; firms make the point that a person employed in a business not offering insurance often can get coverage through a spouse's employer. All these strategies involve major political problems and create incentives for employers to organize and spend resources to oppose the plan, while most beneficiaries individually have little to gain and cannot be inspired to act collectively.

Costs, no matter where they fall, have become much more important than they used to be, especially in health care policy and regardless of whether the budget is in deficit or surplus. For decades, costs were a secondary consideration at best, and even then only for large, expensive projects costing billions of dollars. Costs were of no concern at all for smaller projects of only a few million dollars. Mere thousands have long been rounded off in federal budgets. Debate challenging the feasibility of Medicare in 1965 did address the cost issue, and even President Johnson's staff was concerned about the higher-than-expected rate at which health care costs were rising after its passage, but those concerns were not given the weight that they receive today. Nor were there so many sources of competing cost estimates. Few politicians want to raise taxes, so they must find other programs to cut or must claim that their program will actually save money. An important aspect of the CBO staff's job is validating—or, more likely, rejecting—claims of expected savings, for example, savings from malpractice reform as noted above.

Complexity

Calling a proposal "bureaucratic" is another rallying cry. Fear of bureaucratic red tape can bring a proposal under deep suspicion if opponents are successful in making a plausible case (often laced with exaggeration) that it is likely to spawn bureaucratic growth and replace private decision making with decisions made by bureaucrats. This concern is paramount in health care. It puts proponents on the defensive and can greatly diminish the likelihood of adoption. Proposals that seem to replace physicians' clinical judgment with bureaucratic rules are strongly resisted, as are efforts to direct middle-class patients to specific providers. Likewise, much of the so-called managed care backlash of the late 1990s and early 2000s arose from the requirement for patients to jump through administrative hoops to see a specialist. Ironically, it was principally Republican members of Congress who designed and passed the MMA, one of the more complicated expansions of health care coverage ever adopted, including income-adjusted premiums that change each year, gaps in coverage, availability through managed care firms or competing local pharmacy benefit management plans, penalties for late signup, and the authority of various plan administrators to change the drugs they cover from time to time. If further proof was needed, the MMA showed that it is difficult to write a law and not be "bureaucratic" when it tries to strike a balance between public and private responsibilities, includes incentives for prudence, accommodates regional variations and individual preferences for care delivery, and holds down costs.

Even when restrictions on freedom are minimized, paperwork burdens by themselves cause fierce resistance. Business, particularly small business, is viscerally fearful that any government-mandated compliance, however innocent at first, will eventually prove to be the nose of the camel under the tent, as Congress, bureaucratic regulators, and the courts reinterpret the scope of their authority, the degree of compliance, and, most especially, the scope of reporting required. This fear of paperwork has made businesses unwilling to accept federal subsidies intended to get them started on employee health insurance coverage, even companies that could clearly benefit from the subsidies. That the 2010 PPACA was able to overcome these fears long enough to pass the bill—with no Republican support—is a testimony only to the support of many other interest groups. Once it was passed, business, especially small business, tried to change it, especially the provision that requires all businesses to file a 1099 form with the federal government on all sales over $600—fulfilling an IRS dream of creating a paper trail that would eventually lead to finding many small businesses buying and using equipment, goods, and services but not reporting their existence to the IRS. Talk of modifying or repealing that burdensome new rule began immediately after passage of the law.

Political Action or Legitimation

A proposal that seems appealing on an analyst's slide presentation software may have no chance of passage, or even consideration, in the real political world.

Thus, political action—passage into law, adoption as an executive order or regulation, or, increasingly, an issuance of the courts—is far from a given. Many factors come into play: besides elements of the issue itself, these include saliency and timing and institutional factors.

Saliency and Timing

Public opinion plays an important role in political feasibility. If the public is engaged with an issue, it will be supportive; if the public is in strong opposition, the issue will fade quickly from the agenda.

The saliency of an issue dictates the kind of politics that accompanies it. Salient issues draw heavy press attention and thus provide legislators with the opportunity for credit taking, which encourages individual grandstanding and partisanship. Compromise around a majority position becomes harder. Party discipline tends to break down, because members of Congress know that voters will hold them accountable and may punish them for not protecting district interests. For the president, salient issues involve big stakes, making him vulnerable to demands for concessions by lawmakers willing to bargain for their vote. But if the issue is nonsalient, private interests and lawmakers' attentive constituents are likely to call the shots. An actual or perceived emergency—such as the Medicare trust fund going broke—can help proposals, giving legislators political cover from opposing interest-group pressure and allowing program or budget cuts that would otherwise be impossible.

President George W. Bush found out that even a popular, engaged president cannot necessarily control public opinion. In 2005, Bush introduced and strongly endorsed the idea of private accounts as a substitute for part of the nation's Social Security system. In spite of an all-out personal effort and tireless support from his cabinet, the idea gained little popularity with the American public and therefore met with fierce resistance in Congress.

Timing can easily kill an issue, either because another issue pushes it off the agenda (foreign affairs events, for example) or because the issue has not been resolved as election time approaches. The policy debate becomes grist for campaign debate. Issues that have been the subject of negotiation and compromise become campaign slogans and sound bites, widening rather than narrowing the gap between the parties. Compromise becomes even harder if one party believes it may gain enough seats in the election to change the lineup supporting or opposing a particular proposal. Kingdon (1995) made the point that the policy window opens only briefly. Proposals that are ready to go when the opportunity arises have a better chance of being adopted than ones that still have to be worked out. Downs's issue attention cycle (1972) characterizes the tenuous hold that problems have on the national agenda, especially if they are costly to solve. They enjoy saliency only so long as they are not replaced by another, more interesting problem.

Timing has generally been unkind to national health insurance proposals. They tend to be proposed early in the legislative session, but because of their complexity, serious battles over the most important features—the role of government and financing—often are delayed until well into the first year of a president's term or early in the second year. By then, the congressional midterm elections are looming. Differences of opinion about policy issues become the focus of ideological tirades. Members begin looking to the election and thinking about how to use the health care debate to embarrass the other party or how to delay a vote on the legislation. If things go as hoped, the party will come back with additional seats, thereby improving their bargaining power on the health bill. This political maneuvering has been the death knell of health care reform proposals for decades.

It nearly happened again to the Obama reform. The House passed its reform in early November 2009. But the Senate did not act until Christmas Eve of the same year, leaving too little time before the Christmas recess for a conference committee to reconcile differences between the House and the Senate. When members came back for the second session of the 111th Congress, the Democrats had lost their filibuster-proof Senate majority with the assumption of a seat in the Senate by Scott Brown (R-MA), making it impossible to pass any revised bill that might come out of a conference report. Indeed, few doubted that the Republicans would allow a conference committee to be appointed.

To avoid the second-session-certain-death syndrome, Democrats in the two houses agreed to make changes to the Senate-passed bill in a separate reconciliation act, thus obviating the need for a conference committee to iron out their differences. The heavily Democratic House passed the Senate version of the PPACA, sending it to the president, as well as the Health Care and Education Reconciliation Act of 2010, sending it to the Senate. By Senate rules, reconciliation acts require only a simple 51-vote majority to pass, which was well within the capability of the Democratic Senate. The president signed the PPACA on March 23, 2010, and the reconciliation act on March 30, 2010. When the midterm election was over less than eight months later, Republicans had taken back the House and reduced the Democratic Senate majority by six votes. Had reform not passed when it did, it would have joined the trash heap of legislative history of health reform bills that died when they did not make it into law by the end of the first session. There have been other exceptions, but their scant number tends to prove the rule. Do it early or forget it.

Institutional Factors

Implied in various authors' notions of political feasibility is a set of issues related to the role of institutions in the policy process. Proposals are much more likely to succeed if backed by a president with substantial political capital, including a large majority of his party controlling both houses. In its absence, with two houses and two parties to get through, along with interest-group opposition, a general distrust of government, affordability concerns, and issues as complex as health care policy, the default is policy failure. Any remaining hope must come from a policy entrepreneur, someone—often a president or a member of Congress—pushing the solution forward, bargaining, and making persistent demands for progress. The possibility for success depends on this individual's legislative and policy prowess, placement on key committees, and level of expertise and determination. If the president is the policy entrepreneur, success is more likely if the proposal is one that helps fulfill campaign promises or helps establish his legacy. Prospects rise further if he is a savvy master of the congressional process and is clever enough to court rather than offend powerful interests that wield influence with congressional leaders or delegations. President Obama when first elected, and President Clinton, after learning the hard way, both hired experienced legislators as their chiefs of staff to help push the right buttons, salve the right egos, and make the right offers to key members of Congress in exchange for support of the president's favored proposals.

Legislators must be able to see how the proposal will benefit their reelection prospects, either by giving them an opportunity to claim credit for serving the interests of their attentive constituents or by allowing them to trade their vote on this issue for another that is important to them.

Big plans require big majorities and a powerful policy entrepreneur. Again, for national health insurance this means a president who is popular and whose party commands a large majority in both houses. Medicare slipped through because of the lopsided Democratic victory in 1964. Votes can be lost through the traditional disagreements between the parties but also through the inevitable tension between groups of liberals: those who favor comprehensive change and those who want something more scaled down with a better chance to win. In the Carter years, Democrats split their support for national health care reform over the issue of comprehensive cradle-to-grave versus catastrophic-only coverage: President Carter versus Sen. Edward Kennedy (D-MA) and Big Labor, and then Carter versus labor. In the Clinton years, single-payer advocates versus managed care advocates did the same thing during debates on the health care proposal. Presidents with small majorities are simply not able to muster the votes for large comprehensive proposals. As criticism of their proposal heats up, it tends to cost them support in the polls as well, further depleting their reserve of capital. Even with his substantial majorities in Congress, President Obama was barely able to pass a much-scaled-back national health reform.

A large number of factors impinge on the willingness of members of Congress to provide the votes the president needs. Chief among them are district concerns. Proposals that require members to set aside the interests of their districts are often doomed to failure. So-called sin taxes fall on a small number of industries, usually represented by a block of important legislators such as those representing wineries in California and New York or tobacco interests in the South. Especially ill advised are proposals that offend an industry concentrated in the district of one or more key committee chairs (as did a graduate medical education reform proposal when the Senate Finance Committee was chaired by a senator from New York, a state with many teaching hospitals). Conversely, proposals are likely to succeed by wide margins if they serve the interests of many legislators' districts and allow them to take credit for bringing projects and services, such as subsidies for hospitals, to their districts. Many believe that the true masters of this strategy of marshaling support in many districts are defense contractors, who are likely to hire a subcontractor in every key congressional district, knowing that they will be bringing with the local firm a representative and two senators who are likely to lend their support should the weapons system be threatened with defunding.

Not all these criteria of political feasibility carry equal weight. For some criteria the weight changes with the issue; others are always heavily weighted. Effectiveness is likely to be a less important consideration in a debate on subsidies than in a debate on mandates. Timing and comprehensiveness are less important if the issue is less salient. Concentrated costs and benefits are always important, however, because members of Congress place service to their districts at the top of their priority lists, and members from districts chosen to bear concentrated costs are by definition well financed and likely to use their resources to fight the proposal. The public's support is crucial for salient policies, not so much for narrow, behind-the-scenes deals.

For many issues, the criteria for political feasibility are both additive and interactive in their effect on the probability of success. Appropriateness of the government role is especially debatable if the costs of the proposal are high. Comprehensiveness tends to raise costs, which are likely to be concentrated somewhere. Effectiveness becomes more uncertain with each additional complexity, and complexity means more time and debate—with the likely result that the proposal will be still under debate as election time approaches and the parties are looking for issues useful for defining themselves. These additive and interactive effects highlight the difficulty of getting the planets in the right alignment for successful enactment of comprehensive policy change.

Implementation

Once a policy is put in place, it is rarely self-executing. Rather, federal agencies must issue regulations, write checks, set up oversight committees or boards, and collect data on the process and impact of the new law (see chapter 4). In many instances, states and localities are the implementers, and they must designate or hire staff, develop procedures, select recipients, send checks, and collect data—among many other tasks. Implementation is not the end product of public policy but rather the beginning of feedback to policymakers about the progress of the program, its successes and failures, and any unintended consequences. In the United States, implementation also has a special value in that the 50 states can implement differently even the most stringent program, thanks to differences in institutional arrangements and in the demographic and social makeup of the states. By studying the implementation process and effects across the states, policy analysts and political scientists can gather information that is helpful both to Congress and to frameworks and models of the policy process.

Theories of Policy Change

The policy process framework is important in understanding the process of policymaking, but it fails to answer questions such as why some policies pass and others don't and why policy change does occur. Numerous explanations have been posited as to why policy changes. We briefly summarize three of these theories: the garbage can model, the policy advocacy model, and the punctuated model.

The Garbage Can Model

John Kingdon (1995) argued that policy change occurs in unpredictable ways as separate elements of the policy process intersect, as in a garbage can collecting trash. Three streams—problems, policies, and politics—merge. These streams develop and operate largely independently. Problems are defined and moved to the government agenda; policy solutions are developed, whether or not they respond to a problem; the politics may change suddenly with the election of a new administration, whether or not the policy community is ready or the problems facing the country have changed. The separate streams come together at critical times: a problem is recognized; a solution is available; the political climate makes the time right for change. This critical time, or opening of the policy window, is an opportunity for advocates to push their pet proposals.

A policy window is open but a short time. Precipitating events may be enabling legislation that comes up for renewal or the influx of new members of Congress. The item suddenly becomes "hot" because things come together at the same time: problems, solutions, policymakers' attention, and the desire to act. Kingdon (1995), like Cohen, March, and Olsen (1972), from whom his model is adapted, called this process coupling. Typically coupling comes at the hands of a policy entrepreneur: a president, a cabinet secretary, a senator or a representative, a lobbyist, an academic, a lawyer, a journalist, or a career bureaucrat—inside or outside the formal policy circle—who does the brokering to make things happen. "No one type of participant dominates the pool of entrepreneurs" (Kingdon, 1995, 204). The entrepreneur's job is to push, shape, negotiate, disseminate, and couple the problem to a solution or a pet solution to a problem. "As to problems, entrepreneurs try to highlight the indicators that so importantly dramatize their problems. They push for one kind of problem definition rather than another . . . As to proposals, entrepreneurs are central to the 'softening-up' process" (205). An important contribution of this model is the recognition that solutions sometimes precede problems. The process is anything but well-ordered.

The Advocacy Coalition Framework

A model that recognizes the long-term nature of policy change is the work of Sabatier and Jenkins-Smith (1988, 1993), who argued that policy change should be viewed over a long time horizon—at least a decade. Problems are not "solved" and taken off the policy map. Rather, as Wildavsky (1979) noted, once a solution is implemented, it creates new sets of issues, ensuring that no public problem ever really dies.

The framework developed by Sabatier and Jenkins-Smith, called the advocacy coalition framework, suggests that analysis of policy change requires a time perspective of a decade or more and should focus on policy subsystems, or what they call advocacy coalitions. Policy change, they posit, occurs as a result of competition within the subsystem and events outside the subsystem. This approach differs from the garbage-can model in that it focuses on *coalitions* of interests composed of actors including Congress, the president, interest groups, and the press, rather than on the actors themselves. Advocacy coalitions are composed of people who share a particular belief system and who are committed to working toward a policy over time. These coalitions spend time "venue shopping," or trying to find government entities that might be most amenable to their cause. Policy change occurs following an external shock or intervention or when very solid empirical evidence leads to policy-oriented learning across belief systems.

Punctuated Equilibrium

Baumgartner and Jones (1993) argued that policymaking is generally characterized by long periods of relative stability (equilibrium) punctuated by the occasional major change. Significant policy shifts occur when the balance of forces that generally promote the status quo is disrupted such that the forces protecting the current situation are overwhelmed. One way this can occur is by fashioning a new policy image and exploiting multiple policy venues. Change is most likely when a positive feedback system forms and even those who previously objected to the change conclude that it is inevitable and participate in the change process. This model offers a pretty fair description of how the 2010 PPACA was able to overcome major interest-group opposition: PhRMA saw change coming, its members feared they would lose some major market protections, such as protection from the competition of imported drugs, and so they cut a deal with the White House to limit the damage in exchange for their support of the bill. Once they were on board, other interests saw the train leaving the station and were eager to jump aboard.

Conclusion

Taken together, the various understandings of the policy process framework suggest that problems and solution options must meet certain criteria if they are to reach the political agenda and survive the political process of policymaking. The problem must be (viewed as) appropriate for government action, not usurping state sovereignty or replacing market solutions with government interference. Its solution must seem to be technically feasible and effective and must reflect a general consensus among experts. Costs must not be concentrated on powerful interests and must not be budget-busting, nor should they involve too much redistribution from the haves to the have-nots.

Means testing can be invoked to attract conservative supporters, but such a feature may (or may not) offend liberals. Proposed solutions must not involve (or imply for the future) excessive reporting or other administrative burdens or transaction costs, especially if the burden will fall on states or small business. Burdens on the federal bureaucracy are of interest to no one in Congress. Nobody cares.

The district interests of powerful congressional committee chairs must not be transgressed. Someone who can speak for others, someone who has great political skill, institutional endowments, political capital, and great persistence, must shoulder the duties of policy entrepreneur. Ideally, the other party's turf must not be encroached upon, although President George W. Bush deliberately pushed Medicare drug coverage to steal the issue from the Democrats, so there are clearly exceptions. Members of Congress must be able to claim credit for bringing home the pork or a good policy. Supporters must not be balkanized or uncompromising; opponents must not be well organized, concentrated, moneyed, prestigious, or otherwise well positioned to mount a well-financed and well-orchestrated fight. If they are, they must be bought off with deals that limit the damage to them. Public support is key if the issue is salient.

Health policy is typically, but not always, complex. The exceptions are areas such as abortion and sexual-abstinence education, which are best characterized as morality policies. The health policy domain has long been characterized by incremental change. The PPACA is a case in point. Its individual and employer mandates are bold. Its reform of the insurance industry is thorough, but its control of costs, use patterns, and quality are pretty tame.

Of course, incremental is in the eye of the beholder. Many liberals felt that the 2010 PPACA was a mere incremental step toward national health reform. But many conservatives thought it was a comprehensive and calamitous expansion of the role of the federal government in health care. Perhaps in some ways, both were correct. An individual mandate was more than an incremental step toward universal access. A board to make recommendations on cost control, prohibited from pushing too far or too fast by constraints placed upon its mandate, was pretty much an incremental step. Perhaps the strong influence of ideology on how one views the role of government in health care makes those terms unhelpful. What conservatives view as monumental, liberals view as incremental.

CHAPTER SEVEN

Problem to Policy

Our Health System's Problems and the 2010 Reform

Despite Obama's and the Democratic Congress's valiant efforts, American health care remains woefully inadequate and continues on a downhill path that threatens to pull the country down with it. Costs are enormous, more than twice the average of other industrialized countries. Quality is poor: 12th at best, much lower by some measures (the World Health Organization, or WHO, says we're 37th). We are the 16th among 19 industrialized countries in mortality amenable to health care intervention (Nolte & McKee, 2003, table 1, p. 3).

Health systems around the world are evaluated with three criteria:

—Access: how available they are to meet the health care needs of the population,

—Quality: how well they meet standards of quality in their capacity to render care, the processes of care that they administer, and the outcomes that they produce, and

—Costs: how efficiently they deliver the care—that is, keep costs and expenditures under control.

Here we assess the American system against these criteria. Our system leaves much room for improvement.

Access

Uniquely among comparable nations, we don't cover everybody. Before reform, the number of people who had no health insurance was 45 to 50 million, depending on whose count was taken. The 2010 reform greatly rectifies that problem by adding perhaps 16 million new Medicaid recipients and eventually enrolling another 24 million previously uninsured people in private health insurance plans sold through new health insurance exchanges. The exchanges don't come online until 2014, but state high-risk pools began operating across the nation in 2010, available to individuals who have been turned down for insurance and have been uninsured for six months or more. Their premiums will vary by age and other risk factors but within limits on the number of categories and size of premium differences among the categories. An individual mandate requires every citizen to purchase minimal health insurance. To assist those who have been uninsured for six months and have no other options, subsidies will be made available, based upon income, so that individuals can purchase one of five plan options varying in price and the estimated percentage of their health care costs that will be covered by the policy. Policies are standardized to reduce buyer confusion and assure that a required set of coverages are included. Insurance vendors will have to compete on price and service of that coverage. Employers larger than a minimal size are required to offer substantially subsidized insurance to their employees or pay fines. Small firms are eligible for a subsidy. A new long-term-care insurance policy was to open to enrollment by elderly people willing to buy into the plan while they were still working, but the policy was so poorly designed that the Obama administration decided to forgo its implementation.

Even after the reform, 12 million people living in the United States will lack insurance at least part of the year. Many of those not granted access by the reform will be illegal immigrants, and thus care will be denied to millions of school children, domestic and restaurant workers, truck drivers, farm laborers, and others with the potential to infect others, underperform, or surreptitiously obtain care they can't pay for. Elderly people who need nursing home care will still have to turn to Medicaid when their own funds prove inadequate.

Quality

In most cities, just over half of the care recommended by experts for a given disease is actually delivered. California declared an epidemic after 5 children died of whooping cough in summer 2010, while 910 more Californians were known to be infected and many more cases bore investigation (Mckinley, 2010). The problem was worst in Hispanic neighborhoods where children did not receive recommended vaccinations. Yet by many estimates, one-third or more of care that is delivered is wasted—often unneeded or ineffective and routinely quite expensive. The likelihood of getting the right diagnosis and appropriate care is about

55 percent, according to major national studies by the RAND Corporation, Dartmouth University, and others.

The PPACA approach to quality is essentially to throw money at a bunch of pilot approaches and see what works. This is about the best we can do, given that we can define the problem—too much morbidity, too much mortality, too little mitigation of health-care-amenable premature deaths, too many care-induced injuries and infections, too much wasted and ineffective care—but we simply don't know how to solve it. Reliable outcome data are helpful and are beginning to be collected. But determining what types of practices and choices affect those outcomes and, importantly, ensuring that providers implement those practices and make the appropriate choices and avoid accidents (negligent and otherwise) remain nearly insurmountable barriers in this country. We lag behind the rest of the industrialized world in adoption of electronic medical records, thought by many to be a first step in putting into the physician's hands the means to improve diagnosis and treatment and avoid duplicative and unnecessary care.

Under new Medicare payment policies in the PPACA, hospitals will be penalized for avoidable readmissions and hospital-induced infections and other problems in certain circumstances, and they will be rewarded for quality improvements. Demonstration projects will test "bundled care payments," paying the hospital a fixed sum for both inpatient and subsequent outpatient care (requiring more coordination between doctors and hospitals). Other demonstrations will pay safety-net hospitals with global budgets, leaving it to the hospitals to ration care to get the most value for the money. Accountable-care organizations (ACOs) will be encouraged to form consortia among various providers in a community, meet quality standards, and share in savings if they can deliver care to their Medicare population at lower cost than the amount spent on the same geographic population a year or so earlier. This reform is aimed at reducing the variation in health care spending that researchers have found among cities treating similar patients. Miami and several other high-spending cities cost Medicare nearly half again as much per patient as the rest of the nation or as other large cities such as San Francisco. The differences are in care intensity. Somewhere between the extremes, presumably, is the right amount of care. But the ACO idea is untested, and getting buy-in by providers who are really the problem may be difficult.

Medicaid patients with multiple chronic conditions will be encouraged to seek a "medical home," where care can be better coordinated. The designated provider and the state will receive higher federal Medicaid matching payments, as an incentive to encourage the use of medical homes for Medicaid patients with two or more chronic conditions. Medicare will use its payment clout to discourage physicians from owning and operating their own specialty hospitals to compete with more general hospitals. The effect may be to push physicians to move their care back to the hospital.

Will these changes improve quality of care? Maybe, hopefully; but in reality, it is most likely that they will be implemented by hospitals that are financially well off and already near the top of their game. It is worth noting that, should the new constraints really become binding, there is always the possibility that they may be loosened by Congress in the face of industry opposition. When the forerunner of the Agency for Healthcare Research and Quality synthesized the evidence on back surgery and reported that it typically doesn't work or causes more harm than good, the orthopedic surgeons came within a hair's breadth of closing the agency down. Can we really expect a new advisory agency to make much difference in physician and hospital practice?

Workforce issues are another problem that reform needed to address. Many argue that we have too few primary care physicians; others say that they are simply maldistributed, leaving some areas with few primary care options. Primary care is care that a patient receives—or should receive—on first contact with the health care system. Its practitioners include family physicians, pediatricians, general practitioners, internal medicine physicians, and osteopaths, as well as physician assistants and nurse practitioners; sometimes obstetricians and gynecologists as well as nurses and care coordinators are considered primary care practitioners. The shortage is captured by a few contrasting numbers: just 37 percent of medical professionals practice primary care, but 56 percent of patient visits require it. By one estimate, 60 million Americans lack primary care. But just 8 percent of medical school graduates go into primary care (Kaiser Family Foundation, n.d.).

Relatively lousy pay is one big reason for the shortage: pay gaps between primary care physicians and other specialties offer doctors little encouragement to enter primary care. Three primary care specialties (pediatricians, family practice physicians, and internists) earned starting salaries in 2008 of $125,000, $130,000, and $135,000, while radiologists earned $350,000, anesthesiologists $275,000, and general surgeons $220,000 (Ebell, 2008).

The 2010 reform did some things to redress these workforce problems, but much less than was hoped for. A task force was told to try to solve the problem.

And primary care specialists got a small extra increase in salary, about 10 percent, for five years. Yet research has shown that higher specialist pay leads to lifetime accumulated wealth among specialists that is twice what primary care physicians will accumulate over their careers. A 10 percent increase in primary care pay will do little to address that gap: primary care doctors would go from about 48 percent of cardiologists' 2008 pay to about 56 percent (calculated from Vaughn et al., 2010).

Cost

The new law is estimated to cut costs by approximately $143 billion over a decade (half of it from Medicare cuts to be implemented after 2018 [according to the Congressional Budget Office], assuming Congress has the political backbone to cut fees to hospitals and excess physicians). To put that number in perspective, it's worth remembering that in the bank bailouts of 2009–10, the giant insurer AIG alone got $181 billion. Other banks got billions more. So saving $143 billion would be good but a long way from solving our health care cost problem. Indeed, the financial consulting firm PricewaterhouseCoopers estimated that the health reform will raise premiums more than 100 percent for most insured people, because it will bring into the insurance pool those whose preexisting conditions have previously excluded them, and in addition provider taxes and Medicare cuts will be shifted to private payers (PricewaterhouseCoopers, 2009).

The cuts that are to be made are to come from reducing the excessively high payments to a certain type of Medicare managed care plan, lowering overly generous subsidies to hospitals that serve large numbers of Medicare and Medicaid patients, and reducing payments to hospitals, doctors, nursing homes, home health and other providers, drug and equipment suppliers, and others. Additional revenues to offset costs of the expanded coverage will come from taxes on insurance companies, health care providers and their suppliers, tanning salons, and high-premium employer-sponsored employee insurance plans, plus a 1 percent payroll tax on incomes over $200,000; smaller amounts will come from fines assessed for failing to comply with individual and employer mandates. Yet even with the proposed changes, overall costs will still rise rapidly. Costs are projected to go from $2.6 trillion in 2010 to $4.3 trillion in 2018 (CMS Office of the Actuary, 2010).

In the reform debate, the Senate, in the face of opposition, dropped a provision that would have set up a new agency with clout to ban ineffective procedures.

House proposals to substantially cut costs by imposing a price-setting medical care board were scrapped by the Senate. Indeed, the Senate version protects physicians and hospitals from pay cuts through 2018. And after union demands for relief were made to President Obama, he agreed to delay implementation of an excise tax on high-priced insurance plans through the same period and to raise the threshold at which the tax starts to more than twice 2010 average premiums. The CMS estimates that just two years after the new cuts and taxes are due to kick in (in 2018), health care costs will exceed one-fifth of GDP.

Why Not More?

How did such an earnest—and at the time very popular—leader manage to bite off so little, yet create so much anger, while Congress in fact moved rather modestly in the direction of actually attacking our most critical problem, health care costs, and did rather little to improve quality?

The Strength of Opposing Interest Groups

First, like many Democrats before him, he decided to avoid major political battles with his left wing over expansion of coverage and battles with the many provider and supplier interest groups that would have ensued if he had seriously addressed the cost control issue. He avoided battles with the doctors by not imposing serious quality reforms such as a demand to follow practice protocols. The left pushed him toward expanding coverage and thus increasing costs while the provider lobby pushed back from payment cuts and limits on the use of high-tech care, an aspect of our pattern of health care that differentiates us from the rest of the world. That is, we use more high-tech care than anybody else—and of course we pay dearly for it—and yet have few health outcome benefits to show for it, specifically not in life expectancy or lower morbidity than the rest of the industrialized world.

The problem for the future of our health care system is not simply that costs will go up with expanded coverage but that those additional users of care will enter our inefficient and unbalanced delivery system, further aggravating its shortcomings. Our lack of primary care practitioners and heavy reliance upon specialists will only be aggravated when more patients enter the system.

Expanding access to insurance was clearly necessary, if only to save the rest of us the hidden costs of serving the uninsured even more inefficiently through emergency care. There is also the immorality and embarrassment of being the only industrialized nation to wait so long to expand coverage to most citizens. But putting coverage expansion before cost control means spending even more money on already-too-expensive health care before any meaningful measures can cut costs. Moreover, it's easier politically to expand coverage than it is to cut costs, so it's not at all unlikely that reform will succeed at coverage expansion while cost control continues to fail. Indeed, if past experience is any guide, we are not likely to see health care reform back on the national agenda for at least a decade, probably more, during which time insurance premiums will continue to outstrip wages, Medicare's shortfall will grow, and Medicaid expenditures will continue to consume larger and larger shares of state budgets. Also during that time, providers are likely to seek "morning after" relief of taxes and revenue cuts imposed upon them, as we saw in the years following the 1997 Balanced Budget Act.

But before concluding that Obama failed to learn the lessons of history by failing to address cost control as his first agenda item, it's important to recall that President Jimmy Carter tried it that way and failed. He started with a cost-cutting proposal and was handed his hat in exchange. Republicans were able to take the Carter initiative as their own in the next administration and do just that: cut costs without any coverage expansion. They did much the same in 1997, radically cutting Medicare and substantially cutting Medicaid, adding expansion of coverage to children in the State Children's Insurance Program (S-CHIP) only at the last minute in their mostly cost-cutting Balanced Budget Act. Their cuts dwarfed the S-CHIP expansion, so net savings were huge. But Democrats find that kind of cheap reform harder to pull off.

To his credit, Obama did try something relatively new: he took on the insurance industry. Not that others had not tried—and sometimes succeeded—at least modestly. The Health Insurance Portability and Accountability Act of 1996 is the result of one such effort at insurance industry reform. And all states have adopted modest protections for those unlucky Americans who must buy their health insurance in the small-group or individual market. But those reforms were mostly tinkering around the edges of insurance company abuses. The new reform goes much further, putting an end to the most abusive practices: exclusion from coverage of preexisting conditions; nonrenewal of policies for those who experience above-average costs; annual and lifetime coverage limits; rescissions of coverage for minor errors or omissions on one's insurance application form; and holding onto too much of premiums or paying exorbitant salaries to executives rather than paying an adequate share of premiums for health care.

Reforms do not come easily, especially in the special world of insurance. Since the earliest years of insurance, when merchants sought to cover their losses if their ships sank, sellers of insurance have worried about adverse selection and the resultant "death spiral." They fear that only those who are likely to suffer a loss will buy coverage. When only the sickest buy insurance, payouts rise, and when that happens, insurance premiums rise for the next buyers, so the problem becomes even more aggravated. Those at lowest risk drop out of the too-expensive market, leaving only the most risky in the pool. Eventually no one can afford to join the pool as it spirals down to its demise. For the insurance industry to swallow the proposed reforms and permit people with preexisting conditions to buy insurance, the quid pro quo demanded by the industry was that consumers not be allowed to sort themselves out into high-risk buyers and low-risk nonbuyers of insurance. No one has come up with any alternative way to avoid the death spiral while not enforcing a ban on coverage of preexisting conditions, other than to force everyone to buy insurance, thereby guaranteeing that low-risk buyers are in the risk pool too.

So began the cascade of closed-off options. Once having decided to reform insurance, those shaping the proposal were left with an individual mandate as the only option. But mandating poor people to buy insurance does not work unless you require employers to offer insurance and subsidize both poor people and small business so that they can afford to make the purchase. And you must decide who deserves a subsidy, how much subsidy to offer, and how big a penalty to impose on noncompliers. Next question: how to pay for the subsidies? Enter new taxes and payment cuts and, of course, the costly political choices of whom to tax and what to cut. Of course the cuts have to be in Medicare, because that's where the federal government's money is heavily going, and the taxes have to be on health care providers and suppliers, or high earners, or the health insurance premiums of those who get their insurance through their employers—or all of the above.

It is ironic that the individual mandate raised the most ire—and prompted court suits filed by almost exclusively Republican state attorneys general—since many attribute the idea of an individual mandate to the conservative Heritage Foundation. It was introduced in Republican health reform bills in the 1990s, and it was first adopted in Massachusetts under a Republican governor, although his legislature was Democratic.

Tax proposals always reflect a blending of politics, economics, and revenue potential. The Democratic congressional proposals and Obama's ideas were no exception. The politics reflected Obama's campaign promise to raise no taxes on those with incomes below $200,000. The solution? Adding a nearly 1 percent Medicare payroll tax on earners over $200,000 and imposing a tax on various health care suppliers, including drug companies and labs, on the theory that they would be getting 32 million new customers from the reform. The third tax—on "Cadillac" or high-cost health insurance policies—was politically dicier, since the tax would fall mostly on union members, longtime Democratic stalwarts. Even after adjustments to exclude premiums of "high risk" occupations such as firefighters and those whose premiums are high because they are part of a graying workforce, it was still clear that union members who had fought for generous benefits would bear the brunt of what some economists regard as the single best strategy for cutting health care costs—making consumers more aware of the costs of health care. Under this logic, consumers would think twice about whether or not they really needed that CAT scan a physician had suggested and would at least consider finding a cheaper or less generous insurance policy. Initially, the proposal did not include inflation indexing, which would have made the tax imposed on only high premiums actually a political Trojan horse. That is, it would have eventually applied to everyone. Given the inexorable rise in health insurance premiums, many Americans would have eventually found that their own premiums crossed the threshold for being called "Cadillac." Indeed, the proposal initially called for a 40 percent tax on premiums over $23,000, assuming that an average family premium would be $13,000. President Obama proposed delaying imposition of the tax for several years and raising the threshold to $27,500.

While the president was criticized for cutting deals with the major interest groups (the "bad guys" in the 1994 health care reform attempt), the fact that the president's plan faced no major interest-group opposition should not be underestimated. By promising the drug industry that it would face taxes and price cuts of no more than $83 billion over 10 years (as well as continued patent protection for its brand name biologicals, no call for importation of cheaper drugs from abroad, and no ban on paying generic companies to hold their products off the market for another year or two while brand name profits continued to roll in), the White House was able to move the drug industry lobby—the Pharmaceutical Research and Manufacturers of America—from an extremely powerful and determined opponent that had been helpful in killing the Clinton plan to an actual supporter of the Obama plan, running ads in favor of the reform package and joining in its support with such consumer-oriented liberal groups as Families

USA. There were no negative "Harry and Louise" ads run in 2009 or 2010; in fact, ads showing an older (and wiser?) Harry and Louise now had them supporting the president's plan. The cost of this support was that the plan did not seriously address the spiraling health care cost issue and the interest groups largely benefited from the plans of Obama and the Democrats.

Ideology

A second reason that the proposal is far from comprehensive in addressing costs and quality is ideology—in this case mostly conservative ideology. The reform proposal contained three components that fed ideological differences: the public option, abortion, and subsidies and penalties.

The Public Option

While the public option served as a political lightning rod, the proposal was embedded in a more complicated approach called health insurance exchanges, modeled after the popular Federal Employees Health Benefits System. Exchanges are set up by states to offer standardized policies in five categories, ranging from limited catastrophic cost coverage after a huge deductible to quite generous coverage. (If a state decides not to set up an exchange, the federal government will provide one for that state.) The exchanges are designed to provide individuals and small businesses buying federally subsidized policies an easy-to-use market for comparing private insurance company policies, standardized in their coverage to assure minimum coverage levels, absence of loopholes, and transparency in marketing.

The Senate plan called the five categories "Young Invincibles," Bronze, Silver, Gold, and Platinum. Each is designed to cover a specific percentage of expected health care costs, ranging from 60 percent for the Bronze policy to 90 percent for the Platinum policy. The Young Invincibles policy covers only catastrophic costs. Those who want to offer policies through the exchanges will have to offer all five, both through the exchange and outside it. To induce them to keep prices low, liberal Democrats wanted the government to offer its own set of plans, also in each of these categories. The public option would presumably be cheap, since it would have very low administrative costs and low marketing costs. If private policy premiums got too high, consumers would flock to the public option, creating downward price pressure. But given the high administrative costs of private insurance and the reality that the government would not need to engage in much expensive marketing to get its name around, insurance companies feared that a public option would eventually drive out competitors with its lower prices.

While the proposal called for limiting availability of the public option to only those who had been without private insurance for an extended period and could not get it on their own, companies feared that once in place, the public option would become the nose of the camel under the tent, eventually attracting more and more consumers with its low prices and driving out the entire private industry. Liberals felt the fear was irrational, but its real potential for altering the market actually mattered little. It was the symbolic value of a public option with the theoretical potential to successfully compete with the private market that gave Democratic conservatives and the Republican Party a vulnerable point for attack. Nor was it a great idea from a policy perspective. If we know anything about how Congress makes up its collective mind, it is that bold new ideas have little chance of passing the first Congress into which they are introduced. And for all intents and purposes, this was the first Congress in which the public option had taken anything like center stage. No well-informed bookie would have put the odds of its adoption very high. Sadly, the president and his party seemed not to catch onto that rather obvious reality until they had expended considerable capital on it. Finally President Obama came to understand that the odds of success for the public option were too low for the price he was paying and let it be known that he could live without it.

Coupled with hard-to-combat claims that the entire Obama-House-Senate plan represented a substantial increase in the level of government involvement in health care and that it would cost more than $1 trillion over a decade, the public option offered the ideal target for a cheap shot. That it quickly hit its mark, did substantial damage to public attitudes, and had to be abandoned should have surprised no one. For a savvy bunch of politicians like Rep. Henry Waxman (D-CA), chair of the House Energy and Commerce Committee; Sen. Max Baucus (D-MT), chairman of Senate Finance; and President Obama, the whole idea of a public option seems an odd choice of proposals. Was the juice really worth the squeeze? By most estimates it would have affected no more than 2–5 percent of the population. Would it really have made much difference in costs for the market as a whole? And would future Congresses have voted to remove restrictions that kept it a minor player in the market? It was politically costly, quite unproven—indeed even untested politically, in that it had not been through that cycle of proposal, hearings, debate, amendment, defeat, re-introduction, reshaping, and consensus building that novel ideas often have to experience before they can garner the necessary support to make them politically feasible. Some attribute the pressure to offer and keep pushing the public option idea to the lobbying efforts of a newly emergent and increasingly important union: the Service Employees International Union, a key player in a new coalition called Change to Win, which promoted the public option. A count of White House visitor logs suggests that SEIU and Change to Win (of which SEIU was a founding member) representatives may have visited the White House more than any other single pressure group during the reform debate.

Abortion

And then there was the abortion issue. For Republicans it represented just another opportunity to focus attention on a highly charged wedge issue with potential to fractionate Democratic support, mobilize conservative opposition, and galvanize Republican partisans. Senate Democrats included what seemed on its face to be a moderate proposal aimed at keeping the status quo ante on abortion policy: no public funding for it, but no new restrictions on access to it. Conservative House Democrats and Republicans wanted something potentially more limiting: not just a ban on public financing of abortions, but a ban on policies that offered privately funded abortion coverage to individuals who were also receiving public subsidies for the rest of their insurance coverage. The Senate required identical policies to be sold, offering one without abortion coverage for each policy which covered it, and use of only private funds to pay for abortion coverage. The House, on behalf of its anti-abortion coalition, wanted no coverage of abortion through the exchanges—a ban that liberals claimed would wither the market for policies covering abortion, since no one plans to have an abortion and therefore no one would buy such plans.

Eventually a compromise was struck: the Senate language requiring duplicate policies and sequestration of public and private funds (the only funds that could be used for abortion coverage) was adopted in the law. And to seal the deal, the president signed an executive order banning spending of public moneys to support abortion—regarded by most observers as doing no more than affirming current policy. Prolife House members took that as a victory and signed onto the bill. When their leading spokesperson, author of the now-dropped House abortion language, announced that he was satisfied with the compromise and would support the bill, one Republican shouted out "Baby Killer" on the House floor.

He later apologized, sort of. The sordid little incident was further evidence for members and those who observe them that compromise—particularly compromise on a highly salient matter such as abortion—was even harder to come by than provider pay cuts.

Subsidies and Penalties

Subsidies and penalties also remained controversial throughout the process. Set subsidies too low and no one of low or near-poor income could afford to buy a policy despite the mandate. Set them too high and costs of the whole plan would mushroom, necessitating higher taxes. Maximum premium costs-to-the-subsidized of close to 10 percent of income were appealing to some, while others wanted larger subsidies, limiting consumer payments to as little as 2 percent of income. Similar debates surrounded subsidies to small businesses, as did the definition of small business. Eventually, the House and Senate agreed upon a House modification of the Senate bill. Families would pay from $1,000 to $10,000 out of pocket for deductibles and copayments, depending upon income, ranging from incomes one-third above the poverty level to four times the poverty level. And for premiums they would pay an amount ranging from 2 percent of their incomes to 9.5 percent of their incomes, again in income categories in the same range, up to four times the poverty level (about $88,200 for a family of four in 2009).

Even with generous subsidies, however, it could not be assumed that every American would buy insurance even if the purchase was mandated and subsidized (compliance was less likely for families not eligible for a subsidy). Thus the need arose for penalties on individuals for not choosing to buy insurance and on employers for failing to offer it to employees. Again, a debate ensued between the ideologues, who favored mild penalties, and the pragmatists, who feared that penalties too small would segment the market into those for whom the penalty was less costly than insurance they might feel was unneeded. Here the Senate penalty was lower than the House's, so in the adjustments to the Senate bill after its passage by the House, the penalties were increased somewhat, to a maximum of 2.5 percent of income above the federal tax filing minimum, which in 2009 was $18,700 for couples.

Glass Half Full or Half Empty?

Enormous amounts of political capital, energy, and money were spent on the 2010 health reform measure, dubbed by Republicans Obamacare. Yet above all—

despite all the controversies—little was done to truly reform the health care system. A board to impose mandatory cuts in Medicare spending, which Congress would vote up or down without modification, had real potential to reduce spending for marginally valuable procedures, services, and equipment, but ultimately that measure had most of its teeth pulled at the last minute in the Senate. Rather than create an authority to deny payment for costly low-value care, Congress established a new institute that would simply recommend evidence-based choices to the industry.

Writing in the *New Yorker* magazine in the summer of 2009, Atul Gawande, a Massachusetts surgeon and accomplished author who became one of the policy wonks (two years out of medical school) responsible for the truly comprehensive if politically naive (and, some thought, arrogant) Clinton reform plan, struck an optimistic note about the Obama plan. He noted that the new reform law has many promising demonstration projects in it that in the long run might show one or more paths to cost savings and improved quality. One proposal will try to attack the baffling variation in costs of care among similar patients from city to city mentioned above. Dartmouth researchers have found that even among major highly ranked medical centers, costs can vary by 100 percent. Hence, one demonstration project was offered by those same Dartmouth researchers and adopted into the Senate bill by the Senate bill's principal architect, Sen. Max Baucus (D-MT), which would offer provider-communities a benchmark spending target based on prior years' Medicare spending. Spending below that level would be shared between Medicare and the provider-community, with most of the savings going to the providers—as long as certain quality markers were achieved. Another demonstration would pay Medicare physicians, hospitals, nursing homes, and others for achieving appropriate patient outcomes. Yet another would try to discourage the practice of double-dipping by providers: seeking to push patients discharged from the hospital into acute rehabilitation, home care, and other services to increase revenues. The demonstration would pay providers a flat rate for an episode of care regardless of how much care was needed from onset to resolution of the episode of care.

The *New Yorker* author's source of optimism was that American food production once faced a cost crisis that garnered up to 40 percent of family income. Demonstration projects spawned by the U.S. Agriculture Department eventually led to widespread adoption of innovative practices that cut food production costs to where we enjoy them today. The parallel was what he found attractive: a reform plan that included many demonstration approaches that might ultimately reform the system, cut costs, and improve quality. Yet, a cynic might have focused on a different aspect of the analogy: the fact that reform had to await the swelling of costs to 40 percent of family income. Could that be a more compelling lesson to take from the story? Will health care costs continue to rise, and quality continue to suffer, until costs are 40 percent of consumer spending? If so, we may have to go through another half dozen presidents before we get real cost-saving reform.

In short, Obama's new plan is incomplete reform. Having pulled the thread of an individual mandate, individual subsidies and fines, employer fines and subsidies, and industry reforms, his approach must—of necessity—involve substantial spending, significant cuts, and serious taxes. What he's done is a good start, but in the end it is a down payment on what must eventually change in American health care to make our system as good and as cheap as the rest of the industrialized world: reducing the amount of ineffective care (perhaps 30% of all care) and the variation in intensity of care from city to city; curbing overuse of high-tech care; replacing reliance on specialists with primary care; increasing the supply of primary care physicians; imposing care protocols on physicians; delegating more tasks to less-skilled professionals; pushing for fewer interventions and more cost-effective preventive care (in the limited number of instances when it is actually cost-effective); incentivizing lifestyle changes in the general population; and putting an end to excessive pricing and abusive marketing of drugs, laboratory tests, equipment, and services. Yet, ironically, with each passing decade, the populace and the parties seem to grow more resistant to comprehensive reform. Were disgraced president Richard Nixon to come back today with his Republican Comprehensive Health Insurance Plan (then regarded by liberals as piddling and beneath contempt), it would today get perhaps not a single Republican vote—it would be considered too liberal.

Lessons on Reforming Health Care

In a nutshell, there are at least five reasons reform is hard to pass. First, our history launched us on a path that is hard to veer away from (political scientists call this path dependency). In most cases, even in much of managed care, providers are paid for each service separately, and health care markets are oligopolistic, with entry to both professions and delivery institutions restricted, vitiating the potential benefits of competition. We pay the highest prices in the world.

Insurance premium increases outstrip wage increases every year. Insurance insulates consumers from costs. Consumption patterns create expectations of unrestricted access to the latest technologies. Physicians make consumption decisions—and even too often medical equipment decisions for hospitals—often as imperfect agents of either the patient or the hospital, potentially influenced by impacts on their own incomes and other benefits of practice and use of certain manufacturers' equipment. And as consumers we know next to nothing about how to evaluate our need for care or the quality of the care we are receiving.

Second, our institutional structure makes comprehensive reform very difficult, with so many gatekeepers in Congress, access points for opponents at the subcommittee, committee, and floor venues to effect either damaging modifications or delay that can sap the periodic zeal for reform when it arises in the populace every decade or two. And if Congress were not enough of a challenge, the bureaucracy and the courts are additional barriers once something does pass. One reason conservatives are skeptical of budget estimates for health care programs is that experience has shown that bureaucratic interpretations of new program authorities can be used to broaden their scope. The states too, as independent actors in our federal system, can be both barriers to and distorters of congressional purpose. Waivers are one of the ways Congress lets the states end-run efforts to nationalize the system. States can also sue to block reforms or act in a contrary way in implementation.

Third, the status quo is extremely valuable to powerful interest groups representing hospitals, physicians, drug companies, equipment makers, labs, allied health professionals, nursing homes, home health agencies, and many more. Each of these has a major financial stake in the way things are done, and for members of Congress, these stakes represent constituent and campaign contributors' jobs, businesses, and revenue sources. Health care lobbies are many, well organized, well funded, effectively represented in members' districts, and possessed of large staffs of lobbyists who make their living by keeping open access to key health committee members and floor leaders.

Fourth, health care is an ideal partisan issue. Both parties espouse certain principles that often they honor mostly in the breach. For Democrats it is a certain antibusiness, antifarm bias, accompanied by a prolabor, prowelfare, progreen, proregulatory approach. For Republicans it is a preference for probusiness, antigovernment, antiregulation, antiwelfare principles; state governance over federal governance; lower taxes; and market-based solutions. Each party violates these precepts when the spirit suits them. But usually not on health care. There, the ideological and partisan planks in their platforms rule. Each hews to its first principles, drawing battle lines that make compromise difficult and, inevitably, create opportunities to use policy differences to distinguish one party from the other as the next election cycle draws near. However, as we noted earlier, there is some shifting to the right on these positions.

And finally, there is the budget. Each attempt at reform means sweetening the pot for many interests if support is to be gained. Given the high prices that we pay our health care industry, it is inevitable that deals cut to finance promises to hold harmless or improve the situation of the various interests will be expensive. The interests range from the uninsured to small business and labor, to physicians, hospitals, and drug companies, to elderly patients, people with disabilities or mental illness, and a host of others.

Given these realities of our health care system and our political culture and political institutions, it seems unlikely that we will see comprehensive reform including cost-control and quality assurance in the near or relatively near future. Indeed, Obama and many others regard the 2010 reform and its access improvements as the most significant change in our health care system since Medicare and Medicaid were adopted, more than 50 years ago. And those programs as well as this one were mostly distributive—supposedly the easiest kind of politics. How long will we have to wait until Congress feels sufficient budget pressure to adopt real cuts in health care spending and place curbs on bad private medical care practices? Will it be 50 years?

As a consequence of the political and policy straitjacket in which we find ourselves, we must be prepared to continue to pay for often inferior care reflecting a bias toward high technology, high prices, little preventive effort, and access restricted to those who have insurance or are willing to visit emergency rooms for nonemergency conditions. Perhaps we should take solace that for generations to come, many people are likely to be able to make a comfortable living producing and delivering health care to one another. Unfortunately, Medicare spending will require higher taxes, which, also unfortunately, the current reform has already raised to pay for new enrollees. Perhaps the necessity to pile on additional Medicare payroll taxes—eventually applying to the middle class as well as those in upper income brackets—will bring about a demand for reform much earlier than the above speculation of a half century. Alas, even taking on the provider lobbies to cut providers' fees may be preferable to taking on the middle class with a substantial tax hike.

One Price of Victory: Negotiating with Enemies

Political scientists and political pundits will long speculate upon—and in the end probably settle upon—a few factors that differentiated the success of the Obama national health reform initiative from all the previous false starts of the preceding 45 years since Medicare and Medicaid changed the face of American health care delivery. Surely they will speculate upon the importance of the way in which President Obama—through the brokering of his blunt and pragmatic chief of staff, Rahm Emanuel—negotiated with health care interest groups to turn their potential opposition into support by cutting deals that limited the damage they would suffer in whatever reform passed. This tactic worked for Lyndon Johnson, giving the hospitals essentially no-limit cost-plus reimbursement, giving the physicians usual, customary, and reasonable fee schedules, and giving the insurance carriers all the claims-processing duties that could have been carried out more cheaply by the government itself. Interest groups are critical in health care. President Clinton and his wife started their reform by challenging and castigating them, starting with the drug companies, and then locking the physicians and others out of bill-drafting negotiations.

The Obama approach was to recognize that these powerful players had much to lose, as did he, if they fought it out in Congress and the public arena. Instead, he brought them in one by one and cut deals. He asked each to endure limited cuts over a decade, and in exchange he promised to protect them by limiting the total damage they would incur. For the drug companies, this meant they would not be subjected to competition from drugs reimported from Canada and elsewhere, and their lucrative biological-treatment patents would not be shortened, nor would they be prohibited from colluding with generic makers to withhold competitive products. For the hospitals, cuts in payments would be limited. For the physicians, long-delayed, accumulated payment cuts due to be implemented under the 1997 Balanced Budget Agreement would be permanently delayed. PhRMA was the first to break ranks with fellow reform opponents and as such may have gained the most in its bargaining. Indeed, its decision, which seemed to lead to a cascading collapse of health care delivery group opposition to the Obama plan, so angered the Chamber of Commerce that that group's president made it a personal mission to get the head of PhRMA fired at the end of the legislative process. But by then, the die had been cast. Obama had quieted a critical source of opposition, moving it to the sidelines; PhRMA even ran supportive ads favoring the reform package.

But history is likely to conclude that there were also other factors at work. One was the president's leadership style. Whereas Bill and Hillary Clinton had written a more-than-1,400-page bill and delivered it to Congress, a full year too late—which then failed to pass it out of a single committee, President Obama laid out broad guidelines but left it to Congress to write its own bills. This is a critical difference. When policy wonks write the bill, they make trade-offs based upon effectiveness of policy choices and how the system's parts will work together to move toward the policy goals. When politicians design a program, they count votes: who will favor and oppose this approach, what will it take to get so and so on board, how much will we have to drop from our list of ideal solutions to avoid creating organized opposition from certain groups of members? Furthermore, the choices are made in many one-on-one or small-group sessions targeted at winning support for crucial votes in key committees at critical times. The process is recursive, and so long as promises made are kept, the terms of the deal can be renegotiated on a daily or weekly basis to accommodate new developments. Obama was fundamentally lucky that he had in the House that master legislator and deal crafter Henry Waxman (D-CA) as chair of the key legislative committee, House Energy and Commerce. Waxman seemingly can work with anyone to get to a legislative solution. His style differs radically from that of his predecessor John Dingell (D-MI), longtime national health reform advocate, longtime chair of the House Energy and Commerce Committee before he was unseated by Waxman, and longtime abrupt and abrasive, sometimes bullying legislative leader.

In the Senate, Max Baucus (D-MT) angered his Democratic colleagues when he gave in repeatedly to Republican demands for delay, gave them equal representation on his informal subcommittee of the Senate Finance Committee, which he formed as a task force to write the Senate bill and which ultimately produced a bill that was much more conservative than the House version. But his approach reflected the realities of the Senate, where loss of a single conservative Democrat's vote could sink the entire effort. Baucus is a conservative Democrat. He respects and is respected by fellow conservatives in both parties. And for a time, he seemed to have even a good chance of winning Republican votes for a cheaper, narrowly focused reform effort, but he lost that support largely through no fault of his own but rather because of Republican constituent opposition to any major health reform. Republicans were simply scared off and concluded as a party that they were better off simply opposing everything.

At that point, when the Baucus effort had come considerable distance but ultimately failed, the job of reviving the legislation in the Senate fell to a combination of White House behind-the-scenes negotiations and the one-on-one deal-making efforts of Majority Leader Harry Reid (D-NV). Reid had left most of the bill drafting, negotiating, and deal-making to Baucus, but he kept to his own enterprise a steely determination to do what it took to push the package to fruition. When Nebraska senator Ben Nelson demanded special treatment of his state's Medicaid program, Reid put it in the bill. When independent Joe Lieberman (I-CN) demanded that the public option be dropped from the bill, Reid made sure that it got dropped and that President Obama got on board with the disappointing change.

Finally, when both houses had passed versions that differed in a few key aspects, leaders of both houses and the White House worked together to cut deals with House Blue Dogs, anti-abortion coalition members, and unions to recraft important provisions in the bills through a special reconciliation process that required only a majority vote, since the Senate had by then lost its supermajority and could no longer stop a Republican filibuster.

Conclusion

In the end the legislative process in 2009–10 worked as it should, with the agenda set by the president but the bill crafting and vote garnering done largely within the legislative process by legislative leaders like Waxman and Speaker Nancy Pelosi (D-CA), who were willing to compromise even their own personally most enduring policy preferences to make sure they got the larger legislative goal: passage of the legislation. The Obama administration played key roles at key points, but overall, this was a congressional performance helped along by a president savvy enough to stay out of the way of a powerful and gifted Speaker and an effective majority leader.

From past experiences over the previous four and one half decades of failed reform efforts, Obama and legislative leaders had learned the necessity of fast action, legislative prominence in the bill drafting, and trading policy options for votes. But those failures also contributed to the Obama administration's success. Clinton's opposition came from many quarters but perhaps nowhere more fiercely than from the health insurance industry and from employers opposed to the employer mandate. The passage of time had made it clear that insurance

companies really were abusive and that reform was greatly overdue. Yet the reforms that Obama proposed would largely level the playing field among companies, making them all compete within restrictions on abusive practices. Removing the option to engage in favorable selection, rescissions, annual and lifetime
payouts, and so forth meant that no company needed to worry that a competitor
would undercut its market share of desirable clients—or leave them with a high-
risk pool. The Clinton approach actually would have damaged small insurance
companies by causing them to stretch their coverage beyond their capacity to
avoid unfavorable selection. It was the small insurance companies who most
opposed him. Oddly, the employer mandate—such a third rail in the Clinton
initiative—got barely a mention in the Obama plan debate. Policy analysts call
this "softening up." Policies are easier to pass once they've been through the process a few times. This may, in part, explain the fierce opposition to the public
option, which would have permitted the government to offer a government-run
insurance option to compete with private plans. Since it would likely cost less
because no profits would be taken and operating expenses would likely be low, it
would force private plans to hold their prices down. The industry had good reason to fear it, but the industry also benefited from the fact that it was a brand
new proposal. It had not been vetted in previous legislative sessions. It was a bold
new initiative, little understood and therefore greatly feared. Ultimately it had to
be dropped, after drawing criticism and opposition vastly disproportionate to its
near-term potential to harm the industry; that potential was minimized by the
restrictions on who could access the public plans (only those uninsured for six
months who could not obtain insurance in the private market). Will the public
option draw as much opposition next time it's offered? Will it also be better
fleshed out, its implications and potential effects better estimated, and its potential beneficiaries better organized to support it? Quite likely.

The individual mandate, in contrast, had been discussed in the past but had
not previously been proposed by a president at the national level. Perhaps what
made it work this time was that it was a Republican idea adopted by the Democrats and it had been adopted and successfully implemented in Massachusetts.
And it is noteworthy that, unlike initiatives that hurt concentrated interests like
hospitals or physicians, burdens placed on individuals fall on the disorganized
and noncohesive.

In short, the reform limited the damage it did to powerful interests and fell
most heavily upon the disorganized uninsured and the insurance industry. But it
was also bringing that industry millions of new clients, and in the end the dam-

age would probably be mitigated because the reform would level the playing field within the industry. It placed new but small burdens on high earners and put modest taxes and cuts on the health care industry. Mostly what the reform did was to expand coverage, the cost of which fell most heavily upon people and industries who could afford it. Provisions that caused real opposition were simply dropped along the way. Such is the nature of deal-making in Congress.

Conclusion

There is something special about the politics of health care. Over many decades, a variety of ideological, institutional, and political factors have served to stymie, if not obliterate, dozens of proposals for comprehensive health care reform. But failure to enact a national health insurance system does not mean that health care reform in this country has not occurred. On the contrary, as this book has illustrated, health reform in Washington and the states has blossomed since 1965, often in ways unrecognized by much of the country's population. Irregularly there are bursts of substantial change, as in 2010 when the Obama health reform expanded care to many previously uninsured, imposed health insurance mandates on individuals and employers, reformed the health insurance industry with many consumer protections, and strengthened the powers of the congressional advisory board charged with trying to rein in Medicare and Medicaid spending. This was substantial change but lacked key ingredients to make it comprehensive: a clear method of controlling health care cost inflation and a mechanism for imposing quality reform that relies upon more than physician voluntary interest. Without these fundamental changes in our system, we will continue to pay dearly for inferior care.

Health care is special. Leaving aside traditional economists' concerns with information asymmetry, entrance barriers, and other characteristics of the noncompetitive market that is health care, the health care market is *politically* unique. It combines fear of disease and death, third-party payment, publicly supported biomedical research that continuously fuels demand for new forms of care, and an elderly population that wants unlimited health care through Medicare and votes in great numbers to keep it available. Everyone is a consumer of health care and, in the usual course of events, cares only that new cures are being discovered. This makes medical breakthroughs highly salient and helps fuel their demand. Inventors and medical device makers know that if they build it, their buyers will come.

As long as government stays out of the picture, it is a safe assumption that insurance will cover most care demanded by most people most of the time and the quest for new forms of care will continue.

Yet Americans have been told through mass-media campaigns that reform will always be expensive or disruptive to them, may limit their choices of providers and types of care, and will adversely affect quality. They have also been warned that even if reform works, it is likely to make only very small improvements in access over the status quo, changing from 85 percent to perhaps 95 percent the proportion of the insured population.

While attempts at comprehensive health reform in this country have come up short, they have served an important role in focusing policymakers' attention on health care issues, moving the policy analysis process forward, broadening and deepening policymakers' understanding of the problem and its solution options, sometimes adding new options to the solution list, creating some health policy expertise within the media, and defining the agenda for incremental reform. When the stars align properly, the solutions can be ready to go, and we get the substantial, if not quite comprehensive, reforms of 2010.

At the other extreme of the health care policy continuum, politics is incremental—the kind that goes on day in and day out, year in and year out. In ordinary health politics, those who make their living from health care—the caring professionals, insurance carriers, facility management and support staff, university teaching and training program faculty, drug and equipment suppliers, some very seasoned members of Congress and senators who have made health reform their life project, state Medicaid directors and governors, and a host of others—have learned to get what they want quietly, away from the glare of news coverage and intense public scrutiny. What they want is usually a small change in the status quo: changes in reimbursement policies, for example, that benefit certain urban hospitals or allow physicians to form unions or managed care organizations without fear of antitrust violations. They quietly go after policies that support these, with inside lobbying techniques, and, as often as not, they win.

Occasionally, bipartisan support from seasoned legislators results in a well-crafted incremental improvement in public coverage of health care. The 1997 Children's Health Insurance Plan and its reauthorization and expansion in 2009 is the leading example. S-CHIP makes the point that incremental changes are often predicated on well-defined, quantified problems and are familiar to policymakers who have debated and voted on these or similar issues in previous sessions. Proposals that raise few problems of technical feasibility, are not too expensive, broadly diffuse costs, offend no one's sense of the appropriate limits on the role of the federal government, garner little press and public attention, are complex enough to discourage interlopers, and seem to promise benefits that make them worth their cost are likely to be easiest to pass. A student of health policy who watched only these ordinary day-to-day client and interest-group politics would capture much of what happens in health care policy and over time might witness considerable change. Some of these may include

- a major shift in public and private health policy from defined benefits to defined contributions—government and firms will provide a health premium benefit for minimal managed-care coverage; benefits above that minimum will come from the beneficiary;
- malpractice tort reform and limits on awards;
- capping overall health spending as a percentage of first the public budget and later the gross domestic product;
- heavier reliance on outcomes research studies to guide clinical and coverage decisions, public and then private; and
- gradual incursion of Medicare payment policy into the choices physicians and hospitals can make for patients with certain conditions.

Each of these proposals addresses an important aspect of the health care cost problem. Over time, research and analysis on them will accumulate, and as the budget binds, answers are likely to be seriously sought and variations on these themes are likely to be among those that will pass many tests of political feasibility. The softening-up process for them has already begun.

Politics, too, evolve and change, reflecting the public's ongoing response to economic, social, and political forces. As this book has illustrated, America's institutions are far from moribund but are as dynamic and changing as the people they represent and the policies they initiate, adopt, and implement. Governing health in this country is a major undertaking—one accomplished with care and caution befitting both the country's long-standing distrust of strong government and the tremendous economic impact that health spending has on the nation as a whole. Those who fail to understand how the governing process works are likely to find themselves paying the bill for those who do.

References

Aaron, Henry J. (2009, June 15). *Health Care, Entitlements, and the Federal Budget.* Retrieved July 2, 2009, from Brookings Institution: www.brookings.edu/speeches/2009/0615_youth_entitlement_aaron.aspx.

Abelson, Reed. (2010, Nov. 10). Some Companies Shift Health Costs to Better-Paid. Retrieved 2010, from *New York Times:* www.nytimes.com/2010/11/10/business/10insure.html.

Aberbach, Joel D. (2000). A Reinvented Government, or the Same Old Government? In *The Clinton Legacy,* ed. Colin Campbell and Bert A. Rockman. New York: Chatham House.

Abrahms, Boud. (2006). Lawmakers Seek to Rein in Pork. *Tallahassee Democrat,* Feb. 5, 2A.

Abramson, Jill. (1998). The Business of Persuasion Thrives in Nation's Capital: Issues in Depth: Lobbying—The Influence Industry. *New York Times,* Sept. 29. www.nytimes.com.

AcademyHealth. (2003). State of the States: Bridging the Health Coverage Gap. Jan. www.statecoverage.net.

Adams, Rebecca. (2003a). For First Time, Fighting Odds for Malpractice Awards Cap. *CQ Weekly,* Mar. 1, 484–91.

———. (2003b). Many Skirmishes Lie ahead for Medicare Overhaul as Major Constituencies Remain Billions Apart. *CQ Weekly,* Mar. 1, 481.

———. (2005a). Cries Grow to Increase FDA's Drug Oversight. *CQ Weekly,* Feb. 21, 438–39.

———. (2005b). Heavy Lifting Ahead: Federal and State Outlook on Health. *Governing* and *CQ Weekly,* June 22–23.

Advisory Commission on Intergovernmental Relations (ACIR). 1985. *The Question of State Government Capability.* Washington, DC: Government Printing Office.

Agency for Healthcare Research and Quality (AHRQ). (2006). AHRQ Mission: Mission and Budget. www.ahrq.gov/about/budgtix.htm.

Ainsworth, Scott. (2002). *Analyzing Interest Groups: Group Influence on People and Policies.* New York: W. W. Norton.

Aldrich, John, Brittany N. Perry, and David W. Rohde. (2009, Aug. 29). House Appropriations after the Republican Revolution. Retrieved from Social Science Research Network: http://ssrn.com/abstract=1451207.

Aldrich, John H., and David W. Rohde. (2005). Congressional Committees in a Partisan Era. In *Congress Reconsidered,* 8th ed., ed. Bruce I. Dodd and Lawrence C. Oppenheimer. Washington, DC: CQ Press.

Aligning Incentives in Medicare. (2010, June). Retrieved from Medpac.gov: http://medpac.gov/documents/Jun10_EntireReport.pdf.

Ambinder, Marc. (2010, Feb. 1). The Corporations Already Outspend the Parties. The Atlantic Monthly Group. Retrieved 2010, from *Atlantic:* www.theatlantic.com/politics/archive/2010/02/the-corporations-already-outspend-the-parties/35113/.

American Dental Association (ADA). (2011). Fluoride and Fluoridation. Retrieved Dec. 9, 2011, from www.ada.org/fluoride.aspx.

Anderson, Odin W. (1990). *Health Services as a Growth Enterprise in the United States since 1875.* 2nd ed. Ann Arbor, MI: Health Administration Press.

Andres, Gary. (2004). Lobbying's Changed, So Why Haven't Our Perceptions of It? *Roll Call,* May 17. www.rollcall.com.

Ansolabehere, Stephen, James M. Snyder Jr., and Charles Stewart III. (2001). The Effects of Party and Preferences on Congressional Roll-Call Voting. *Legislative Studies Quarterly* 26 (4): 533–72.

Anton, Thomas. (1989). *American Federalism and Public Policy.* New York: Random House.

Appleby, Julie, Mary A. Carey, and Phil Galewitz. (2010, May 14). Lobbyists Have Long Wishlist for New Health Rules. Retrieved from www.kaiserhealthnews.org/Stories/2010/May/14/Health-Lobbying.aspx.

Appleby, Paul H. (1945). *Big Democracy.* New York: Knopf.

Arnold, R. Douglas. (1990). *The Logic of Congressional Action.* New Haven, CT: Yale University Press.

As Elections Loom, GOP Ardor Gives Way to Pragmatism. (1997). In *CQ Almanac 1996,* 52nd ed. Washington, DC: Congressional Quarterly. http://library.cqpress.com.proxy.lib.umich.edu/cqalmanac/cqal96-841-24595-1091346.

Associated Press. (2009, Feb. 9). Economic Stimulus Bill Passes Senate Hurdle. Retrieved from MSNBC.com, Feb. 9, 2009: www.msnbc.msn.com/id/29106540.

Babington, Charles. (2009, June 20). Outsourcing Healthcare Debate to Congress May Prove Untenable for Obama. Retrieved July 16, 2009, from *Washington Examiner:* http://washingtonexaminer.com/politics/2009/06/outsourcing-healthcare-debate-congress-may-prove-untenable-obama.

Bach, Stanley, and Steven Smith. (1988). *Managing Uncertainty in the House of Representatives: Adaptation and Innovation in Special Rules.* Washington, DC: Brookings Institution.

Baker, Peter. (2009, July 27). A Presidential Pitfall: Speaking One's Mind. Retrieved 2009, from *New York Times:* www.nytimes.com/2009/07/27/us/politics/27memo.html?ref=us&pagewanted=print.

Balla, Steven J. (1998). Administrative Procedures and Political Control of the Bureaucracy. *American Political Science Review* 92:663–73.

———. (2001). Interstate Professional Associations and the Diffusion of Policy Innovations. *American Politics Research* 29 (3): 221–45.

Barber, James David. (1985). *The Presidential Character: Predicting Performance in the White House.* Englewood Cliffs, NJ: Prentice-Hall.

Barnes, Robert, and Dan Eggen. (2010). Supreme Court Affirms Fundamental Right to Bear Arms. *Washington Post,* June 29.

Baumgartner, Frank R., Jeffrey M. Berry, Marie Hojnacki, David C. Kimball, and Beth L. Leech. (2009). *Lobbying and Policy Change: Who Wins, Who Loses, and Why.* Chicago: University of Chicago Press.

Baumgartner, Frank R., and Bryan D. Jones. (1993). *Agendas and Instability in American Politics.* Chicago: University of Chicago Press.

Baumgartner, Frank R., and Beth L. Leech. (2001). Interest Niches and Policy Bandwagons: Patterns of Interest Group Involvement in National Politics. *Journal of Politics* 63:1191–1213.

Bazelon, Emily. (2011). The Reincarnation of Pro-Life. *New York Times Magazine,* May 27.

Beamer, Glenn. (2004). State Health Care Reform Politics and the Unfortunate End of the 1990s. *Journal of Health Politics, Policy, and Law* 29:293–304.

Beckel, Michael. (2009, Nov. 10). House Democrats Backing Abortion Restrictions Received Significant Campaign Cash from Pro-Life Groups. Retrieved from *OpenSecrets.org* blog: www.opensecrets.org/news/2009/11/house-democrats-backing-abortion.html.

Becker, Elizabeth. (1999). V.A. Chief, under Fire, Is Said to Plan an Early Departure. *New York Times,* July 9. www.nytimes.com.

Begala, Paul. (2009). Grassroots Lobbying, Health Care Reform Front-and-Center. Speech delivered at the 2009 National Chiropractic Association. Press Release, Mar. 10, p. 1.

Beitsch, Les, Robert G. Brooks, Nir Menachemi, and Patrick M. Libbey. (2006). Public Health at Center Stage: New Roles, Old Props. *Health Affairs* 25 (4): 911–22. doi:10.1377/hlthaff.25.4.911.

Benda, Peter, and Charles Levine. (1986). OMB and the Central Management Problem: Is Another Reorganization the Answer? *Public Administration Review* 46:379–91.

Bendavid, Naftali, T. R. Goldman, and Sheila Kaplan. (1993). Handicapping Health Care's Major Players. *Legal Times,* Oct. 11, S28–S45.

Bengali, Shashank. (2010, June 18). Obama Officials Still Approving Flawed Gulf Drilling Plans. Retrieved 2010, from McClatchy Newspapers: www.mcclatchydc.com/2010/06/18/96185/federal-approval-still-flowing.html#storylink=misearch.

Ben Nelson's Medicaid Deal. (2009, Dec. 19). Retrieved from Politico: www.politico.com/livepulse/1209/Ben_Nelsons_Medicaid_deal.html.

Berry, Emily. (2009, Sept. 24). United, Wellpoint Accused of Creating Artificial Grassroots Lobbying Efforts. Retrieved July 13, 2010, from American Medical News: www.ama-assn.org/amednews.

Berry, Jeffrey M. (1984). *The Interest Group Society.* Boston: Little, Brown.

Beyle, Thad. (1989). From Governor to Governors. In *The State of the States,* ed. Carl Van Horn. Washington, DC: Congressional Quarterly Press.

Binder, Sarah A. (1999). The Dynamics of Legislative Gridlock, 1947–96. *American Political Science Review* 93:519–33.

———. (2003). *Stalemate: Causes and Consequences of Legislative Gridlock.* Washington, DC: Brookings Institution Press.

Binder, Sarah A., Eric D. Lawrence, and Forrest Maltzman. 1999. Uncovering the Hidden Effect of Party. *Journal of Politics* 61:815–31.

Binder, Sarah A., Thomas Mann, and Molly Reynolds. (2008). *One Year Later: Is Congress Still the Broken Branch?* Governance Studies at Brookings, vol. 2, Jan. Washington DC: Brookings Institution.

Birnbaum, Jeffrey H. (2004). Capitol Hill Listens to Coalitions. *Washington Post,* May 3, E1.

Black Man Given Nation's Worst Job. (2008). *Onion,* Nov. 5, 44–45. www.theonion.com/articles/black-man-given-nations-worst-job,6439/.

Blue Dog Days: The Democratic Party's Centrists. (2009, Aug. 1). *Economist* 392 (864): 25.

Blumenthal, Sidney. (1994). The Education of a President. *New Yorker,* Jan. 24, 31–43.

Bond, Jon R., and Richard Fleisher. (1990). *The President in the Legislative Arena.* Chicago: University of Chicago Press.

Boodman, Sandra G. (1994). Health Care's Power Player. *Washington Post,* National Weekly Edition, Feb. 14–20, 6–7.

Borins, Sandford. (1999). *Innovating with Integrity: How Local Heroes Are Transforming American Government.* Washington, DC: Georgetown University Press.

Bosso, Christopher. (1994). The Contextual Bases of Problem Recognition. In Rochefort & Cobb, 1994.

Bosso, Christopher J., and Michael Thomas Collins. (2002). Just Another Tool? How Environmental Groups Use the Internet. In *Interest Group Politics,* 6th ed., ed. Allan J. Cigler and Burdett A. Loomis. Washington, DC: CQ Press.

Bottom, William P., Cheryl L. Eavey, Gary J. Miller, and Jennifer Nicoll Victor. (2000). The Institutional Effect on Majority Rule Instability: Bicameralism in Spatial Policy Decisions. *American Journal of Political Science* 44:523–40.

Bowler, M. Kenneth. (1987). Changing Politics of Federal Health Insurance Programs. *PS* 20:202–11.

Bozeman, Barry, and Leisha DeHart-Davis. (1999). Red Tape and Clean Air: Title V Air Pollution Permitting Implementation as a Test Bed for Theory Development. *Journal of Public Administration Research and Theory* 9:141–77.

Brinkley, Joel. (1993). Cultivating the Grass Roots to Reap Legislative Benefits. *New York Times,* Nov. 11, A1.

Brisbin, Richard A., Jr. (1998). The Reconstitution of American Federalism? The Rehnquist Court and Federal-State Relations, 1991–1997. *Publius* 28 (1): 189–215.

Broder, David S. (1993). Who Does the Senate Represent? *Washington Post,* National Weekly Edition, Aug. 23–29, 4.

———. (1994a). Congress Cranks Up Its Health Reform Sausage-Maker. *Washington Post,* National Weekly Edition, Apr. 25–May 1, 10.

———. (1994b). Congressional Staffers Wield Power in Health Care Reform. *Ann Arbor News,* July 13, A9.

Broder, David S., and Stephen Barr. (1993). Going over the Top on Oversight? *Washington Post,* National Weekly Edition, Aug. 2–8, 31.

Broder, John. (2009, July 1). With Something for Everyone, Climate Bill Passed. Retrieved from *New York Times:* www.nytimes.com/2009/07/01/us/politics/01climate .html?pagewanted=print.

Brodie, Mollyann, and Robert J. Blendon. (1995). The Public's Contribution to Congressional Gridlock on Health Care Reform. *Journal of Health Politics, Policy, and Law* 20:403–10.

Brown, Clyde, and Herbert Waltzer. (2002). Lobbying the Press: "Talk to the People Who Talk to America." In *Interest Group Politics,* 6th ed., ed. Allan J. Cigler and Burdett A. Loomis. Washington, DC: CQ Press.

Browne, William. (1991). Issue Niches and the Limits of Interest Group Influence. In *Interest Group Politics,* 3rd ed., ed. Allan J. Cigler and Burdett A. Loomis. Washington, DC: Congressional Quarterly Press.

———. (1993). Group Leaders, Grassroots Confidants, and Congressional Responses. Paper presented at the annual meeting of the Midwest Political Science Association, Chicago, Apr. 6–8.

Brownlow, Louis. (1949). *The President and the Presidency.* Chicago: University of Chicago Press.

Brudnick, Ida A. (2008, Oct. 1). *Congressional Salaries and Allowances.* Congressional Research Service, Report RL30064. Retrieved 2011, from Congressional Research Service: http://opencrs.com/document/RL30064/2008-10-01/.

Burgin, Eileen. (2003). Congress, Health Care, and Congressional Caucuses: An Examination of the Diabetes Caucus. *Journal of Health Politics, Policy, and Law* 28:789–820.

Burns, James MacGregor. (1984). *The Power to Lead.* New York: Simon and Schuster.

Bush, George W. (2004). Speech Accepting Republican Nomination for President at the Republican National Convention, Sept. 2. *CQ Weekly,* Sept. 4, 2072.

Butler, Patricia A. (2004). *ERISA Update: The Supreme Court Texas Decision and Other Recent Developments.* Washington, DC: National Academy for State Health Policy.

Byrne, P. (2011). Labeling of Genetically Engineered Foods. Colorado State University Extension. Retrieved Dec. 11, 2011, from www.ext.colostate.edu/pubs/foodnut/ 09371.html.

Califano, Joseph A. (1994). Imperial Congress. *New York Times Magazine,* Jan. 23, 40–41.

Calmes, Jackie. (2010, Nov. 11). Panel Seeks Social Security Cuts and Tax Increases. Retrieved 2010, from *New York Times:* www.nytimes.com/2010/11/11/us/politics /11fiscal.html.

Calvert, Randall L., Mark J. Moran, and Barry R. Weingast. (1987). Congressional Influence over Policymaking: The Case of the FTC. In *Congress: Structure and Policy,* ed. Mathew D. McCubbins and Terry Sullivan. New York: Cambridge University Press.

Campbell, John C. (1992). *How Policies Change: The Japanese Government and the Aging Society.* Princeton, NJ: Princeton University Press.

Campion, Frank D. (1984). *The AMA and U.S. Health Policy.* Chicago: Chicago Review Press.

Canes-Wrone, Brandice, and Scott de Marchi. (2002). Presidential Approval and Legislative Success. *Journal of Politics* 64:491–509.

Canham, Matt. (2011). Insurance Mandate Has Politicians Flipping, Flopping. *Salt Lake Tribune,* June 19.

Carey, John M., Richard Niemi, and Lynda Powell. (2000). *Term Limits in the State Legislatures.* Ann Arbor: University of Michigan Press.

Carey, Mary Agnes. (2003). Small Issues Add Up to Big Headaches for Medicare Prescription Drug Conference. *CQ Weekly,* Oct. 11, 2508–10.

Carney, Eliza Newlin. (1998). The Ailing AMA. *National Journal,* Oct. 3. www .nationaljournal.com.

Carter, Jimmy. (1981, Jan. 17). President Jimmy Carter's Farewell Address. *Congressional Quarterly Weekly Report* 39:196.

———. (1982). *Keeping the Faith: Memoirs of a President.* New York: Bantam Books.

Casamayou, Maureen Hogan. (2001). *The Politics of Breast Cancer.* Washington, DC: Georgetown University Press.

Ceaser, Douglass. (1988). The Reagan Presidency and American Public Opinion. In *The Reagan Legacy: Promise and Performance,* ed. Charles O. Jones. Chatham, NJ: Chatham House.

Center for Responsive Politics. (2005). Influence and Lobbying: PACs: What Is a PAC? Retrieved Dec. 21, 2011, from OpenSecrets.org: www.opensecrets.org/pacs/ pacfaq.php.

———. (2010a). Influence and Lobbying: 527s: Advocacy Group Spending in the 2008 Elections. Retrieved July 28, 2010, from OpenSecrets.org: www.opensecrets.org/527s/index.php.

———. (2010b). Influence and Lobbying: 527s: Advocacy Group Spending in the 2010 Elections. Retrieved July 28, 2010, from OpenSecrets.org: www.opensecrets .org/527s/index.php.

———. (2010c). Influence and Lobbying: 527s: Introduction: Advocacy Group Spending. Retrieved from OpenSecrets.org: www.opensecrets.org/527s/index.php.

———. (2010d). Influence and Lobbying: Lobbying: Top Industries, 1998 and 2010. Retrieved from OpenSecrets.org: www.opensecrets.org/lobby/top.php?showYear =2010&indexType=i.

———. (2010e). Politicians and Elections: Outside Spending. Retrieved 2011, from Open Secrets.org: www.opensecrets.org/outsidespending/index.php, www.opense crets.org/outsidespending/summ.php?disp=O.

———. (2011a). House Reelection Rates, 1964–2020, and Senate Reelection Rates 1964–2010: Politicians and Elections. Retrieved 2011, from OpenSecrets.org;- www.opensecrets.org/bigpicture/reelect.php.

———. (2011b). Influence and Lobbying: Lobbying: Lobbying Database, Number of Lobbyists. Retrieved Dec. 21, 2011, from OpenSecrets.org: www.opensecrets .org/lobby/index.php.

———. (2011c). Influence and Lobbying: PACs: PAC Overview, Political Action Committees, Health, PAC Contributions to Federal Candidates. Retrieved Dec. 21, 2011, from OpenSecrets.org: www.opensecrets.org/pacs/sector.php?txt=H01 &cycle=2012.

———. (2011d). Influence and Lobbying: PACs: Top PACs, Total Expenditures, 2010. Retrieved Dec. 21, 2011, from OpenSecrets.org: www.opensecrets.org/pacs /toppacs.php?cycle=2010&Type=E&filter=P.

———. (2011e). Influence and Lobbying: Ranked Sectors. Retrieved Dec. 4, 2011, from OpenSecrets.org: www.opensecrets.org.lobby/top.php?showYear=a+indexType=c.

———. (2011f). Politicians and Elections: Historical Elections: Incumbent Advantage, 2010. Retrieved Dec. 21, 2011, from OpenSecrets.org: www.opensecrets. org/bigpicture/incumbs.php.

———. (2011g). Politicians and Elections: Overview; Incumbent Advantage. Retrieved 2011, from OpenSecrets.org: www.opensecrets.org/overview/incumbs.php.

Center on Budget and Policy Priorities. (2011). Policy Basics: Where Do Our Federal Dollars Go? Retrieved April 2011, from Center on Budget and Policy Priorities: www.cbpp.org.

Centers for Disease Control and Prevention (CDC). (2011a). About CDC: CDC Organization, CDC's Mission and Vision. www.cdc.gov/about/organization/mission .htm.

———. (2011b). About CDC: Our History Our Story. www.cdc.gov/about/history/ ourstory.htm.

Centers for Medicare and Medicaid Services (CMS). (2005). CMS Oral History Interview with Donna Shalala. www.cms.hhs.gov/about/historyshalala.asp.

———. (2011). *Center for Medicare and Medicaid Innovation*. Retrieved 2011, from Centers for Medicare and Medicaid Services: http://innovations.cms.gov.

Centers for Medicare and Medicaid Services (CMS), Office of the Actuary, National Health Statistics Group. (2010). Table 127: National Health Expenditures— Summary, 1960 to 2007. Retrieved from Centers for Medicare and Medicaid Services: www.cms.hhs.gov/NationalHealthExpendData; www.census.gov/compen dia/statab/2010/tables/10s0127.pdf.

Cigler, Allan J., and Burdett A. Loomis. (1991). Organized Interests and the Search for Certainty. In *Interest Group Politics*, 3rd ed., ed. Allan J. Cigler and Burdett A. Loomis. Washington, DC: Congressional Quarterly Press.

———. (2002). Introduction: The Changing Nature of Interest Group Politics. In *Interest Group Politics*, 6th ed. Burdett Loomis and Allan Cigler. Washington, DC: CQ Press.

Clapp, Charles L. (1963). *The Congressman: His Work as He Sees It.* Garden City, NY: Anchor Books.

Clark, Peter B., and James Q. Wilson. (1961). Incentive Systems: A Theory of Organizations. *Administrative Science Quarterly* 6:129–66.

Clarke, Gary J. (1981). The Role of the States in the Delivery of Health Services. *American Journal of Public Health* 71:59–69.

Clauser, Steven B., and Brant E. Fries. (1992, Summer). *Nursing Home Resident Assessment and Case-Mix Classification: Cross-National Perspectives.* Retrieved Sept. 14, 2010, from Centers for Medicare and Medicaid: www.cms.gov/health carefinancingreview/pastarticles/itemdetail.asp?itemid=CMS1191217.

Clymer, Adam, Robert Pear, and Robin Toner. (1994). For Health Care, Time Was a Killer. *New York Times,* Aug. 29, A1.

Cobb, Roger W., and Charles D. Elder. (1972). *Participation in American Politics: The Dynamics of Agenda-Building.* Boston: Allyn and Bacon.

Cochran, John. (2004). George W. Bush: Another Shot at His Legacy. *CQ Weekly,* Aug. 28, 1944–55.

Code of Regulations. (2011). Retrieved Dec. 11, 2011, from Electronic Code of Federal Regulations: http://ecfr.gpoaccess.gov/cgi/t/text/text-idx?c=ecfr&tpl=/ecfrbrowse /Title42/42tab_02.tpl.

Cohen, Jeffrey. (1994). Presidential Rhetoric and the Public Agenda. *American Journal of Political Science* 39:87–107.

Cohen, Michael D., James G. March, and Johan O. Olsen. (1972). A Garbage Can Model of Organizational Choice. *Administrative Science Quarterly* 17:1–25.

Cohen, Richard E., and Brian Friel. (2010, Feb. 26). 2009 Vote Ratings: Politics as Usual. Retrieved 2011, from *National Journal:* www.nationaljournal.com/2009vote ratings.

Cohn, Peter. (2005). House Considers Budget Cuts Package. *National Journal,* Nov. 19, 3638.

Colamosca, Anne. (1979). The Trade Association Hustle. *New Republic,* Nov. 3, 16–19.

Collier, Ken. (1995). The President, the Public, and the Congress. Paper presented at the annual meeting of the Midwest Political Science Association, Chicago, Apr. 6–8.

Committee on House Administration. (2009). Retrieved from Committee on House Administration: Congressional Member Organizations: http://gop.cha.house.gov /index.php?option=com_content&view=article&id=333&Itemid=373.

Congressional Budget Office (CBO). (2009a, Oct. 9). Letter to Honorable Orin Hatch, U.S. Senator from Elmendorf, Douglas, Director CBO. Retrieved from Congressional Budget Office: www.cbo.gov/publications/bysubject.cfm?cat=9.

———. (n.d.). CBO's Role in the Budget Process. Retrieved Dec. 15, 2011 from Congressional Budget Office: www.cbo.gov/aboutCBO/budgetprocess.cfm.

Congressional Quarterly. (1997). *Congressional Quarterly Almanac.* Washington, DC: CQ Press.

Congressional Research Service (CRS). (2010). About CRS. Retrieved Dec. 11, 2011, from www.loc.gov/crsinfo/.

Conlan, Timothy J., and Francosi Vergniolle De Chantal. (2001). The Rehnquist Court and Contemporary American Federalism. *Political Science Quarterly* 116:253–75.

Conlan, Timothy, and Paul Posner. (2011). Inflection Point? Federalism and the Obama Agenda. *Publius* 41 (3): 421–46. doi:10.1093/publius/pjr020.

Connolly, Ceci. (2009, Aug. 9). Seniors Remain Wary of Health-Care Reform. Retrieved Sept. 30, 2009, from *Washington Post:* www.washingtonpost.com/wp-dyn/content/article/2009/08/08/AR2009080802367_pf.html.

Connolly, Ceci, and Michael D. Shear. (2009, July 9). Discord on Health Care Dulls Luster of New Pacts. Retrieved from *Washington Post:* www.washingtonpost.com/wp-dyn/content/article/2009/07/08/AR2009070804184.html?sid=ST2009070901798.

Cowan, Richard, and Andy Sullivan. (2011, June 22). Republicans Walk out of Budget Talks over Taxes. Retrieved from Reuters.com: www.reuters.com/article/2011/06/23/us-usa-debt-cantor-idUSTRE75M3SA20110623.

Cox, Gary W., and Mathew D. McCubbins. (1993). *Legislative Leviathan: Party Government in the House.* Berkeley: University of California Press.

———. (2002). Agenda Power in the U.S. House of Representatives, 1877–1986. In *Party, Process, and Political Change in Congress: New Perspectives on the History of Congress,* ed. David W. Brady and Mathew D. McCubbins. Palo Alto, CA: Stanford University Press.

CQ Weekly. (2011, Jan. 3). *Party Unity History.* Retrieved 2011, from CQ Weekly: http://library.cqpress.com.proxy.lib.umich.edu/cqweekly/document.php?id=weeklyreport112-000003788817&type=hitlist&num=3.

Crabtree, Susan. (2011). White House: Obama's Signing Statements are Legit—Unlike Bush's. Retrieved from TPM (Talking Points Media): http://tpmdc.talkingpointsmemo.com/2011/04/white-house-obamas-signing-statements-are-legit-unlike-bushs.php.

Crawford, Craig. (2005). Craig Crawford's 1600: A Fortified White House. *CQ Weekly,* May 23, 1406.

Cronin, Thomas, and Michael A. Genovese. (1998). *The Paradoxes of the American Presidency.* New York: Oxford University Press.

Davidson, Roger H. (1984). The Presidency and the Congress. In *The Presidency and the Political System,* ed. Michael Nelson. Washington, DC: Congressional Quarterly Press.

Davidson, Roger H., and Walter J. Oleszek. (1994). *Congress and Its Members.* Washington, DC: Congressional Quarterly Press.

Davis, Aaron. (2009, Nov. 10). *Groups Redirect Health-Care Ads to Cheer and Jeer Democrats.* Retrieved from *Washington Post:* www.washingtonpost.com/wp-dyn/content/article/2009/11/09/AR2009110903452.html.

Davis, Christopher M., and David Newman. (2010, Nov. 30). *The Independent Payment Advisory Board.* CRS Report R41511. Congressional Research Service: www .crs.gov.

DeGregorio, Christine A. (2000). Leaders and Advocates in Pursuit of Policy: Some Consequences of Changing Majorities in the U.S. House of Representatives. Paper presented at the annual meeting of the Midwest Political Science Association, Chicago, Apr. 26–30.

Derthick, Martha. (1975). *Uncontrollable Spending for Social Services Grants.* Washington, DC: Brookings Institution.

———. (1990). *Agency under Stress.* Washington, DC: Brookings Institution.

Dery, David. 1984. *Problem Definition in Policy Analysis.* Lawrence: University Press of Kansas.

De Tocqueville, Alexis. ([1835] 1956). *Democracy in America.* Ed. Richard D. Heffner. New York: Mentor Books.

Diamond, Martin. (1985). What the Framers Meant by Federalism. In *American Intergovernmental Relations: Foundations, Perspectives, and Issues,* ed. Laurence O'Toole Jr. Washington, DC: Congressional Quarterly Press.

Dickerson, John. (2009, June 1). The Honeymoon Is Not Over. Retrieved July 17, 2009, from *Slate:* www.slate.com/toolbar.aspx?action=print&id=2220798.

Dinan, John. (2011). Shaping Health Reform: State Government Influence in the Patient Protection and Affordable Care Act. *Publius* 41 (3): 395–420. doi:10.1093/ publius/pjr005.

Dodd, Lawrence C., and Bruce I. Oppenheimer. (2005). A Decade of Republican Control: The House of Representatives, 1995–2005. In *Congress Reconsidered,* 8th ed., ed. Bruce I. Dodd and Lawrence C. Oppenheimer. Washington, DC: CQ Press.

———, eds. (2009). *Congress Reconsidered.* 9th ed. Washington, D.C.: CQ Press.

Dodd, Lawrence C., and Scot Schraufnagel. (2009). Reconsidering Party Polarization and Policy Productivity: A Curvilinear Perspective. In Dodd & Oppenheimer, 2009.

Dorroh, Jennifer. (2009). Statehouse Exodus. *American Journalism Review,* April– May. www.ajr.org/article.asp?id=4721.

Downs, Anthony. (1972). Up and Down with Ecology: The "Issue-Attention Cycle." *Public Interest* 28:38–50.

Drew, Christopher, and Richard Oppel Jr. (2004). How Power Lobby Won Battle of Pollution Control at E.P.A. *New York Times,* Mar. 6, A1.

Drew, Elizabeth. (2005). Selling Washington. *New York Review of Books,* June 23, 11. www.nybooks.com/articles/18075.

Duncan, Phil. (1993). *Politics in America, 1994: The 103d Congress.* Washington, DC: Congressional Quarterly Press.

Dwyre, Diana. (2002). Campaigning outside the Law: Interest Group Issue Advocacy. In *Interest Group Politics,* 6th ed., ed. Allan J. Cigler and Burdett A. Loomis. Washington, DC: CQ Press.

Eaton, Sabrina, and Stephen Koff. (2009, Feb. 26). Ohioans in Congress Add Earmarks to $410 Billion Spending Bill. Retrieved July 22, 2009, from Plain Dealer Bureau: www.cleveland.com/news/plaindealer/index.ssf?/base/news/123564081863660.xml&coll=2.

Ebell, Mark H. (2008). Future Salary and US Residency Fill Rate Revisited. *Journal of the American Medical Association* 300 (10): 1131–32.

Eckholm, Eric. (2011). Several States Forbid Abortion after 20 Weeks. *New York Times*, June 26.

Edelman, Murray. (1964). *The Symbolic Uses of Politics*. Urbana: University of Illinois Press.

Editorial: Majority Rule on Health Care Reform. (2009). *New York Times*, Aug. 30. www.nytimes.com/2009/08/30/opinion/30sun1.html?pagewanted=print.

Edney, Anna, and Drew Armstrong. (2011). Obama Says He Backs Sebelius's Morning-After Pill Restrictions for Teens. Bloomberg, *Businessweek*, Dec. 8. www.businessweek.com/news/2011-12-08/Obama-says-he-backs-morning-after-pill-for-teens/html.

Edsall, Thomas B. (1996). Issue Coalitions Take On Political Party Functions: Alliances on Left, Right Gain Power. *Washington Post*, Aug. 8, A1.

Edwards, George C. (1980). *Presidential Influence in Congress*. San Francisco: W. H. Freeman.

———. (1989). *At the Margins: The Presidential Leadership of Congress*. New Haven, CT: Yale University Press.

———. (2000). Campaigning Is Not Governing: Bill Clinton's Rhetorical Presidency. In *The Clinton Legacy,* ed. Colin Campbell and Bert A. Rockman. New York: Chatham House.

Edwards, George, and B. Dan Wood. (1999). Who Influences Whom? The President, the Congress, and the Media. *American Political Science Review* 93:327–45.

Eggen, Dan. (2009, July 31). Industry Is Generous to Influential Bloc. Retrieved from *Washington Post:* www.washingtonpost.com/wp-dyn/content/article/2009/07/30/AR2009073004267.html.

———. (2010a, Feb. 28). Expecting Final Push on Health-Care Reform, Interest Groups Rally for Big Finish. Retrieved July 28, 2010, from *Washington Post:* www.washingtonpost.com/wp-dyn/content/article/2010/02/27/AR2010022703253.html.

———. (2010b, July 25). Hospital Lobbyists Try to Minimize Damage. Retrieved from *Washington Post:* www.washingtonpost.com/wp-dyn/content/article/2009/07/24/AR2009072403255.html.

Eggen, Dan C., and Philip Rucker. (2009, Aug. 16). Loose Network of Activists Drives Reform Opposition. Retrieved from *Washington Post:* www.washingtonpost.com/wp-dyn/content/article/2009/08/15/AR2009081502696.html.

Eisen, Norm. (2009, May 29). Update on Recovery Act Lobbying Rules: New Limits on Special Interest Influence. Retrieved from the White House: www.whitehouse

.gov/blog/2009/05/29/update-recovery-act-lobbying-rules-new-limits-special -interest-influence.

Eisler, Kim Isaac. (1999). Almost Every Business Has Its Man—or Woman—in Washington: Here Are the 50 Association Heads with Real Clout. *Washingtonian Magazine,* Sept., 97.

Ellwood, John, and James Thurber. (1977). The New Congressional Budget Process. In *Congress Reconsidered,* ed. Lawrence Dodd and Bruce Oppenheimer. New York: Praeger.

Epstein, David, and Sharyn O'Halloran. (1994). Administrative Procedures, Information, and Agency Discretion. American Journal of Political Science 38:697–722.

Epstein, Samuel. (1979). The Politics of Cancer. Garden City, NY: Anchor Press.

Estimates of Mentally Ill Too High, Study Says. (2002, Feb. 2). Retrieved 2010, from *New York Times:* www.nytimes.com/2002/02/17/us/estimates-of-mentally-ill-too -high-study-says.html.

Ethridge, Emily. (2009, Dec. 28). Drug Imports Blocked, Preserving Obama Pact. Retrieved Jan. 4, 2010, from *CQ Weekly:* http://library.cqpress.com.proxy.lib.umich .edu/cqweekly/weeklyreport111-000003273504.

Eyestone, Robert. (1978). *From Social Issues to Public Policy.* New York: John Wiley.

Farnam, T. W., and Carol Leonnig. (2010, May 22). Corporate PACs Betting on Republicans to Regain Control of Congress. Retrieved July 9, 2010, from *Washington Post:* www.washingtonpost.com/wp-dyn/content/article/2010/05/21/AR2010052102513.

Feder, Judith, John Holahan, Randall Bovbjerg, and Jack Hadley. (1982). Health. In *The Reagan Experiment,* ed. John L. Palmer and Isabel V. Sawhill. Washington, DC: Urban Institute Press.

Federal Election Commission. (2005). FEC Issues Semi-Annual Federal PAC Count. www.fec.gov.

———. (n.d.). Top 50 Nonconnected PACs. Retrieved from Federal Election Commission: www.fec.gov/press/press2009/20090415PAC/documents/20top50non connectedreceipts2008.pdf.

Feldstein, Paul J. (1977). *Health Associations and the Demand for Legislation.* Cambridge, MA: Ballinger.

Fenno, Richard. (1973). *Congressmen in Committees.* Boston: Little, Brown.

———. (1978). *Home Style: House Members in Their Districts.* Boston: Little, Brown.

Fiorina, Morris. (1981). Congressional Control of the Bureaucracy: A Mismatch of Incentives and Capabilities. In *Congress Reconsidered,* 2nd ed., ed. Lawrence C. Dodd and Bruce Oppenheimer. Washington, DC: Congressional Quarterly Press.

Fiscella, Kevin. (2003). Assessing Health Care Quality for Minority and Other Disparity Populations. Washington DC: Agency for Healthcare Research and Quality. www.ahrq.gov/qual/qdisprep.

Fluoridation Action Network. 2011. Breaking News Nov. 2011. Retrieved Dec. 10, 2011, from www.fluoridealert.org.

Food and Drug Administration. (2011). About the FDA. Retrieved Dec. 11, 2011, from www.fda.gov/AboutFDA/default.htm.

Ford, Julie L., Beth H. Olson, and Amy J. Baumer. (2004). Michigan Residents "Weigh In" on Health Issues. IPPSR-SOSS Bull. 04-01. http://ippsr.msu.edu /Publications/b0401.pdf.

Foreman, Christopher. (1995). Grassroots Victim Organizations: Mobilizing for Personal and Public Health. In *Interest Group Politics*, 4th ed., ed. Allan J. Cigler and Burdett A. Loomis. Washington, DC: Congressional Quarterly Press.

Forgette, Richard, and Lindsey Scruggs. (2005). Committee Assignments and House Republicans: Have Party Effects Increased? Paper presented at the 2005 Southern Political Science Association Meeting, New Orleans, Jan. 6–9.

Fortier, John. (2008, Nov. 25). Dingell's Ouster Reveals Democrats' New Order. Retrieved July 1, 2009, from Politico: www.politico.com/news/stories/1108/15934 .html.

Fox, Daniel, and Daniel Schaffer. (1989). Health Policy and ERISA: Interest Groups and Semipreemption. *Journal of Health Politics, Policy, and Law* 14:239–60.

Foxhall, Kathryn. (2005). Managed Care in It for the Long Term. *State Legislatures*, June, 32–34.

Frates, Chris. (2010, Mar. 22). Intense Lobbying behind Health Reform. Retrieved from Politico: www.politico.com/news/stories/0310/34831.html.

Fritsch, Jane. (1995). The Grass Roots, Just a Free Phone Call Away. *New York Times*, June 23, A1.

Furlong, Scott R. (2005). Exploring Interest Group Participation in Executive Policymaking. In *The Interest Group Connection: Electioneering, Lobbying, and Policymaking in Washington*, 2nd ed., ed. Paul S. Herrnson, Ronald G. Shaiko, and Clyde Wilcox. Washington, DC: CQ Press.

Gais, Thomas, and James Fossett. (2005). Federalism and the Executive Branch. In *The Executive Branch*, ed. Joel D. Aberbach and Mark A. Peterson. Institutions of American Democracy Series, ed. Jaroslav Pelikan. New York: Oxford University Press, 2005.

Gawande, Atul. 2009. Getting There from Here: How Should Obama Reform Health Care? *New Yorker*. Retrieved Dec. 11, 2011, from www.newyorker.com/reporting /2009/01/26/090126fa_fact_gawande#ixzz1gAUpXk5Q.

Gerber, Elisabeth. (1999). *The Populist Paradox*. Princeton, NJ: Princeton University Press.

Gibson, William E., and Bob LaMendola. (2010, Nov. 14). Florida GOP Looks to Stymie Health-Care Overhaul. Retrieved 2010, from *Orlando Sentinel*: www.orland osentinel.com/health/os-health-care-repeal-florida-20101114-10,0,2575392.story.

Gilmour, John B. (2002). Institutional and Individual Influences on the President's Veto. *Journal of Politics* 64:198–218.

Glick, Henry R., and Amy Hutchinson. (2001). Physician-Assisted Suicide: Agenda Setting and the Elements of Morality Policy. In *The Public Clash of Private Values: The Politics of Morality Policy*, ed. Christopher Z. Mooney. New York: Chatham House.

Goldstein, Amy. (2003). For GOP Leaders, Battles and Bruises Produce Medicare Bill. *Washington Post*, Nov. 30, A08, final edition.

———. (2009, Dec. 16). Hospital, Physician Lobbyists Fought Medicare Buy-In Plan. Retrieved from *Washington Post:* www.washingtonpost.com/wp-dyn/content /article/2009/12/15/AR2009121505083.html.

Goldstein, Amy, and Helen Dewar. (2003). Congress Poised to Pass Medicare Bills: Prescription Drug Benefit Is Centerpiece of Biggest Revamp in 28 Years. *Washington Post,* June 27, A6.

Goldstein, Jacob. (2009, Mar. 4). Supreme Court Rules in Wyeth v. Levine. Retrieved 2011, from *Wall Street Journal, Health Blog:* http://blogs.wsj.com/health/2009/03 /04/supreme-court-rules-in-wyeth-v-levine/.

Goldstein, Kenneth M. (1999). *Interest Groups, Lobbying, and Participation in America.* New York: Cambridge University Press.

Goode, Erica. (2001). Nine Million Gaining Upgraded Benefit for Mental Care. *New York Times,* Jan. 1, www.nytimes.com.

Gordon, Joshua. (2005). The (Dis)Integration of the House Appropriations Committee: Revisiting the Power of the Purse in a Partisan Era. In *Congress Reconsidered,* 8th ed., ed. Lawrence C. Dodd and Bruce I. Oppenheimer. Washington, DC: CQ Press.

Gormley, William T., Jr. (1982). Alternative Models of the Regulatory Process: Public Utility Regulation in the States. *Western Politics Quarterly* 25:297–317.

Government Accountability Office / General Accounting Office (GAO). (2000). *Medicaid and SCHIP: Comparisons of Outreach, Enrollment Practices, and Benefits.* GAO/ HEHS-00-86. Washington, DC: Government Printing Office.

———. (2005). GAO at a Glance. www.gao.gov/about/gglance.html.

———. (2009). Fiscal Year 2010 Performance Plan, April 13, 2009. Retrieved Dec. 10, 2011, from Fiscal Year 2010 Performance Report GAO-09-304SP: www.gao .gov/htext/d09304sp.htm.

Grant, Daniel, and Lloyd Omdahl. (1993). *State and Local Government in America.* 6th ed. Madison, WI: WCG Brown and Benchmark.

Grassroots Lobbying / AA Advocacy. (n.d.). Retrieved July 9, 2010, from American Academy of Anesthesiologist Assistants: www.anesthetist.org/lobby; www.aca today.org/press_css.cfm?CID=3319.

Gray, Virginia, David Lowery, James Monogan, and Erik K. Godwin. (2009). Incrementing toward Nowhere: Universal Health Care Coverage in the States. *Publius* 40 (1): 82–113.

Greenhouse, Linda. (2007, Apr. 3). Justices Say E.P.A. Has Power to Act on Harmful Gases. Retrieved Sept. 30, 2009, from *New York Times:* www.nytimes.com/2007 /04/03/washington/03scotus.html?sq=Court Rules EPA auth.

Greenstein, Fred. (2004). *The Presidential Difference: Leadership Style from FDR to George W. Bush.* Princeton, NJ: Princeton University Press.

Grier, Kevin B., and Michael Munger. (1993). Comparing Interest Group Contributions to House and Senate Incumbents, 1980–86. *Journal of Politics* 55:615–43.

Grim, R. (2010, Mar. 24). *GOP Senators Refusing to Work Past 2PM, Invoking Obscure Rule.* Retrieved 2010, from *Huffington Post:* www.huffingtonpost.com/2010/03/24 /gop-senators-refusing-to_n_511639.html?view=print.

Gutermuth, Karen. (1999). The American Medical Political Action Committee: Which Senators Get the Money and Why? *Journal of Health Politics, Policy, and Law* 24:357–82.

Haass, Richard N. (1994). Bill Clinton's Adhocracy. *New York Times Magazine*, May 29, 40–41.

Hackey, Robert B. (2001). State Health Policy in Transition. In *The New Politics of State Health Policy*, ed. Robert B. Hackey and David A. Rochefort. Lawrence: University Press of Kansas.

Hall, Richard L. (1996). *Participation in Congress*. Ann Arbor: University of Michigan Press.

Hall, Richard L., and Kris C. Miler. (1999). Paying the Costs of Costly Signaling: Legislators as Group Agents in Agency Rulemaking. Paper presented at the annual meeting of the Midwest Political Science Association, Chicago, Apr. 15–18.

Hall, Richard, and Frank Wayman. (1990). Buying Time: Moneyed Interests and the Mobilization of Bias in Congressional Committees. *American Political Science Review* 84:797–820.

Halloran, Liz. (2009, Oct. 22). Framing Health Care Debate as Battle of Sexes. Retrieved from NPR.org: www.npr.org/templates/story/story.php?storyId=114011389.

Hamburger, Tom. (2010, Jan. 1). New Tactics Alter Flavor of Lobbying. Retrieved from *Chicago Tribune*: www.chicagotribune.com/business/chi-fri-obama-business-0101-jan01,0,344028,print.story.

Hammond, Thomas, and Jack Knott. (1996). Presidential Power, Congressional Dominance, Legal Constraints, and Bureaucratic Autonomy in a Model of Multi-Institutional Policymaking. *Journal of Law, Economics, and Organization* 12:121–68.

Hammond, Thomas H., and Gary J. Miller. (1987). The Core of the Constitution. *American Political Science Review* 81:1155–74.

Harris, Gardiner. (2009a, Jan. 28). U.S. Peanut Plant Knew of Contamination, Inspectors Say. Retrieved from *New York Times*: www.nytimes.com/2009/01/28/world/americas/28iht-29peanut.19758851.html?_r=1.

———. (2009b, Mar. 14). President Promises to Bolster Food Safety. *New York Times*. Retrieved Dec. 11, 2011, from www.nytimes.com/2009/03/15/us/politics/15address.html.

———. (2009c, Mar. 20). Drug Maker Told Studies Would Aid It, [Court] Papers Say. Retrieved from *New York Times*: www.nytimes.com/2009/03/20/us/20psych.html.

Harris, Gardiner, and David M. Halbfinger. (2009, Sept. 25). F.D.A. Reveals It Fell to a Push by Lawmakers. Retrieved from *New York Times*: www.nytimes.com/2009/09/25/health/policy/25knee.html.

Harris, Gardiner, and William Neuman. (2010, Sept. 14). Salmonella at Egg Farm Traced to 2008. Retrieved 2010 from *New York Times*: www.nytimes.com/2010/09/15/business/15egg.html.

Harris, Richard. (1966). *A Sacred Trust.* New York: New American Library.

Hart, Alexander C. (2009, Oct. 10). Medical Malpractice Reform Savings Would Be Small, Report Says. Retrieved Nov. 9, 2010, from *Los Angeles Times:* http://articles .latimes.com/2009/oct/10/nation/na-malpractice10.

Hartocollis, Anemona. (2010, July 2). Failure of State Soda Tax Plan Reflects Power of an Antitax Message. Retrieved from *New York Times:* www.nytimes.com/2010 /07/03/nyregion/03sodatax.html.

Hayes, Michael T. (1992). *Implementation and Public Policy.* White Plains, NY: Longman.

Health and Human Services, Department of (HHS). (2011). HHS: What We Do. Retrieved from Health and Human Services: www.hhs.gov/ocio/about/whatwedo /what.html.

Health Care Reforms Proposed during the Obama Administration. (n.d.). Retrieved from Wikipedia: http://en.wikipedia.org/wiki/Health_care_reforms_proposed _during_the_Obama_administration.

Heaney, Michael T. (2004a). Outside the Issue Niche: The Multidimensionality of Interest Group Identity. *American Politics Research* 32 (6): 611–51.

———. (2004b). Reputation and Leadership inside Interest Group Coalitions. Paper presented at the annual meeting of the American Political Science Association, Chicago, Sept. 2–5.

Heclo, Hugh. (1977). *A Government of Strangers.* Washington, DC: Brookings Institution.

———. (1978). Issue Networks and the Executive Establishment. In *The New American Political System,* ed. Anthony King. Washington, DC: American Enterprise Institute.

Heilprin, John. (2004). EPA to Pursue Clean-Air Lawsuits. *Tallahassee Democrat,* Jan. 10, 5A.

Heinz, John P., Edward O. Laumann, Robert L. Nelson, and Robert H. Salisbury. (1993). *The Hollow Core: Private Interests in National Policy Making.* Cambridge, MA: Harvard University Press.

Heinz, John P., Edward O. Laumann, Robert H. Salisbury, and Robert L. Nelson. (1990). Inner Circles or Hollow Cores? Elite Networks in National Policy Systems. *Journal of Politics* 52:356–90.

Herbert, Bob. (2004). Malpractice Myths. *New York Times,* June 21, A19.

Herrick, Rebekah, and Michael K. Moore. (1993). Political Ambition's Effect on Legislative Behavior: Schlesinger's Typology Reconsidered and Revised. *Journal of Politics* 55:765–76.

Herszenhorn, David. (2009, July 16). Baucus: On Paying for Healthcare, Obama Isn't Helping. Retrieved 2009, from *New York Times:* http://thecaucus.blogs.nytimes .com/2009/07/16/baucus-on-health-care-debate-obama-isnt-helping/.

Herszenhorn, David, and Robert Pear. (2009a, July 20). Democrats May Limit Tax Increase for Health Plan. Retrieved 2009, from *New York Times:* www.nytimes .com/2009/07/21/health/policy/21health.html?fta=y&pagewanted=print.

———. (2009b, July 23). Concerns on Plan Show Clashing Goals. Retrieved 2009, from *New York Times:* www.nytimes.com/2009/07/23/health/policy/23center.html ?fta=y&pagewanted=print.

Hill, Jeffrey, and Carol S. Weissert. (1995). Implementation and the Irony of Delegation: The Politics of Low-Level Radioactive Waste Disposal. *Journal of Politics* 57:344–69.

Hinckley, Barbara. (1990). *The Symbolic Presidency.* New York: Routledge.

Hojnacki, Marie, and David C. Kimball. (1998). Organized Interests and the Decision of Whom to Lobby in Congress. *American Political Science Review* 92:775–90.

———. (1999). The Who and How of Organizations' Lobbying Strategies in Committee. *Journal of Politics* 61:999–1024.

Horn, Murray. (1995). *The Political Economy of Public Administration.* New York: Cambridge University Press.

Hulse, Carl, and Philip Shenon. (2006, Apr. 5). The DeLay Resignation: The Overview; Continuing Legal Troubles Reportedly Left DeLay Dispirited. *New York Times.* Retreived Jan. 28, 2011, from http://query.nytimes.com/gst/fullpage.html ?res=9D00E6DC1030F936A35757C0A9609C8B63&scp=4&sq=Tom+Delay+ resigns&st=cse&pagewanted=all.

Human Rights Watch. (2011). US: Court Overrules Anti-Prostitution Gag Rule for US Groups. July 8. Retrieved Dec. 11, 2011, from http://www.hrw.org/news/2011 /07/08/us-court-overrules-anti-prostitution-gag-rule-us-groups.

Iglehart, John K. (1977). The Hospital Lobby Is Suffering from Self-inflicted Wounds. *National Journal,* Oct. 1, 1526–31.

Inglehart, John. (2009, June 18). Interview—Doing More with Less: A Conversation with Kerry Weems. Retrieved from *Health Affairs:* doi:10.1377/hlthaff.28.4 .w688–w696.

Ingram, Helen. (1977). Policy Implementation through Bargaining. *Public Policy* 25:449–501.

Initiative and Referendum Institute. (2010). Election Results 2010: Tea Party Spillover? Retrieved from Initiative and Referendum Institute: http://iandrinstitute .org.

Jacobs, Lawrence R. (1993). Health Reform Impasse: The Politics of American Ambivalence toward Government. *Journal of Health Politics, Policy, and Law* 18:629–55.

Jacobs, Lawrence R., and Robert Y. Shapiro. (1995). Don't Blame the Public for Failed Health Care Reform. *Journal of Health Politics, Policy, and Law* 20:411–23.

———. (2000). *Politicians Don't Pander: Political Manipulation and the Loss of Democratic Responsiveness.* Chicago: University of Chicago Press.

Jacobson, Gary C. (1987). *The Politics of Congressional Elections.* 2nd ed. Boston: Little, Brown.

Janiskee, Brian. (1995). Bicameralism and Health Legislation in Michigan. Paper presented at the annual meeting of the Midwest Political Science Association, Chicago, Apr. 6–8.

Johnson, Cathy Marie. (1992). *The Dynamics of Conflict between Bureaucrats and Legislators.* Armonk, NY: M. E. Sharpe.

Johnson, Linda. (2005). Abstinence Advocates Want Condom Correction. *Tallahassee Democrat,* June 30, 6A.

Johnson, Lyndon Baines. (1971). *The Vantage Point.* New York: Holt, Rinehart, and Winston.

Jones, Charles O. (1984). *An Introduction to the Study of Public Policy.* Monterey, CA: Brooks/Cole.

———. 1994. *The Presidency in a Separated System.* Washington, DC: Brookings Institution.

Jones, Mark P., and Wonjae Hwang. (2005). Party Government in Presidential Democracies: Extending Cartel Theory beyond the U.S. Congress. *American Journal of Political Science* 49:267–82.

Joondeph, Bradley W. (2011). Federalism and Health Care Reform: Understanding the States' Challenges to the Patient Protection and Affordable Care Act. *Publius* 41 (3): 447–70. doi:10.1093/publius/pjr010.

Jost, Kenneth. (2003). Medical Malpractice: Are Lawsuits out of Control? *CQ Researcher* 13 (6, Feb. 14): 129–52.

Joyce, Amy. (2005). Bill Targets Wal-Mart's Health Care. *Tallahassee Democrat,* June 23, 4A.

Just 8% Approve of Job Congress Is Doing. (2011, June 22). Retrieved 2011, from Rasmussen Reports: www.rasmussenreports.com/public_content/politics/mood_of_america/congressional_performance.

Justice, Glen. (2005). Ads Will Seek to Turn DeLay's Powerful Network into His Downfall. *New York Times,* Mar. 20, A11.

Kaiser Commission on Medicaid and the Uninsured (KCMU). (2011). Enrollment Data for 1998–2008: Medicaid Enrollment in 50 States; Conducted by Health Management Associates, September 2009. Retrieved from Kaiser Commission on Medicaid and the Uninsured: www.kff.org/about/kcmu.cfm.

Kaiser Family Foundation. (2011a). Enhanced Medicaid Match Rates Expire in June 2011. Retrieved from Kaiser Family Foundation: www.kff.org.

———. (2011b). Focus on Health Reform. Summary of the New Health Reform Law. Retrieved 2011, from Kaiser Family Foundation: www.kff.org.

———. (2011c). Medicaid Facts: Medicaid Enrollment; June 2010 Data Snapshot. Retrieved 2011, from Kaiser Family Foundation: www.kff.org.

———. (2011d). State Medicaid Fact Sheets. Retrieved 2011, from Kaiser Family Foundation: www.kff.org.

———. (n.d.). Primary Care Shortage: Background Brief. Retrieved Dec. 10, 2011, from KaiserEDU.org: www.kaiseredu.org/Issue-Modules/Primary-Care-Shortage/Background-Brief.aspx.

Kaiser Health News Staff. (2011, Apr. 4). Understanding Rep. Ryan's Plan for Medicare. Retrieved from Kaiser Health News: www.kaiserhealthnews.org/Stories/2011/April/05/ryan-plan-for-medicare-vouchers-vs-premium-support.aspx.

Kane, Paul. (2010, Feb. 18). Value of Congressional Earmarks Increased in Fiscal 2010. Retrieved from *Washington Post:* www.washingtonpost.com/wp-dyn/content/article/2010/02/17/AR2010021705110.html.

Kaufman, Herbert. (1977). *Red Tape.* Washington, DC: Brookings Institution.

Kearns, Doris. (1976). *Lyndon Johnson and the American Dream.* New York: Harper and Row.

Keefe, William J. (1984). *Congress and the American People.* 2nd ed. Englewood Cliffs, NJ: Prentice-Hall.

Keiser, K. Robert, and Woodrow Jones Jr. (1986). Do the American Medical Association's Campaign Contributions Influence Health Care Legislation? *Medical Care* 24:761–66.

Kelly, Michael. (1993). David Gergen, Master of the Game. *New York Times Magazine,* Oct. 31, 62.

Kennedy, Edward M. (2005). Perspective: The Role of the Federal Government in Eliminating Health Disparities: Strong Federal Action Is Crucial to Marshaling the Resources and Political Will to End Minority Health Disparities. *Health Affairs* 24 (2): 452–58.

Kernell, Samuel. (1984). The Presidency and the People. In *The Presidency and the Political System,* ed. Michael Nelson. Washington, DC: Congressional Quarterly Press.

———. (1991). Facing an Opposition Congress: The President's Strategic Circumstance. In *The Politics of Divided Government,* ed. Gary Cox and Samuel Kernell. Boulder, CO: Westview Press.

Kernell, Samuel, Peter W. Spelich, and Aaron Wildavsky. (1975). Public Support for Presidents. In *Perspectives on the Presidency,* ed. Aaron Wildavsky. Boston: Little, Brown.

Kersh, Rogan, and James Morone. (2002). The Politics of Obesity: Seven Steps to Government Action. *Health Affairs* 21 (6): 142–53.

Kerwin, Cornelius M. 2003. *Rulemaking: How Government Agencies Write Law and Make Policy.* 3rd ed. Washington, DC: CQ Press.

Kiewiet, Roderick, and Mathew McCubbins. (1991). *The Spending Power: Congress, the President, and the Appropriations Process.* Chicago: University of Chicago Press.

Kingdon, John. (1977). *Congressmen's Voting Decisions.* New York: Harper and Row.

———. (1995). *Agendas, Alternatives, and Public Policies.* 2nd ed. New York: Harper Collins.

Kirkpatrick, David. (2009a, Aug. 6). David D. Kirkpatrick: White House Affirms Deal on Drug Cost. Retrieved from *New York Times:* www.nytimes.com/2009/08/06/health/policy/06insure.html.

———. (2009b, Nov. 7). Pelosi Faces Competing Pressures on Health Care. Retrieved from *New York Times:* www.nytimes.com/2009/11/07/health/policy/07pelosi.html.

———. (2009c, Dec. 26). Catholic Group Supports Senate on Abortion Aid. Retrieved from *New York Times:* www.nytimes.com/2009/12/26/health/policy/26abort.html.

Kirkwood, R. Cort. (2011). Georgia's Law Sends Illegals Fleeing; Leftists File Suit. *U.S. News and World Report,* June.

Klein, Ezra. (2010, Mar. 18). Andy Stern: "We Need to Make Ourselves More Involved in These People's Career Planning." Retrieved from *Washington Post:* http://voices.washingtonpost.com/ezra-klein/2010/03/andy_stern_we_need_to _make_our.html.

Knott, Jack, and Gary Miller. (1987). *Reforming Bureaucracy: The Politics of Institutional Choice.* Englewood Cliffs, NJ: Prentice-Hall.

Knowlton, Brian, and Derrick Henry. (2009, July 26). Democrats Disagree on State of Health Reform Bill. Retrieved July 27, 2009, from *New York Times:* www.ny times.com/2009/07/27/health/policy/27talkshows.html?ref=us&pagewanted.

Kosterlitz, Julie. (1994). The Big Sell. *National Journal,* May 14, 1118–23.

Krane, Dale. (2003). The State of American Federalism, 2002–03: Division Replaces Unity. *Publius* 33 (1): 1–44.

Krehbiel, Keith. (1992). *Information and Legislative Organization.* Ann Arbor: University of Michigan Press.

———. (1998). *Pivotal Politics: A Theory of U.S. Lawmaking.* Chicago: University of Chicago Press.

Kuraitis, Vince. (2010, Mar. 28). Pilots, Demonstrations, and Innovation in the PPACA Healthcare Reform Legislation. Retrieved 2010, from e-CareManagement blog: http://e-caremanagement.com/pilots-demonstrations-innovation-in-the -ppaca-healthcare-reform-legislation/.

Kurtz, Howard. (1994). Rolling with the Punches from the Press Corps. *Washington Post,* National Weekly Edition, Jan. 24–30, 10.

Kurtz, Karl. (1989). State Legislatures in the 1990s. In *Handbook on State Government Relations.* Washington, DC: Public Affairs Council.

Lacy, Marc. (2000). Blocked by Congress, Clinton Wields a Pen. *New York Times,* July 5, A11.

Ladenheim, Kala. (1997). Health Insurance in Transition: The Health Insurance Portability and Accountability Act of 1996. *Publius* 27 (2): 33–51.

Lambert, David A., and Thomas McGuire. (1990). Political and Economic Determinants of Insurance Regulation in Mental Health. *Journal of Health Politics, Policy, and Law* 15:169–89.

Lamm, Richard D. (1990). The Ten Commandments of Health Care. In *The Nation's Health,* 3rd ed., ed. Philip R. Lee and Carroll L. Estes. Boston: Jones and Bartlett.

Landes, William, and Richard Posner. (2008, May 2). Legal Theory Blog: "*All the theory that fits.*" Retrieved July 14, 2009, from Landes and Posner on Rational Judicial Behavior: http://lsolum.typepad.com/legaltheory/2008/05/landes-posner-0.html.

Lasker, Eric G. (2005). Position on Federal Preemption Consistent with Law and Public Health. *Legal Backgrounder* 20:9. www.web.lexis-nexis.com.proxy.lib.fsu .edu.

Layton, Charles, and Mary Walton. (1998). Missing the Story at the Statehouse. *American Journalism Review,* July–Aug., 42–63.

Lee, Christopher. (2006). Bush Seeks to Increase Health Savings Accounts. *Washington Post*, Feb. 6, A13.

Leonhardt, David. (2009, June 10). America's Sea of Red Ink Was Years in the Making. Retrieved Dec. 1, 2010, from *New York Times:* www.nytimes.com/2009/06/10/business/economy/10leonhardt.html.

Levi, Jeffrey, Rebecca St. Laurent, Laura M. Segal, and Serena Vinter. (2009). *Shortchanging America's Health*. Issue Report from Trust for America's Health. Washington D.C.: Trust for America's Health and Robert Wood Johnson Foundation, www.rwjf.org/files/research/tfahshortchanging2009fnlrv2.pdf.

Lichtblau, Eric. (2010a, June 24). Across from White House, Coffee with Lobbyists. Retrieved from *New York Times:* www.nytimes.com/2010/06/25/us/politics/25caribou.html.

———. (2010b, July 1). Lobbyist Says It's Not about Influence. Retrieved from *New York Times:* www.nytimes.com/2010/07/02/us/02podesta.html.

———. (2010c, July 13). Beyond Guns: N.R.A. Expands Political Agenda. Retrieved from *New York Times:* www.nytimes.com/2010/07/13/us/politics/13nra.html.

Light, Paul. (1984). The Presidential Policy Stream. In *The Presidency and the Political System*, ed. Michael Nelson. Washington, DC: Congressional Quarterly Press.

———. (1991). *The President's Agenda: Domestic Policy Choice from Kennedy to Reagan*. Rev. ed. Baltimore: Johns Hopkins University Press.

Lindblom, Charles. (1980). *The Policy-Making Process*. Englewood Cliffs, NJ: Prentice-Hall.

Lipinski, Daniel. (2009). Navigating Congressional Policy Processes: The Inside Perspective on How Laws Are Made. In Dodd & Oppenheimer, 2009.

Liptak, Adam. (2009, Feb. 1). To Nudge, Shift, or Shove the Supreme Court Left. Retrieved Feb. 3, 2009, from *New York Times:* www.nytimes.com/2009/02/01/weekinreview/01liptak.html?_r=1&.

———. (2010a, Jan. 22). Justices, 5-4, Reject Corporate Spending Limit. Retrieved July 13, 2010, from *New York Times:* www.nytimes.com/2010/01/22/us/politics/22scotus.html.

———. (2010b, July 24). Court under Roberts Is Most Conservative in Decades. Retrieved 2011, from *New York Times:* www.nytimes.com/2010/07/25/us/25roberts.html?

———. (2011a). Justices Reject Ban on Violent Video Games for Children. *New York Times*, June 27.

———. (2011b). Justices Strike Down Arizona Campaign Finance Law. *New York Times*, June 26.

Locker, Richard. (2005). A True Tennessee Titan. *State Legislatures* 31 (7): 56–59.

Loepp, Daniel. (1999). *Sharing the Balance of Power: An Examination of Shared Power in the Michigan House of Representatives, 1993–1994*. Ann Arbor: University of Michigan Press.

Lohmann, Susanne. (1998). An Information Rationale for the Power of Special Interests. *American Political Science Review* 92:809–27.

Long, Mark, and Angel Gonzalez. (2010, May 13). Transocean Seeks Limit on Liability. Retrieved from *Wall Street Journal:* http://online.wsj.com/article/SB10001424052748704635204575241852606380696.html.

Long, Norton E. (1949). Power and Administration. *Public Administration Review* 9:257–64.

Loomis, Burdett A. (1988). *The New American Politician.* New York: Basic Books.

Loven, Jennifer. (2005). Bush Says He Would Veto Changes to New Medicare Drug Plan. *Tallahassee Democrat,* Feb. 12, A4.

Lovern, Ed. (2002). Ready, Aim, Litigate: AHA Takes Feds to Court to Stop HHS from Eliminating Medicaid Loophole. *Modern Healthcare,* Mar. 11, 8–11.

Lowi, Theodore J. (1964). American Business, Public Policy, Case-Studies, and Political Theory. *World Politics* 16:677–715.

Lozano, Juan A. (2010). Tom DeLay Guilty: Jury Convicts Republican in Money Laundering Trial. Retrieved November 24, 2010, from *Huffington Post:* www.huffingtonpost.com/2010/11/24/tom-delay-guilty-money-laundering_n_788325.html.

MacKuen, Michael B., and Calvin Mouw. (1992). The Strategic Configuration, Personal Influence, and Presidential Power in Congress. *Western Political Quarterly* 45:579–608.

Mann, Thomas E., and Norman J. Ornstein. 2006. *The Broken Branch.* New York: Oxford University Press.

———. (2009). Is Congress Still the Broken Branch? In *Congress Reconsidered,* 9th ed., ed. Lawrence C. Dodd and Bruce Oppenheimer. Washington, DC: CQ Press.

Manning, Jennifer. (2010, Nov. 21). Membership of the 111th Congress: A Profile. Retrieved Dec. 1, 2010, from Congressional Research Service: www.senate.gov/CRSReports/crs-publish.cfm?pid=%260BL%29PL%3B%3D%0A.

March, William. (2010, June 22). *Tampa Bay Online Tampa Tribune.* Retrieved Dec. 1, 2010, from *Tampa Bay Online Tampa Tribune:* www2.tbo.com/content/2010/jun/22/220947/candidates-finding-success-spending-millions-own-c/.

Marcus, Ruth. (1998). Big Tobacco Quietly Tries to Grow Grass Roots: Industry's Sophisticated Lobbying Tactics Strike Some Critics as Deceptive. *Washington Post,* May 16, A1.

Marini, John. (1992). *The Politics of Budget Control: Congress, the Presidency, and the Growth of the Administrative State.* Washington, DC: Crane, Russak.

Marmor, Theodore. (1970). *The Politics of Medicare.* Chicago: Aldine.

Martin, Andrew D. (2001). Congressional Decision Making and the Separation of Powers. *American Political Science Review* 95:361–78.

Martinez, Barbara. (2009, Dec. 22). Cosmetic Surgeons Get Reid to Tax Tanning Salons Instead. Retrieved from *Wall StreetJournal:* http://online.wsj.com/article/SB126144830913601141.html.

Martinez, Gebe, and Mary Agnew Carey. (2004). Erasing the Gender Gap Tops Republican Playbook. *CQ Weekly,* Mar. 6, 564–70.

"Mary Landrieu Defends 'Louisiana Purchase' Medicaid Deal for Louisiana." (2010, Feb. 5). Retrieved 2010, from *Huffington Post:* www.huffingtonpost.com/2010/02/05/mary-landrieu-defends-lou_n_450476.html.

Matlack, Carol, James A. Barnes, and Richard E. Cohen. (1990). Quid with Quo? *National Journal* 22:1473.

Mayer, Kenneth R. (2001). *With the Stroke of a Pen: Executive Orders and Presidential Power.* Princeton, NJ: Princeton University Press.

Mayer, Lindsay R., Michael Beckel, and Aaron Kiersh. (2009, June 17). Diagnosis: Reform. Retrieved from *OpenSecretsBlog:* www.opensecrets.org/news/2009/06/diagnosis-reform.html.

Mayhew, David. (1974). *Congress: The Electoral Connection.* New Haven, CT: Yale University Press.

———. (1987). The Electoral Connection and the Congress. In *Congress: Structure and Policy,* ed. Mathew McCubbins and Terry Sullivan. New York: Cambridge University Press.

———. (1991). *Divided We Govern: Party Control, Lawmaking, and Investigations, 1946–1990.* New Haven, CT: Yale University Press.

McCarty, Nolan, Keith T. Poole, and Howard Rosenthal. (2006, June). Polarized America. Retrieved July 1, 2009, from Polarized America: The Dance of Ideology and Unequal Riches: http://polarizedamerica.com/#POLITICALPOLARIZATION.

———. (2011). Polarized America: The Dance of Ideology and Unequal Riches. Retrieved 2011, www.voteview.com/Polarized_America.htm#POLITICALPOLARIZATION.

McCaughan, Michael. (2010, Apr. 19). Who Will Run PhRMA? AZ's Chip Davis, for Now. Retrieved from *In Vivo:* http://invivoblog.blogspot.com/2010/04/who-will-run-phrma-azs-chip-davis-for.html.

McCoy, Kevin. (2000). Flurry of Regulations Set to Kick in as Clinton Exits: New Rules Affect Many Industries. *USA Today,* Nov. 27, 4B.

McCubbins, Mathew, and Thomas Schwartz. (1984). Congressional Oversight Overlooked: Police Patrols vs. Fire Alarms. *American Journal of Political Science* 28:165–79.

McFarlane, Deborah R., and Kenneth J. Meier. (2001). *The Politics of Fertility Control: Family Planning and Abortion Policies in the American States.* New York: Chatham House.

McGrane, Victoria. (2009, Dec. 22). Lobbyists on Pace for Record Year. Retrieved from Politico: www.politico.com/news/stories/1209/30882.html.

McGrory, Mary. (1999). The Corner on Caring. *Washington Post,* Aug. 26, A3.

McKinley, Jesse. (2009, Nov. 30). A Tax on Nips and Tucks Angers Patients, Surgeons. Retrieved from *New York Times:* www.nytimes.com/2009/11/30/health/policy/30cosmetic.html.

———. (2010, June 23). Whooping Cough Kills 5 in California. Retrieved 2010, from *New York Times:* www.nytimes.com/2010/06/24/us/24cough.html?sq=epidemic&st=cse&scp=1&page.

Meier, Kenneth. (1985). *Regulation: Politics, Bureaucracy, and Economics*. New York: St. Martin's.

Meier, Markus H., Bradley S. Albert, and Saralisa C. Brau. (2010, June). *Overview of FTC Antitrust Actions in Health Care Services and Products*. Retrieved from US Federal Trade Commission, Washington, DC, June 2010. www.ftc.gov/bc/0610hcup date.pdf.

Meinke, Scott R. (2005). Long-Term Change and Stability in House Voting Decisions: The Case of the Minimum Wage. *Legislative Studies Quarterly* 30:103–26.

Memmott, Mark. (2011, June 29). Coincidence? Their Pay Withheld, California Lawmakers Strike Budget Deal. Retrieved 2011, from National Public Radio: www .npr.org.

Michigan Consumer Health Care Coalition. (2005). *Facts about Drug Advertising* 5 (1): 2.

Miller, Gary J. (1993). Formal Theory and the Presidency. In *Researching the Presidency*, ed. George C. Edwards III, John H. Kessel, and Bert A. Rockman. Pittsburgh: University of Pittsburgh Press.

Moe, Terry. (1985). The Politicized Presidency. In *The New Direction in American Politics*, ed. John E. Chubb and Paul E. Peterson. Washington, DC: Brookings Institution.

Montgomery, Lori. (2009a, July 16). CBO Chief Criticizes Democrats' Health Reform Measures. Retrieved 2009, from *Washington Post:* www.washingtonpost .com/wp-dyn/content/article/2009/07/16/AR2009071602242.html.

———. (2009b, Nov. 7). Democrats to Resolve Abortion Impasse on the House Floor. Retrieved 2011, from *Washington Post:* http://voices.washingtonpost.com/capitiol briefing/2009/11/democrats_to_resolve_abortion.html.

Mooney, Christopher Z. (2001). The Public Clash of Private Values. In *The Public Clash of Private Values: The Politics of Morality Policy*, ed. Christopher Z. Mooney. New York: Chatham House.

Morone, James A. (1990). *The Democratic Wish: Popular Participation and the Limits of American Government*. New York: Basic Books.

———. (1993). The Health Care Bureaucracy: Small Changes, Big Consequences. *Journal of Health Politics, Policy, and Law* 18:723–39.

———. (1995). Nativism, Hollow Corporations, and Managed Competition: Why the Clinton Health Care Reform Failed. *Journal of Health Politics, Policy, and Law* 20:391–98.

Mosk, Matthew. (2010, Mar. 17). ABC News Exclusive: Study Shows Money Flooding into Campaigns for State Judgeships. Retrieved from ABC News: http://abc news.go.com/Blotter/study-shows-money-flooding-campaigns-state-judgeships /story?id=1012004.

Moss, Michael. (2010, May 29). The Hard Sell on Salt. Retrieved from *New York Times:* www.nytimes.com/2010/05/30/health/30salt.html.

Moy, Ernest, Elizabeth Dayton, and Carolyn M. Clancy. (2005). Compiling the Evidence: The National Healthcare Disparities Reports: These Important Reports

Contribute to the Infrastructure Needed to Track Progress toward Eliminating Disparities. *Health Affairs* 24 (2): 376–87.

Mueller, Keith J. (1992). State Government Policies and Rural Hospitals: Facilitating Change. *Policy Studies Journal* 20:168–81.

Murray, Shailagh, and Lori Montgomery. (2009). On Health Care, the Prognosis Is Compromise. *Washington Post,* July 6. www.washingtonpost.com/wp-dyn/con tent/article/2009/07/05/AR2009070502517.html.

Nagourney, Adam. (2009, July 26). Partisan or Not, a Tough Course on Health Care. Retrieved July 26, 2009, from *New York Times:* www.nytimes.com/2009/07/26/us /politics/26partisan.html?_r=1&hp=&pagewanted=.

Nathan, Richard P. (1983). *The Administrative Presidency.* New York: John Wiley.

———. (1993). *Turning Promises into Performance.* New York: Twentieth Century Fund.

Nather, David. (2004). Congress as Watchdog: Asleep on the Job? *CQ Weekly,* May 22, 1190–95.

National Association of State Budget Officers (NASBO). (2002). *Budget Processes in the States.* Washington, DC: NASBO. www.nasbo.org/Publications/PDFs/bud pro2002.pdf.

———. (2008). Budget Process in the States: State Expenditure Report. Retrieved from National Association of State Budget Officers: www.nasbo.org.

———. (2010). *State Expenditure Report.* Washington DC: National Association of State Budget Officers.

———. (2011). The Fiscal Survey of the States. Retrieved Dec. 11, 2011, from National Association of State Budget Officers: www.nasbo.org.

National Commission on the State and Local Public Service. (1993). *Frustrated Federalism: Rx for State and Local Health Care Reform.* Albany, NY: Nelson A. Rockefeller Institute of Government.

National Conference of State Legislatures (NCSL). (2005). The Term Limited States. www.ncsl.org/programs/legman/about/states.htm.

———. (2011). *State Legislation and Actions on Health Savings Accounts (HSAs) and Consumer-Directed Health Plans, 2004–2010.* Retrieved 2011, from National Conference of State Legislatures: www.ncsl.org.

National Health Council (NHC). (2010). National Health Council: Welcome. Retrieved 2010, from NationalHealthCouncil.org: www.nationalhealthcouncil.org.

National Health Policy Forum. (2009, June 15). Medicaid Disproportionate Share Hospital (DSH) Payments. Retrieved Oct. 28, 2010, from National Health Policy Forum: www.nhpf.org/library/the-basics/Basics_DSH_06-15-09.pdf.

National Public Radio (NPR). (2000). *Morning Edition,* Nov. 3. www.npr.org.

National Right to Life Press Releases. (n.d.). Retrieved July 9, 2010, from National Right to Life: www.nrlc.org/press_releases_new/index.html; www.mdrtl.org /mediaarchives.html.

Neal, Rebecca. (2009, Feb. 25). House Passes $410 Billion 2009 Omnibus Spending Bill. Retrieved Dec. 1, 2010, from *Federal Times:* www.federaltimes.com/article /20090225/CONGRESS01/902250306/.

Nelson, Suzanne. (2000). Brooks Voted Out but Not Silenced. *Roll Call*, Dec. 14. http://rollcall.com.

Neuman, William. (2010, Sept. 22). An Iowa Egg Farmer and a History of Salmonella. Retrieved 2010, from *New York Times*: www.nytimes.com/2010/09/22/business/22eggs.html.

Neustadt, Richard E. (1960). *Presidential Power*. New York: John Wiley.

———. 1990. *Presidential Power and the Modern Presidents*. New York: Free Press.

Nixon, Ron. (2010, Dec. 27). Lawmakers Finance Pet Projects without Earmarks. Retrieved from *New York Times*: www.nytimes.com/2010/12/28/us/politics/28earmarks.html?pagewanted=print.

Noah, Timothy. (1993). AMA Lavishly Courts Congressional Staffers Who Will Affect Outcome of Clinton's Health Plan. *Wall Street Journal*, June 30, A16.

Nolte, Ellen, and Martin McKee. (2003). Measuring the Health of Nations: Analysis of Mortality Amendable to Health Care. *British Medical Journal* 327:1–5, Table 1.

Norrander, Barbara, and Clyde Wilcox. (2001). Public Opinion and Policymaking in the States: The Case of Post-Roe Abortion Policy. In *The Public Clash of Private Values: The Politics of Morality Policy*, ed. Christopher Z. Mooney. New York: Chatham House.

NPR Staff. (2010, Nov. 11). Texas Gov. Rick Perry Is "Fed Up!" Retrieved 2010, from NPR *Morning Edition*: www.npr.org/templates/story/story.php?storyId=131048009.

Obama Cites His Agenda in Holiday Address. (2009). *CBS News*, July 4.

Obama Interview with Steve Kroft. (2008). CBS, *60 Minutes*, Nov. 16.

Office of History and Preservation, Office of the Clerk. (2010). *Women in Congress*. Retrieved Dec. 1, 2010, from Women in Congress: http://womenincongress.house.gov/historical-data/.

Office of Management and Budget (OMB). (2011a). *Analytical Perspectives, Budget of the United States Government, Fiscal Year 2012*. Retrieved 2011, from Office of Management and Budget: www.whitehouse.gov/sites/default/files/omb/budget/fy2012/assets/spec.pdf.

———. (2011b). Table 8.5: Outlays for Mandatory and Other Related Programs, 1962–2016. In *Tables: United States Federal Budget FY 2012*. Retrieved 2011, from Office of Management and Budget: www.whitehouse.gov/omb/budget/Historicals.

———. (2011c). Table 32-1: Budget Authority and Outlays by Function, Category, and Program. In *Analytical Perspectives, Budget of the United States Government, Fiscal Year 2012*. Retrieved July 2011, from Office of Management and Budget: www.whitehouse.gov/omb/budget/Analytical_Perspectives.

———. (2011d). Summary Table S-4. In *Tables: United States Federal Budget FY 2012*. Retrieved 2011, from Office of Management and Budget: www.whitehouse.gov/sites/default/files/omb/budget/fy2012/assets/tables.pdf.

———. (2011e). 2011 Report to Congress on the Benefits and Costs of Federal Regulations and Unfunded Mandates on State, Local, and Tribal Entities. Office of Information and Regulatory Affairs, Office of Management and Budget, Washing-

ton, DC. Retrieved 2011, from Office of Management and Budget: www.whitehouse
.gov/sites/default/files/omb/inforeg/2011_cb/2011_cba_report.pdf.

The Official Alphabetical List of the House of Representatives of the United States
One Hundred Twelfth Congress. (2011). Retrieved July 19, 2011, from Office of
the Clerk U.S. House of Representativies: http://clerk.house.gov/committee_info
/oal.pdf.

Oleszek, Walter J. (1989). *Congressional Procedures and the Policy Process.* 3rd ed.
Washington, DC: Congressional Quarterly Press.

———. 2004. *Congressional Procedures and the Policy Process.* 6th ed. Washington,
DC: CQ Press.

Olson, Laura K. (2010). *The Politics of Medicaid.* New York: Columbia University
Press.

Olson, Mancur, Jr. (1968). *The Logic of Collective Action.* New York: Schocken.

OMB Director Lew Calls GOP Budget a "Bankrupt Approach," Threatens Vetoes.
(2000). *Tax Management Financial Planning Journal,* May 16, 137–38.

111th United States Congress. (2010, Nov. 30). Retrieved Dec. 1, 2010, from Wikipedia:
http://en.wikipedia.org/wiki/111th_United_States_Congress.

Ornstein, Norman. (2004). Lobbyists Often Get More Shakedowns Than They Give.
Roll Call, Feb. 25. www.rollcall.com.

Ornstein, Norman J., Thomas E. Mann, and Michael J. Malbin. (2002). *Vital Statistics on Congress, 2001–2002.* Washington, DC: AEI Press.

———. 2008. *Vital Statistics on Congress 2008.* Washington, DC: Brookings Institution Press.

Ostrom, Elinor. (1999). Institutional Rational Choice: An Assessment of the Institutional Analysis and Development Framework. In *Theories of the Policy Process,* ed.
Paul A. Sabatier. Boulder, CO: Westview Press.

Overby, Peter. (2009, Dec. 16). Natural Gas Fights for Position in Climate Bill. *Morning Edition.* Retrieved from National Public Radio: www.npr.org/templates/story
/story.php?storyId=121419226.

Pal, Leslie A., and Kent R. Weaver. (2003). Conclusions. In *The Government Taketh
Away: The Politics of Pain in the United States and Canada,* ed. Leslie A. Pal and R.
Kent Weaver. Washington, DC: Georgetown University Press.

Parker, Glenn. (1989). *Characteristics of Congress.* Englewood Cliffs, NJ:
Prentice-Hall.

Patterson, Samuel. (1983). Legislators and Legislatures in the American States. In
Politics in the American States, 4th ed., ed. Virginia Gray, Herbert Jacob, and Kenneth Vines. Boston: Little, Brown.

Paul-Sheehan, Pamela. (1998). The States and Health Care Reform: The Road Traveled and Lessons Learned from Seven That Took the Lead. *Journal of Health Politics, Policy, and Law* 23:319–61.

Pear, Robert. (1993). Drug Industry Gathers a Mix of Voices to Bolster Its Case. *New
York Times,* July 7, A1.

———. (2000a). Clinton to Order Medicare to Pay New Costs. *New York Times,* June 7. www.nytimes.com.

———. (2000b). One Step at a Time: Clinton Seeks More Help for Poor and Elderly. *New York Times,* Feb. 7. www.nytimes.com.

———. (2003). Bill on Medicare Drug Benefit Is Stalled by House-Senate Republican Antagonism. *New York Times,* Aug. 27, 15.

———. (2004). In a Shift, Bush Moves to Block Medical Suits. *New York Times,* July 24. www.nytimes.com.

———. (2005). Panel Seeks Better Disciplining of Doctors. *New York Times,* Jan. 5, A21.

———. (2009a, July 27). Reach of Subsidies Is Critical Issue for Health Plan. Retrieved July 27, 2009, from *New York Times:* www.nytimes.com/2009/07/27/health/policy/27health.html?_r=1&hp=&pagewanted.

———. (2009b, Nov. 16). In House, Many Spoke with One Voice: Lobbyists'. Retrieved from *New York Times:* www.nytimes.com/2009/11/15/us/politics/15health.html.

———. (2010a, May 15). Health Insurance Companies Try to Shape Rules. Retrieved from *New York Times:* www.nytimes.com/2010/05/16/health/policy/16health.html.

———. (2010b, June 21). Confirmation Fight on Health Chief. Retrieved from *New York Times:* www.nytimes.com/2010/06/22/health/policy/22medicare.html.

———. (2010c, July 18). Standards Issued for Electronic Health Records. Retrieved 2010, from *New York Times:* www.nytimes.com/2010/07/14/health/policy/14health.html.

———. (2010d, Aug. 22). Tighter Medical Privacy Rules Sought. Retrieved 2010, from *New York Times:* www.nytimes.com/2010/08/23/health/policy/23privacy.html.

———. (2010e, Sept. 21). Short of Repeal, G.O.P. Will Chip at Health Law. Retrieved 2010, from *New York Times:* www.nytimes.com/2010/09/21/health/policy/21repeal.html.

———. (2010f, Sept. 23). States Ask for Phase-In on Insurance Change. Retrieved from *New York Times:* www.nytimes.com/2010/09/23/business/23states.html.

Pear, Robert, and David Herszenhorn. (2009, July 25). Democrats' Divide Fuels Turmoil on Health Care. Retrieved July 25, 2009, from *New York Times:* www.nytimes.com/2009/07/25/us/politics/25health.html?hpw=&pagewanted=print.

Pelofsky, Jeremy. (2007, May 7). US Companies Launch New Group to Lobby Health Care. Retrieved Oct. 1, 2009, from AlertlNet: www.alertnet.org/thenews/newsdesk/N07347041.htm.

Perine, Keith. (2004). "Heightened Tensions" Fray Judicial-Legislative Relations. *CQ Weekly,* Sept. 13, 2148–53.

Perrin, Paul C., Hala N. Madanat, Michael D. Barnes, Athena Carolan, Robert B. Clark, Nathan Ivins, Steven R. Tuttle, Heidi A. Vogeler, and Patrick N. Williams. (2008). Health Education's Role in Framing Pornography as a Public Health Issue: Local and National Strategies with International Implications. Retrieved from *Promotion and Education:* http://ped.sagepub.com/cgi/content/short/15/1/11.

Pershing, Ben. (2009a, Aug. 5). Groups Take Health-Reform Debate to Airwaves. Retrieved from *Washington Post:* www.washingtonpost.com/wp-dyn/content /article/2009/08/04/AR2009080401447.htm.

———. (2009b, Nov. 11). New Campaign Targets Democrats for Health Vote, Nov. 11, 2009. Retrieved July 28, 2010, from *Washington Post:* http://voices.washing tonpost.com/capitol-briefing/2009/11/new_campaign_targets_democrats.html.

Peters, B. Guy. (1981). The Problem of Bureaucratic Government. *Journal of Politics* 43:56–82.

Peters, Charles. (1994). Tilting at Windmills. *Washington Monthly* 26 (Jan.–Feb.): 5.

Peterson, Mark. (1990). *Legislating Together: The White House and Capitol Hill from Eisenhower to Reagan.* Cambridge, MA: Harvard University Press.

———. (2000). Clinton and Organized Interests: Splitting Friends, Unifying Enemies. In *The Clinton Legacy,* ed. Colin Campbell and Bert A. Rockman. New York: Chatham House.

Peterson, Paul. (1995). *The Price of Federalism.* Washington, DC: Brookings Institution.

Pfiffner, James P. (1987). Political Appointees and Career Executives: The Democracy-Bureaucracy Nexus in the Third Century. *Public Administration Review* 47:57–65.

———. (2001, Dec. 12). *Recruiting Executive Branch Leaders: The Office of Presidential Personnel.* Retrieved from Brookings Institution: www.brookings.edu/articles /2001/spring_governance_pfiffner.

Pharmaceutical Research and Manufacturers of America (PhRMA). (2004). In the Courts: Overview. Retrieved from Pharmaceutical Research and Manufacturers of America: www.phrma.org/issues/courts.

———. (2009). Families USA Jointly Promote Measures to Ensure Quality, Affordable Healthcare Coverage. 2009, April 21. Retrieved from Pharmaceutical Research and Manufacturers of America: www.phrma.org/media/releases/phrma -families-usa-jointly-promote-measures-ensure-quality-affordable-healthcare -cove.

Phillips, Kate, and Jeff Zeleny. (2010, Feb. 25). White House Blasts Shelby Hold on Nominees. Retrieved 2010, from *New York Times:* http://thecaucus.blogs.nytimes .com/2010/02/05/white-house-blasts-shelby-hold-on-nominees.

Pierson, Paul. (2000). The Limits of Design: Explaining Institutional Origins and Change. *Governance* 13:475–99.

Pollack, Andrew. (2010, June 25). Genetically Altered Salmon Get Closer to the Table. Retrieved 2010, from *New York Times:* www.nytimes.com/2010/06/26/busi ness/26salmon.html.

Pollan, Michael. (2002). *The Botany of Desire: A Plant's-Eye View of the World.* New York: Random House.

Posner, Paul. (1997). Unfunded Mandates Reform Act: 1996 and Beyond. *Publius* 27 (2): 53–71.

Price, David E. (1971). Professionals and "Entrepreneurs": Staff Orientations and Policy Making on Three Senate Committees. *Journal of Politics* 33:316–36.

———. (1978). Policy Making in Congressional Committees: The Impact of "Environmental" Factors. *American Political Science Review* 72:548–74.

Price, Raymond. (1977). *With Nixon*. New York: Viking Press.

PricewaterhouseCoopers. (2009, Oct.). Potential Impact of Health Reform on the Cost of Private Health Insurance Coverage. Retrieved from American Health Solutions:www.americanhealthsolution.org/assets/Reform-Resources/AHIP -Reform-Resources/PWC-Report-on-Costs-Final.pdf.

Priest, Dana, and David S. Broder. (1994). The Pen as a Mighty Sword. *Washington Post*, National Weekly Edition, Jan. 31–Feb. 6, 11.

Provider Conference Call Wednesday to Focus on MDS, RUGs, Nursing Home Payment Changes. (2010, Aug. 27). Retrieved 2010, from McKnight's Long Term Care News: www.mcknights.com/provider-conference-call-wednesday-to-focus-on-mds -rugs-nursing-home-payment-changes/printarticle/177643/.

Publius [Alexander Hamilton, James Madison, and John Jay]. ([1787–88] 1961). *The Federalist Papers*. New York: New American Library.

Pugh, Tony. (2005). Ex-Cabinet Official Slams White House. *Tallahassee Democrat*, Mar. 25, 4A.

Quirk, Paul. (1981). *Industry Influence in Federal Regulatory Agencies*. Princeton, NJ: Princeton University Press.

Quirk, Paul J., and William Cunion. (2000). Clinton's Domestic Policy: The Lessons of a "New Democrat." In *The Clinton Legacy*, ed. Colin Campbell and Bert A. Rockman. New York: Chatham House.

Rand, A. Barry. (2009, Dec.). Health Care Reform Marches On. Retrieved from *AARP Bulletin:* www.salisburymass.com/forums/AARP_Dec09.

Rawls, John. (1971). *A Theory of Justice*. Cambridge, MA: Harvard University Press.

Reich, Robert B., ed. (1988). *The Power of Public Ideas*. Cambridge, MA: Harvard University Press.

Relman, Arnold. (1980). The New Medical-Industrial Complex. *New England Journal of Medicine* 303:963–70.

Rich, Robert F., and William D. White. (1996). Health Care Policy and the American States: Issues of Federalism. In *Health Policy, Federalism, and the American States*, ed. Robert F. Rich and William D. White. Washington, DC: Urban Institute Press.

Richtel, Matt. (2009, July 21). U.S. Withheld Data on Risks of Distracted Driving. Retrieved from *New York Times:* www.nytimes.com/2009/07/21/technology /21distracted.html.

———. (2010, July 6). Lobbyists Try to Reframe Distracted Driving Issue. Retrieved from *New York Times:* http://bits.blogs.nytimes.com/2010/07/06/lobbyists-try-to -reframe-distracted-driving-issue/.

Riddlesperger, James W., Jr. (2005). Redistricting Politics in Texas, 2003. Paper presented at the meeting of the Southern Political Science Association, New Orleans, Jan. 8–10.

Ripley, Randall B., and Grace A. Franklin. (1986). *Policy Implementation and Bureaucracy*. 2nd ed. Chicago: Dorsey Press.

Rivers, Douglas, and Nancy L. Rose. (1985). Passing the President's Program: Public Opinion and Presidential Influence in Congress. *American Journal of Political Science* 29:183–96.

Robinson, Chester A. (1991). *The Bureaucracy and the Legislative Process: A Case Study of the Health Care Financing Administration.* Lanham, MD: University Press of America.

Rochefort, David A., and Roger W. Cobb, eds. (1994). *The Politics of Problem Definition.* Lawrence: University Press of Kansas.

Rockman, Bert. (1984). Legislative-Executive Relations and Legislative Oversight. *Legislative Studies Quarterly* 9:387–440.

Rogers, David. (1999). Speaking Up: Hastert Finds Leading in House Isn't the Same as Being in Charge—GOP Rifts, Tough Rivals, and His Own Low Profile Have Bred Frustration—The Budget Brings Limelight. *Wall Street Journal,* Nov. 8, A1.

Rohde, David. (1990). Divided Government, Agenda Change, and Variations in Presidential Support in the House. Paper presented at a conference in honor of William H. Riker, Rochester, NY, Oct. 12–13.

———. (1991). *Parties and Leaders in the Postreform House.* Chicago: University of Chicago Press.

Rohde, David, and Dennis Simon. (1985). Presidential Vetoes and Congressional Response: A Study of Institutional Conflict. *American Journal of Political Science* 29:397–427.

Romer, Thomas, and James Snyder. (1994). An Empirical Investigation of the Dynamics of PAC Contributions. *American Journal of Political Science* 38:745–69.

Rosenberg, Gerald N. (1991). *The Hollow Hope: Can Courts Bring About Social Change?* Chicago: University of Chicago Press.

Rosenbloom, David H. (1981). The Judicial Response to the Bureaucratic State. *American Review of Public Administration* 50:29–51.

Rosenthal, Alan. (1993). *The Third House: Lobbyists and Lobbying in the States.* Washington, DC: Congressional Quarterly Press.

Roth, Bennett. (2005). Experts Sound Medicare Alarm. *Houston Chronicle,* Feb. 6, 1.

Rourke, Francis. (1984). *Bureaucracy, Politics, and Public Policy.* 3rd ed. Boston: Little, Brown.

———. (1991). American Bureaucracy in a Changing Political Setting. *Journal of Public Administration Research and Theory* 2:111–29.

Rubin, Alissa. (1993). Special Interests Stampede to Be Heard on Overhaul. *Congressional Quarterly,* May 1, 1081–84.

Sabatier, Paul, and Hank Jenkins-Smith. (1988). Special Issue: Policy Changes and Policy-Oriented Learning: Exploring an Advocacy Coalition Framework. *Policy Sciences* 21:123–278.

———. (1993). *Policy Change and Learning: An Advocacy Approach.* Boulder, CO: Westview Press.

Sabato, Larry. (1985). *PAC Power.* New York: W. W. Norton.

———. (1991). *Feeding Frenzy: How Attack Journalism Has Transformed American Politics.* New York: Free Press.

Sack, Kevin. (2009, Dec. 4). Doctors Divide on Bill. Retrieved from *New York Times:* http://query.nytimes.com/gst/fullpage.html?res=9403E2DE113FF937A35751C1A96 F9C8B63.

Sack, Kevin, and Herszenhorn, David. (2009, July 30). Texas Hospital Flexing Muscle in Health Fight. Retrieved from *New York Times:* www.nytimes.com/2009/07 /30/us/politics/30mcallen.html.

Salamon, Lester M., and Alan J. Abramson. (1984). Governance: The Politics of Retrenchment. In *The Reagan Record,* ed. John L. Palmer and Isabel V. Sawhill. Washington, DC: Urban Institute Press.

Salisbury, Robert H. (1969). An Exchange Theory of Interest Groups. *Midwest Journal of Political Science* 13:1–32.

Salisbury, Robert H., John P. Heinz, Edward O. Laumann, and Robert L. Nelson. (1987). Who Works with Whom? Interest Group Alliances and Opposition. *American Political Science Review* 81:1217–34.

Salisbury, Robert, and Kenneth Shepsle. (1981). U.S. Congressman as Enterprise. *Legislative Studies Quarterly* 6:559–76.

Sanford, Terry. (1967). *Storm over the States.* New York: McGraw-Hill.

Sardell, Alice, and Kay Johnson. (1998). The Politics of EPSDT Policy in the 1990s: Policy Entrepreneurship, Political Streams, and Children's Health Benefits. *Milbank Quarterly* 76 (2): 175–205.

Savage, David. (2001). Judgment Call: The Supreme Court Steps In. *State Legislatures,* Feb. 21–23.

———. (2011). Supreme Court Kills Global Warming Suit. *Los Angeles Times,* June 26.

Schattschneider, E. E. (1960). *The Semi-Sovereign People.* New York: Holt, Rinehart, and Winston.

Schatz, Joseph J. (2004). Presidential Support Vote Study: With a Deft and Light Touch, Bush Finds Ways to Win. *CQ Weekly,* Dec. 11, 2900–2904.

Schickler, Eric, and Kathryn Pearson. (2005). The House Leadership in an Era of Partisan Warfare. In *Congress Reconsidered,* 8th ed., ed. Lawrence C. Dodd and Bruce I. Oppenheimer. Washington, DC: CQ Press.

Schlesinger, Joseph A. (1966). *Ambition and Politics.* Chicago: Rand McNally.

———. 1985. The New American Political Party. *American Political Science Review* 79:1152–69.

Schlesinger, Mark, and Richard R. Lau. (2000). The Meaning and Measure of Policy Metaphors. *American Political Science Review* 94:611–26.

Schon, Donald. (1971). *Beyond the Stable State: Public and Private Learning in a Changing Society.* Hammondsworth, UK: Penguin.

Schram, Sanford, and Carol S. Weissert. (1999). The State of U.S. Federalism: 1998–1999. *Publius* 29 (2): 1–34.

Schuler, Kate. 2004. Weighing Promise and Perils of Drug Importation. *CQ Weekly,* July 24, 1788–91.

Schull, Steven A. (1989). *The President and Civil Rights Policy: Leadership and Change.* Westport, CT: Greenwood Press.

Schulman, Bruce J. (2010, Apr. 10). The Costs of Crossing the President. Retrieved December 1, 2010, from Politico: http://dyn.politico.com/printstory.cfm?uuid =175D24E0-18FE-70B2-A8116A00CFD94C58.

Schwitzer, Gary. (2009, Mar.). *The State of Health Journalism in the U.S.: A Report to the Kaiser Family Foundation.* Retrieved from Kaiser Family Foundation: www.kff .org/entmedia/upload/7858.pdf.

Scott, Ruth K., and Ronald J. Hrebenar. (1979). *Parties in Crisis.* New York: Wiley.

Seelye, Katharine Q. (1994). Lobbyists Are the Loudest in the Health Care Debate. *New York Times,* Aug. 16, A1.

———. (2009, Oct. 29). Insurers: Costs Would Skyrocket under House Health Bill. Retrieved from *New York Times:* http://prescriptions.blogs.nytimes.com/2009/10 /29/insurers-costs-would-skyrocket-under-house-health-bill.

———. (2010a, Jan. 30). Pro or Con, Lobbying Thrived. Retrieved from *New York Times:* http://prescriptions.blogs.nytimes.com/2010/01/30/pro-or-con-lobbying-thrived.

———. (2010b, Feb. 12). Lobbying in 2009: A Final Tally. Retrieved from *New York Times:* http://prescriptions.blogs.nytimes.com/2010/02/12/lobbying-in-2009-a -final-tally/.

Shear, Michael. (2009, July 31). Polling Helps Obama Frame Message in Health-Care Debate. Retrieved from *Washington Post:* www.washingtonpost.com/wp-dyn /content/article/2009/07/30/AR2009073001547.html.

Shepsle, Kenneth A. (1991). Penultimate Power: Conference Committees and the Legislative Process. In *Home Style and Washington Work,* ed. Morris P. Fiorina and David W. Rohde. Ann Arbor: University of Michigan Press.

Shepsle, Kenneth A., and Barry R. Weingast. (1984). Legislative Politics and Budget Outcomes. In *Federal Budget Policy in the 1980s,* ed. Gregory Mills and John Palmer. Washington, DC: Urban Institute Press.

———. (1987). The Institutional Foundations of Committee Power. *American Political Science Review* 81:85–104.

———. (1994). Positive Theories of Congressional Institutions. *Legislative Studies Quarterly* 19:149–79.

Shineman, Meghan. (2010, May 27). PHI Responds to CMS on Health Reform Nursing Home Provisions. Retrieved 2010, from PHI: http://phinational.org/archives/ phi-responds-to-cms-on-health-reform-nursing-home-provisions/.

Shrieves, Linda. (2011). Florida Rejects Millions More in Federal Health-Care Grants. *Orlando Sentinel,* June 29.

Silva, Chris. (2009, Aug. 24). Medicare Pay for Services by Nonphysicians Comes under Scrutiny. Retrieved from American Medical News: www.e-healthcaresolu-tions.com/AMA/aricept-amn-0710-inter.php?url=http://www.ama-assn.org /amednews/2009/08/24/gvsb0824.htm.

Silver, George A. (1991). The Route to a National Health Policy Lies through the States. *Yale Journal of Biology and Medicine* 64:443–53.

Simon, Herbert. (1945). *Administrative Behavior: A Study of Decision-Making Processes in Administration Organization.* New York: Free Press.

——. (1960). *The New Science of Management Decision.* New York: Harper and Row.

——. (1976). *Administrative Behavior: A Study of Decision-Making Processes in Administration Organization.* 2nd ed. New York: Free Press.

Sinclair, Barbara. (2005). The New World of U.S. Senators. In *Congress Reconsidered,* 8th ed., ed. Lawrence C. Dodd and Bruce I. Oppenheimer. Washington, DC: CQ Press.

——. (2009). The New World of U.S. Senators. In Dodd & Oppenheimer, 2009.

Singer, Natasha. (2009a, Feb. 10). A Birth Control Pill That Promised Too Much. Retrieved Mar. 24, 2009, from *New York Times:* www.nytimes.com/2009/02/11/business/11pill.html retr 3.24.09.

——. (2009b, Mar. 24). Contraception Pill Strictures are Eased by a Judge. Retrieved from *New York Times:* www.nytimes.com/2009/03/24/health/24pill.html.

——. (2009c, July 17). Harry and Louise Return, with a New Message. Retrieved from *New York Times:* www.nytimes.com/2009/07/17/business/media/17adco.html.

——. (2009d, Aug. 19). Senator Moves to Block Medical Ghostwriting, August 19, 2009. Retrieved from *New York Times:* www.nytimes.com/2009/08/19/health/research/19ethics.html.

Skocpol, Theda. (1992). *Protecting Soldiers and Mothers: The Political Origins of Social Policy in the United States.* Cambridge, MA: Harvard University Press.

——. (1996). *Boomerang: Health Care Reform and the Turn against Government.* New York: W. W. Norton.

Skrzycki, Cindy. (2000a). The Regulators: Paying by the Rules, OMB's Cost Analyses Questioned. *Washington Post,* Feb. 4, E1.

——. (2000b). The Regulators: System Overhaul? Business Groups Hope for a New Era. *Washington Post,* Dec. 19, E1.

Slackiman, Michael. (2009, Sept. 20). Belatedly, Egypt Spots Flaws in Wiping out Pigs. Retrieved from *New York Times:* www.nytimes.com/2009/09/20/world/africa/20cairo.html.

Smith, Ben. (2009a, July 17). Health Reform Foes Plan Obama's "Waterloo." Retrieved Dec. 11, 2011, from Politico: www.politico.com/blogs/bensmith/0709/Health_reform_foes_plan_Obamas_Waterloo.html.

——. (2009b, Aug. 21). The Summer of Astroturf. Retrieved from Politico: politico.com/news/stories/0809/26312.htm.

Smith, David G. (2002). *Entitlement Politics: Medicare and Medicaid, 1995–2001.* New York: Aldine de Gruyter.

Smith, Hedrick. (1988). *The Power Game: How Washington Works.* New York: Random House.

Smith, Richard A. (1995). Interest Group Influence in the U.S. Congress. *Legislative Studies Quarterly* 20:89–139.

Smith, Steven, and Christopher Deering. (1990). *Committees in Congress.* 2nd ed. Washington, DC: Congressional Quarterly Press.

Snyder, James M., Jr., and Tim Groseclose. (2000). Estimating Party Influence in Congressional Roll-Call Voting. *American Journal of Political Science* 44:193–211.

Sonner, Molly W., and Clyde Wilcox. (1999). Forgiving and Forgetting: Public Support for Bill Clinton during the Lewinsky Scandal. *PS* 32 (554–57): 294.

Soraghan, Mike. (2009, July 15). Blue Dogs Threaten to Bring Down Pelosi's Healthcare Bill. Retrieved July 17, 2009, from *The Hill:* http://thehill.com/homenews/house/50377-blue-dogs-threaten-to-bring-down-pelosis-healthcare-bill.

SourceWatch.org: 60 Plus Association. (n.d.). Retrieved July 28, 2010, from 60 Plus Association: www.sourcewatch.org/index.php?title=60_Plus_Association.

Sparer, Michael. (1996). *Medicaid and the Limits of State Health Reform.* Philadelphia: Temple University Press.

Spill, Rorie, Michael J. Licari, and Leonard Ray. (2001). Taking on Tobacco: Policy Entrepreneurship and the Tobacco Litigation. *Political Research Quarterly* 54 (3): 605–22.

Spitzer, Robert J. (1983). *The Presidency and Public Policy: The Four Arenas of Presidential Power.* Tuscaloosa: University of Alabama Press.

Squire, Peverill. (2007). Measuring Legislative Professionalism. *State Politics and Policy Quarterly* 7 (2): 211–27.

Starr, Paul. (1982). *The Social Transformation of American Medicine.* New York: Basic Books.

Stein, M. Robert, and N. Kenneth Bickers. (1995). *Perpetuating the Pork Barrel: Policy Subsystems and American Democracy.* New York: Cambridge University Press.

Steinmo, Sven, and Jon Watts. (1995). It's the Institutions Stupid! Why Comprehensive National Health Insurance Always Fails in America. *Journal of Health Politics, Policy, and Law* 20:329–72.

Stevenson, Richard W. (2005). For This President, Power Is There for the Taking. *New York Times,* May 15, 3.

Stolberg, Sheryl Gay. (2002). Bush Urges a Cap on Medical Liability. *New York Times,* July 26, A16.

———. (2003). Drug Lobby Pushed Letter by Senators on Medicare. *New York Times,* July 30, A13.

———. (2009). Obama Lifts Bush's Strict Limits on Stem Cell Research. *New York Times,* Mar. 10. Retrieved Dec. 11, 2011, from *New York Times:* www.nytimes.com/2009/03/10/us/politics/10stem.html.

Stone, Deborah A. (1988). *Policy Paradox and Political Reason.* Glenview, IL: Scott Foresman.

———. (1989). Causal Stories and the Formation of Policy Agendas. *Political Science Quarterly* 104:281–300.

———. (1993). The Struggle for the Soul of Health Insurance. *Journal of Health Politics, Policy, and Law* 18:287–317.

Stone, Peter H. (1994). Back Off! *National Journal* 26 (Dec. 3): 2840–44.

Sullivan, Terry. (1987). Presidential Leadership in Congress: Security Commitments. In *Congress: Structure and Policy*, ed. Mathew McCubbins and Terry Sullivan. Cambridge: Cambridge University Press.

———. (1991). The Bank Account Presidency: A New Measure and Evidence on the Temporal Path of Presidential Influence. *American Journal of Political Science* 35:686–723.

Tackett, Michael. (2005). The Business of Influence in Washington. *Chicago Tribune*, Apr. 10, 1.

Tannenwald, Robert. (1998). Implications of the Balanced Budget Act of 1997 for the "Devolution Revolution." *Publius* 28 (1): 23–48.

Taxpayers for Common Sense. (2010). Retrieved Dec. 1, 2010, from Taxpayers for Common Sense: www.taxpayer.net/resources.

Taylor, Andrew J. (2004). Denied Their Smoke and Mirrors, Appropriators Hold to Limits. *CQ Weekly*, Nov. 27, 2778–80.

———. (2005). Chambers Spar over Spending Panels. *CQ Weekly*, Feb. 7, 306–7.

Thaemert, Rita. (1994). Twenty Percent and Climbing. *State Legislatures* 20:28–32.

Thomas, Helen. (1999). *Front Row at the White House: My Life and Times*. New York: Scribner.

Thomaselli, Rich. (2010). Big Pharma's Deal with White House Threatened despite $100 Mil Ad Outlay. *Advertising Age* 81 (11). Retrieved Dec. 11, 2011, from *Advertising Age:* http://adage.com/article/news/pharma-deal-white-house-threatened-100m-outlay/142799/.

Thompson, Frank J. (1983). *Health Policy and the Bureaucracy*. Cambridge, MA: MIT Press.

Tierney, John T. (1987). Organized Interests in Health Politics and Policy-Making. *Medical Care Review* 44:89–118.

Toner, Robin. (1994). Gold Rush Fever Grips Capital as Health Care Struggle Begins. *New York Times*, Mar. 13, 1, 10.

Toner, Robin, and Robert Pear. (2003). Bush Seeks Medicare Drug Bill That Conservatives Oppose. *New York Times*, June 23, A18.

Torres-Gil, Fernando. (1989). The Politics of Catastrophic and Long-Term Care Coverage. *Journal of Aging and Social Policy* 1:61–86.

Truman, David B. (1951). *The Governmental Process: Political Interests and Public Opinion*. New York: Knopf.

Tully, Shawn. (2011, Apr. 7). In Defense of Paul Ryan's Medicare Plan. Retrieved 2011, from CNNMoney.com: http://finance.fortune.cnn.com/2011/04/07/in-defense-of-paul-ryans-medicare-plan/.

Urbina, Ian. (2010, May 23). Despite Moratorium, Drilling Projects Move Ahead. Retrieved 2010, from *New York Times:* www.nytimes.com/2010/05/24/us/24moratorium.html.

U.S. Census Bureau. (2011). State Government Finances Summary: 2009. Retrieved Dec. 11, 2011, from www2.census.gov/govs/state/09statesummaryreport.pdf.

U.S. Government Printing Office. (2011). Table 6.1—Composition of Outlays: 1940–2016. In *Budget of the United States Government: Historical Tables Fiscal Year 2012.* Retrieved 2011, from www.gpoaccess.gov/usbudget/fy12/hist.html.

U.S. House. (2011). Office of the Clerk. Retrieved Dec. 11, 2011, from Office of the Clerk, U.S. House of Representatives: http://artandhistory.house.gov/house_history/speakers.aspx.

U.S. Senate. (2011a). Majority and Minority Leaders and Party Whips. Retrieved Dec. 11, 2011, from www.senate.gov/artandhistory/history/common/briefing/Majority_Minority_Leaders.htm.

———. (2011b). Caucus on International Narcotics Control. www.drugcaucus.senate.gov.

Vaida, Bara. (2010, Apr. 3). The Envy List. Retrieved 2010, from *National Journal Magazine:* www.nationaljournal.com/njmagazine/print_friendly.php?ID=cs_20100403_9562.

Vaughn, Bryan T., Steven R. DeVrieze, Shelby D. Reed, and Kevin A. Schulman. (2010). Can We Close the Income and Wealth Gap between Specialists and Primary Care Physicians? *Health Affairs* 29 (5): 933–40.

Wald, Matthew L. (2000, Mar. 10). Safety: On the Road. On the Web. In Danger? Retrieved from *New York Times:* www.nytimes.com/2000/03/10/automobiles/autos-on-friday-safety-on-the-road-on-the-web-in-danger.html.

———. (2005). Senate Version of Bill Pushes States to Adopt Stiff Drunken Driving Penalties. *New York Times,* June 17, A11.

———. (2010, May 1). Tax on Oil May Help Pay for Cleanup. Retrieved from *New York Times:* www.nytimes.com/2010/05/02/us/02liability.html?pagewanted=print.

Waldo, Dwight. (1955). *The Study of Administration.* New York: Random House.

Walker, David B. (2000). *The Rebirth of Federalism: Slouching toward Washington.* 2nd ed. New York: Chatham House.

Walker, David M. (2004). GAO Answers the Question: What's in a Name? *Roll Call,* July 19. http://rollcall.com.

Walker, Jack. (1969). The Diffusion of Innovations among the American States. *American Political Science Review* 63:880–99.

———. (1991). *Mobilizing Interest Groups in America.* Ann Arbor: University of Michigan Press.

Wawro, Gregory. (2000). *Legislative Entrepreneurship in the U.S. House of Representatives.* Ann Arbor: University of Michigan Press.

Waxman, Henry, and Joshua Green. (2009). *The Waxman Report: How Congress Really Works.* New York: Twelve.

Wayne, Leslie, and David Herszenhorn. (2009, July 27). A Bid to Tax Health Plans of Executives. Retrieved July 27, 2009, from *New York Times:* www.nytimes.com/2009/07/27/health/policy/27insure.html?ref=us&pagewanted=print.

Weingast, Barry, and Mark Moran. (1983). Bureaucratic Discretion or Congressional Control? Regulatory Policymaking by the Federal Trade Commission. *Journal of Political Economy* 91:765–800.

Weissert, Carol S. (1992). Medicaid in the 1990s: Trends, Innovations, and the Future of the "PAC-Man" of State Budgets. *Publius* 22 (3): 93–109.

Weissert, Carol S., Jack H. Knott, and Blair S. Stieber. (1994). Education and the Health Professions: Explaining Policy Choice. *Journal of Health Politics, Policy, and Law* 19:361–92.

Weissert, William G., and Edward Alan Miller. (2005). Punishing the Pioneers: The Medicare Modernization Act and State Pharmacy Assistance Programs. *Publius* 35 (1): 115–42.

Weissert, William G., and Carol S. Weissert. (2010). Why Major Health Reform in 2009–10 Won't Solve Our Problems. *Forum* 8 (1). www.bepress.com/forum/vol8/iss1/art9/.

Weisskopf, Michael. (1995). To the Victors Belong the PAC Checks. *Washington Post, National Weekly Edition*, Jan. 2–8, 13.

West, William. (1984). Structuring Administrative Discretion: The Pursuit of Rationality and Responsiveness. *American Journal of Political Science* 28:340–60.

West, William, and Joseph Cooper. (1989–90). Legislative Influence v. Presidential Dominance: Competing Models of Bureaucratic Control. *Political Science Quarterly* 104:581–606.

White, Joseph. (1995). The Horses and the Jumps: Comments on the Health Care Reform Steeplechase. *Journal of Health Politics, Policy, and Law* 20:373–83.

White House. (2011). Report to Congress on the Benefits and Costs of Federal Regulations and Unfunded Mandates on State, Local, and Tribal Entities. Retrieved Dec. 11, 2011, from www.whitehouse.gov/sites/default/files/omb/legislative/reports/2010_Benefit_Cost_Report.pdf.

Whiteman, David. (1987). What Do They Know and When Do They Know It? Health Staff on the Hill. *PS* 20:221–25.

Wildavsky, Aaron. (1966). The Two Presidencies. *Trans-Action* 4:7–14.

———. (1979). *Speaking Truth to Power*. Boston: Little, Brown.

Wilkerson, John D., and David Carrell. (1999). Money, Politics, and Medicine: The American Medical PAC's Strategy of Giving in U.S. House Races. *Journal of Health Politics, Policy, and Law* 24:335–55.

Wilson, Duff. (2009, Dec. 24). Health Bill Doesn't Change Drug Ads. Retrieved from *New York Times:* http://prescriptions.blogs.nytimes.com/2009/12/24/health-bill-doesnt-change-drug-ads/.

Wilson, James Q. (1989). *Bureaucracy: What Government Agencies Do and Why They Do It*. New York: Basic Books.

Wilson, Rick. (1992). Review of *Parties and Leaders in the Postreform House*, by David Rohde. *American Political Science Review* 86:806–7.

Wilson, Woodrow. ([1885] 1913). *Congressional Government*. Boston: Houghton Mifflin.

Wines, Michael. (1994). Clinton Puts Onus for Health Care on Republicans. *New York Times*, Aug. 4, A1.

Wood, Bruce. (1999). The Politics of Disease-Related Patients' Associations: An Anglo-American Comparison. Paper presented at the annual meeting of the American Political Science Association, Atlanta, Sept. 3.

Woodward, Bob. (1994). *The Agenda: Inside the Clinton White House.* New York: Simon and Schuster.

Wright, John R. (1985). PACs, Contributions, and Roll Calls: An Organizational Perspective. *American Political Science Review* 79:400–414.

———. (1990). Contributions, Lobbying, and Committee Voting in the U.S. House of Representatives. *American Political Science Review* 84:417–38.

———. (1996). *Interest Groups and Congress.* Boston: Allyn and Bacon.

Yadron, Danny. (2011, Apr. 19). Democrats Use Ryan Budget for Attack Ads. Retrieved 2011, from *The Wall Street Journal Blog:* http://blogs.wsj.com/washwire/2011/04 /19/democrats-use-ryan-budget-for-attack-ads/?mod=google_news_blog.

York, Anthony. (2008, June 10). Carly Fiorina Wins GOP Senate Nomination. Retrieved Dec. 1, 2010, from *Los Angeles Times:* http://latimesblogs.latimes.com /california-politics/2010/06/do-not-publish—fiorina-wins-us-senate-primary.html.

Index

Page numbers in *italics* refer to figures and tables.